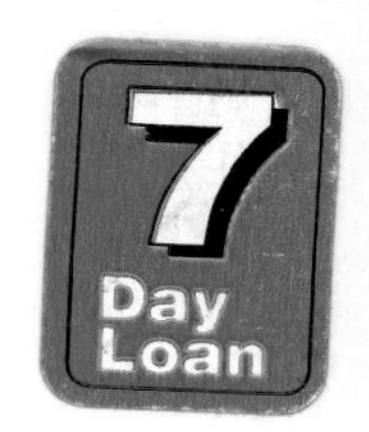

Get ahead!

Medicine

150 EMQs for finals

Get ahead!
Medicine
150 EMQs for finals

David Capewell
Foundation Year House Officer
Emergency Medicine
St. James' Hospital, Leeds, UK

Saran Shantikumar
Foundation Year House Officer
Academic Vascular Surgery
Leeds General Infirmary, Leeds, UK

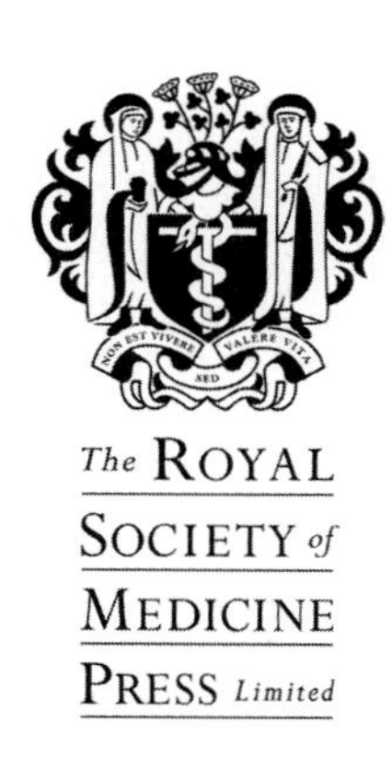

The ROYAL SOCIETY of MEDICINE PRESS Limited

Published by the Royal Society of Medicine Press Ltd
1 Wimpole Street, London W1G 0AE, UK
Tel: +44 (0)20 7290 2921
Fax: +44 (0)20 7290 2929
Email: publishing@rsm.ac.uk
Website: www.rsmpress.co.uk

British Library Cataloguing in Publication Data
A catalogue record for this book is available from the British Library

ISBN 978-1-85315-717-2

Distribution in Europe and Rest of World:

Marston Book Services Ltd
PO Box 269
Abingdon
Oxon OX14 4YN, UK
Tel: +44 (0)1235 465500
Fax: +44 (0)1235 465555
Email: direct.order@marston.co.uk

Distribution in the USA and Canada:

Royal Society of Medicine Press Ltd
c/o BookMasters Inc
30 Amberwood Parkway
Ashland, OH 44805, USA
Tel: +1 800 247 6553/+1 800 266 5564
Fax: +1 419 281 6883
Email: orders@bookmasters.com

Distribution in Australia and New Zealand:

Elsevier Australia
30–52 Smidmore Street
Marrickville NSW 2204, Australia
Tel: +61 2 9517 8999
Fax: +61 2 9517 2249
Email: service@elsevier.com.au

Typeset by IMH(Cartrif), Loanhead, Scotland
Printed by Bell & Bain, Glasgow

Contents

Contents

Preface

Welcome to *Get ahead! Medicine*. This book contains 150 EMQ themes, each with five stems, covering clinical medicine. The EMQs are arranged as 10 practice papers, each containing 15 themes. Allow yourself 90 minutes to two hours for each paper. You can either work through the practice papers systematically or dip in and out of the book using the EMQ index as a guide to where questions on a specific topic can be found. We have tried to include all the main conditions about which you can be expected to know, as well as some more detailed knowledge suitable for candidates aiming at distinction. As in the real exam, these papers have no preset pass mark. Whether you pass or fail depends on the distribution of scores across the whole year group, but around 60% should be sufficient.

We hope that this book fulfils its aim in being a useful, informative revision aid. If you have any feedback or suggestions, please let us know (RevisionForMedicalFinals@gmail.com).

We would like to acknowledge the help of Sarah Vasey and Sarah Burrows, both of the Royal Society of Medicine Press, for their guidance throughout this project, and to Mac Clarke for his careful copyediting and helpful suggestions throughout the *Get ahead!* series.

Finally, we would like to thank our families, Anoushka (DC) and Mary (SS) for their continuing support.

This book is dedicated to Geoff Hall (David's grandfather), who sadly passed away last year.

David Capewell
Saran Shantikumar

Introduction to *Get ahead!*

Get ahead!

Extended matching questions (EMQs) are becoming more popular as a method of assessment in summative medical school examinations. EMQs have the advantage of testing candidates' knowledge of clinical scenarios rather than their ability at detailed factual recall. However, they do not always parallel real-life situations and are no comparison to clinical decision-making. Either way, the EMQ is here to stay.

The *Get ahead!* series is aimed primarily at undergraduate finalists. Much like the real exam, we have endeavoured to include commonly asked questions as well as a generous proportion of harder stems, appropriate for the more ambitious student aiming for honours. The Universities Medical Assessment Partnership (UMAP) is a collaboration of 14 medical schools in the UK that is compiling a bank of EMQs to be used in summative examinations. The questions in the *Get ahead!* series are written to closely follow the 'house-style' of the UMAP EMQs, and hence are of a similar format to what many of you can expect in your exams. All the questions in the *Get ahead!* series are accompanied by explanatory answers, including a succinct summary of the key features of each condition. Even when you get an answer right, I strongly suggest that you read these – I guarantee that you'll learn something. For added interest, we have included some details of eponymous conditions ('eponymous' from Greek *epi* = upon + *onyma* = name; 'giving name'), and, as you have just seen, some derivations of words from the original Latin or Greek.

How to pass your exams

Exam EMQs are intended to be based on 'house officer knowledge'. Sadly, this is not always the case, and you shouldn't be surprised when you get a question concerning the management of various stages of prostate cancer (as I was). So start revising early and don't restrict yourself to the given syllabus if you can avoid it. If your exam is only two weeks away then CRAM, CRAM, CRAM – you'll be surprised at how much you can learn in a fortnight.

During the exam ...

1. Try to answer the questions without looking at the responses first – the questions are written such that this should be possible.

2. Take your time to read the questions fully. There are no bonus marks for finishing the paper early.

3. If you get stuck on a question then make sure that you mark down your best guess before you move on. You may not have time to return to it at the end.

4. Answer all the questions – there is no negative marking. If you are unsure, go with your instinct – it's probably going to be your best guess.

5. Never think that the examiner is trying to catch you out. Red herrings are not allowed, so don't assume that there is one. If a question looks easy, it probably is!

But all this is obvious and there is no substitute for learning the material thoroughly and practising as many questions as you can. With this book, you're off to a good start!

A final word ...

The *Get ahead!* series is written by junior doctors who have recently finished finals and who have experience teaching students. As such, I hope that the books cover information that is valuable and relevant to you as undergraduates who are about to sit finals.

I wish you the best of luck in your exams!

Saran Shantikumar
Series Editor, *Get ahead!*

Practice Paper 1: Questions

Theme 1: Causes of collapse

Options

A. Acute myocardial infarction
B. Cerebrovascular accident
C. Dissecting aortic aneurysm
D. Drug allergy
E. First-dose hypotension
F. Left ventricular failure
G. Ruptured abdominal aortic aneurysm
H. Stable angina
I. Stokes–Adams attack
J. Supraventricular tachycardia
K. Vasovagal syncope
L. Ventricular rupture
M. Wolff–Parkinson–White syndrome

For each of the following scenarios, select the most appropriate diagnosis. Each option may be used once, more than once or not at all.

1. A 45-year-old woman collapses during a church service in summer. Her husband states that she turned pale and collapsed shortly after standing up. She did not jerk or lose urinary continence. She denies chest pain, shortness of breath and palpitations. She recovered after 30 seconds and now feels back to her usual self. All observations – including blood tests, ECG, and lying and standing blood pressure – are normal.

2. A 25-year-old man collapses suddenly while visiting his grandmother in hospital. There appears to be no pulse. The crash team is called, and manage to resuscitate him after identifying ventricular fibrillation on the cardiac monitor. The attending anaesthetist records a repeat ECG and notes that the QRS complexes are broad with slurred upstroke of the R wave.

3. A 75-year-old woman is brought to the emergency department after collapsing. On examination, her heart rate is 80 beats/min and irregular, with a blood pressure of 150/90 mmHg. She has difficulty in moving her left arm and leg.

4. A 67-year-old man presents to the emergency department following a collapse. He has a history of ischaemic heart disease and had been diagnosed with hypertension only last week. He remembers feeling dizzy when he got out of his chair to go to the toilet before fainting. He regained consciousness almost immediately and had fully recovered within 5 minutes.

5. A 57-year-old man is found collapsed at work. On arrival at the emergency department, he is complaining of mild epigastric discomfort that started at rest. He appears pale and sweaty and has vomited once. He is on insulin for type 1 diabetes mellitus.

Theme 2: Nerve lesions of the upper limb

Options

A. Accessory nerve
B. Anterior interosseous nerve
C. Axillary nerve
D. Distal median nerve
E. Distal ulnar nerve
F. Long thoracic nerve
G. Lower brachial plexus
H. Posterior interosseous nerve
I. Proximal median nerve
J. Proximal ulnar nerve
K. Radial nerve
L. Upper brachial plexus

For each of the following scenarios, select the most likely nerve lesion. Each option may be used once, more than once or not at all.

1. A 28-year-old man is involved in a motorcycle accident. He has fractured both his femurs and complains of pain in his neck. On examination, his right arm is hanging by his side, is fully extended at the elbow and is rotated inwards. There is loss of sensation on the outer edge of the right arm and forearm.

2. A 67-year-old woman attends follow-up clinic following a right mastectomy for invasive breast cancer. Her husband has pointed out that her right shoulder blade occasionally sticks out more than the left. On examination, there is no evidence of sensory loss.

3. A 72-year-old man attends the emergency department following a fall. On examination, there is bruising on the right upper arm and the man is unable to extend his metacarpals on the same side. There is loss of sensation over the lateral dorsal aspect of the hand.

4. An 18-year-old woman who recently had neck surgery attends a follow-up clinic. She complains of pain in the left side of her neck. On examination, she is unable to shrug her left shoulder. There is no evidence of sensory loss.

5. A 24-year-old man presents with severe right shoulder pain following a tackle during a rugby match. On examination, the contour of the affected shoulder is flattened and the humeral head is palpable. There is also sensory loss at the upper outer aspect of the arm.

Theme 3: Complications of diabetes mellitus

Options

A. Atherosclerosis
B. Autonomic neuropathy
C. Charcot's joint
D. Connective tissue disease
E. Diabetes dermopathy
F. Lipoatrophy
G. Lipohypertrophy
H. Peripheral vascular disease
I. Neuropathic ulcer
J. Nephropathy
K. Necrobiosis lipoidica
L. Osteoarthritis
M. Venous ulcer

For each of the following scenarios, select the most appropriate complication. Each option may be used once, more than once or not at all.

1. A 66-year-old man with a long history of poorly controlled type 2 diabetes is found to have a foot lesion during his podiatry appointment. The lesion is located on the ball of his left foot. It is small and well circumscribed and appears punched out. The patient denies any pain.

2. A 55-year-old woman with poorly controlled diabetes has collapsed several times over the previous 2 months. All collapses have occurred when she stands from a lying position, and she recovers within minutes. Her husband says that she has never fitted or lost urinary continence during an episode.

3. A 50-year-old type 1 diabetic man presents to his GP with 'unstable' ankle joints. On examination, both ankles are significantly deformed, hypermobile and cold, but are not painful.

4. A 46-year-old type 1 diabetic man attends a routine follow-up clinic. A urine dipstick analysis demonstrates 3+ protein, 1+ blood, no nitrates and no leucocytes. His annual blood tests show a sodium of 135 mmol/L, a potassium of 4.9 mmol/L, a creatinine of 130 μmol/L and a urea of 8.9 mmol/L.

5. A 37-year-old type 1 diabetic man presents to his GP complaining of a painless discoloured lesion over the lateral aspect of his right lower leg. It began as a well-circumscribed red nodule, but enlarged and flattened over time. The surface is brownish-yellow and scaly and has a number of telangiectatic vessels.

Theme 4: Diagnosis of respiratory conditions 1

Options

A. Asbestos-related lung disease
B. Asthma
C. Bronchiectasis
D. Chronic obstructive pulmonary disease
E. Cryptogenic fibrosing alveolitis
F. Cystic fibrosis
G. Extrinsic allergic alveolitis
H. Mesothelioma
I. Non-small cell lung tumour
J. Open pneumothorax
K. Sarcoidosis
L. Secondary lung metastases
M. Sleep apnoea
N. Small cell lung tumour
O. Tuberculosis

For each of the following scenarios, select the most appropriate diagnosis. Each option may be used once, more than once or not at all.

1. A 68-year-old retired accountant has a 3-week history of small haemoptysis. He has also noticed that he is not passing as much urine as normal, although he is otherwise well. On examination, a monophonic wheeze is heard over the left lobe.

2. A 12-year-old boy is brought to the GP by his mother. Over the last couple of years, he has suffered from repeated chest infections, and his mother is worried that he is not putting on any weight. On examination, there are coarse crepitations throughout both lung lobes.

3. A 58-year-old builder complains of left-sided chest discomfort that has been progressing over the last fortnight. He is otherwise well. On examination, the left lower lobe is dull to percussion. A pleural tap is performed, and reveals blood-stained fluid.

4. A 53-year-old shopfitter is admitted to hospital for an elective inguinal hernia operation. A routine chest X-ray shows white lesions over both lungs that cross the lobar boundaries. The patient feels well and auscultation reveals no abnormality.

5. A 16-year-old boy presents to his GP with a 6-month history of night cough and intermittent wheeze. He has previously been well and has never had a chest infection. Examination of the chest is unremarkable.

Theme 5: Glomerulonephritis

Options

A. Drug-induced glomerulonephritis
B. Focal segmental glomerulosclerosis
C. Goodpasture's syndrome
D. IgA nephropathy
E. Membranous glomerulonephritis
F. Mesangiocapillary glomerulonephritis
G. Minimal-change glomerulonephritis
H. Post-streptococcal glomerulonephritis
I. Rapidly progressive glomerulonephritis
J. Rhabdomyolysis

For each of the following scenarios, select the most likely cause of glomerulonephritis. Each option may be used once, more than once or not at all.

1. A 4-year-old boy presents with facial and ankle swelling. He is found to have 3+ of protein in his urine on dipstick analysis. Blood tests reveal an albumin of 16 g/L.

2. A 25-year-old man presents with facial and ankle swelling. He is found to have 3+ of protein in his urine on dipstick analysis. Blood tests reveal an albumin of 16 g/L.

3. A 37-year-old man presents with a 2-week history of coughing up blood. He is found to have 2+ of protein in his urine on dipstick analysis. Blood tests show a urea of 9.5 mmol/L and a creatinine of 148 μmol/L. Further tests confirm that he is positive for the anti-glomerular basement membrane antibody.

4. A 7-year-old boy presents to the emergency department 2 days after developing an upper respiratory infection. He has blood in his urine and flank pain. A renal biopsy is organized, and shows a proliferative glomerulonephritis with antibody deposition.

5. A 15-year-old girl presents to the GP 2 weeks after being diagnosed with tonsillitis. She is generally unwell and puffy and complaining of dark urine. Urine dipstick analysis shows 3+ of protein and 3+ of blood. She is found to have high titres of antistreptolysin O antibody.

Theme 6: Management of hypertension

Options

A. Admit to high-dependency unit for monitoring and intravenous antihypertensive medication
B. Admit to hospital for oral antihypertensive medication
C. Ambulatory blood pressure monitoring
D. Confirm over 4 weeks and treat if persistent
E. Confirm over 12 weeks and treat if persistent
F. Lifestyle advice only
G. No further assessment required
H. Prescribe a single oral antihypertensive agent as an outpatient
I. Prescribe two oral antihypertensive agents as an outpatient
J. Provide lifestyle advice and reassess annually
K. Sublingual nifedipine

For each of the following scenarios, select the most appropriate management option. Each option may be used once, more than once or not at all.

1. A 63-year-old man is shown to have a blood pressure of 135/60 mmHg by his GP. He is otherwise fit and well and has no significant past medical history.

2. A 63-year-old man with newly diagnosed type 2 diabetes is noticed to have a blood pressure of 155/89 mmHg during his initial outpatient appointment. Fundoscopy demonstrates silver wiring, arteriovenous nipping and cotton-wool spots.

3. A 65-year-old woman is found to have a blood pressure persistently over 160/90 mmHg during a 2-month assessment period by her GP. Lifestyle advice has been provided on several occasions. She is otherwise fit and well and is asymptomatic.

4. A 67-year-old man presents to the emergency department complaining of headaches. A routine set of observations shows a blood pressure of 220/120 mmHg. Fundoscopy reveals some arteriovenous nipping but is otherwise normal.

5. A 62-year-old man is brought to the emergency department by his wife. He is complaining of headaches and blurred vision. He is orientated in time and person but not in place. A routine set of observations shows a blood pressure of 240/140 mmHg and a heart rate of 84 beats/min. Fundoscopy shows bilateral papilloedema and flame haemorrhages. Neurological examination is otherwise normal. An emergency head CT highlights no neurological explanation for the symptoms.

Theme 7: Interpretation of cerebrospinal fluid results

Options

A. *Cryptococcus neoformans*
B. *Haemophilus influenzae*
C. Malignancy
D. Multiple sclerosis
E. Mumps
F. *Mycobacterium tuberculosis*
G. *Neisseria meningitidis*
H. *Streptococcus pneumoniae*

For each of the following scenarios, select the most appropriate diagnosis. Each option may be used once, more than once or not at all.

1. A 45-year-old man is admitted with headache and neck stiffness. A lumbar puncture is performed and reveals the following results: clear fluid, lymphocytes 2/mm^3, neutrophils 1/mm^3, low glucose, high protein, positive India ink stain.

2. A 45-year-old man is admitted with headache and neck stiffness. A lumbar puncture is performed and reveals the following results: clear fluid, lymphocytes 340/mm^3, neutrophils 3/mm^3, normal glucose, normal protein, no organisms seen.

3. A 45-year-old man is admitted with headache and neck stiffness. A lumbar puncture is performed and reveals the following results: clear fluid, lymphocytes 4/mm^3, neutrophils 1/mm^3, normal glucose, normal protein, no organisms seen, oligoclonal bands present.

4. A 45-year-old man is admitted with headache and neck stiffness. A lumbar puncture is performed and reveals the following results: cloudy fluid, lymphocytes 21/mm^3, neutrophils 1546/mm^3, low glucose, high protein, Gram-negative diplococcus seen.

5. A 45-year-old man is admitted with headache and neck stiffness. A lumbar puncture is performed and reveals the following results: clear fluid, lymphocytes 1329/mm^3, neutrophils 12/mm^3, low glucose, high protein, positive Ziehl–Neelsen stain.

Theme 8: Thyroid disease

Options

A. De Quervain's thyroiditis
B. Graves' disease
C. Hashimoto's thyroiditis
D. Hypopituitarism
E. Hypothyroidism secondary to amiodarone therapy
F. Hypothyroidism secondary to lithium therapy
G. Sick euthyroid syndrome
H. Single toxic nodule goitre
I. Thyroid cancer
J. Toxic multinodular goitre

For each of the following scenarios, select the most likely diagnosis. Each option may be used once, more than once or not at all.

1. A 26-year-old woman presents to her GP with a history of fever, neck pain and general lethargy. On examination, she has a painful goitre affecting both lobes of the thyroid gland. Blood tests show a raised T_4 level, a low TSH level, a CRP of 67 mg/L and a white cell count of 14.3×10^9/L.

2. A 47-year-old woman presents to the GP with a 4-month history of weight loss, fever and diarrhoea. She describes a gritty feeling in her eyes and feels that they are protruding.

3. A 43-year-old man with a long history of bipolar disorder presents to his GP complaining of weight gain, lethargy and feeling cold all the time. Blood tests show a low T_4 level and a high TSH level.

4. A 49-year-old woman presents to her GP complaining of a neck swelling and tiredness. On examination, she has a symmetrical goitre. Blood tests show a low T_4 level, a raised TSH level and a high titre of antithyroid peroxidase antibodies.

5. A 38-year-old man who is currently in hospital being treated for a severe chest infection is shown to have low T_4 and TSH levels.

Theme 9: Transfusion reactions

Options

A. Begin immunosuppressant therapy with ciclosporin
B. Irradiate the blood products
C. Prescribe another unit of packed red cells
D. Prescribe calcium supplements
E. Prescribe intravenous calcium gluconate followed by subcutaneous insulin

F. Prescribe intravenous calcium gluconate, intravenous insulin and glucose
G. Prescribe potassium supplements
H. Speed up the transfusion
I. Speed up the transfusion and prescribe paracetamol
J. Slow the transfusion and prescribe furosemide
K. Slow the transfusion and prescribe paracetamol
L. Stop the transfusion and prescribe chlorphenamine and adrenaline
M. Stop the transfusion and exclude a haemolytic reaction. Send blood cultures and prescribe broad-spectrum antibiotics
N. Stop the transfusion and inform the blood bank. Take blood for full blood count, clotting screen and Coombs' testing, and begin fluid resuscitation

For each of the following scenarios, select the most appropriate management plan. Each option may be used once, more than once or not at all.

1. Twenty minutes after beginning a blood transfusion, a 29-year-old woman develops a temperature of 37.5°C. She has no other complaints. Her other observations are heart rate 86 beats/min, blood pressure 128/84 mmHg and oxygen saturations 98% in air.

2. Five minutes after beginning a blood transfusion, a 45-year-old man begins to complain of chest and abdominal pain. There is also oozing of blood from his cannulation site. His observations are temperature 38.0°C, heart rate 106 beats/min, blood pressure 108/68 mmHg and respiratory rate 18/min.

3. Forty minutes after beginning a blood transfusion, a 32-year-old woman develops a temperature of 40.2°C and starts shivering. Her heart rate is 126 beats/min and her blood pressure is 96/62 mmHg. It is confirmed that the blood product was cross-matched appropriately and there have been no mistakes in delivery, although there was a delay before it could be administered, as the patient required cannulation.

4. A 70-year-old man with known ischaemic heart disease required a blood transfusion following a lower gastrointestinal bleed. Halfway through his third unit, he became breathless. On examination, his jugular venous pressure was 6 cm and crackles were heard at both lung bases.

5. A 45-year-old man received 15 units of packed red cells during emergency abdominal surgery after rupturing his spleen in a motorcycle accident. A routine postoperative ECG demonstrates wide QRS complexes and tall T-waves.

Theme 10: Dementia 1

Options

A. Alzheimer's disease
B. Creutzfeldt–Jakob disease
C. Depression
D. HIV dementia
E. Huntington's disease
F. Lewy body dementia
G. Normal-pressure hydrocephalus
H. Parkinson's disease
I. Pick's disease
J. Vascular dementia
K. Wernicke–Korsakoff syndrome

For each of the following scenarios, select the most appropriate cause of dementia. Each option may be used once, more than once or not at all.

1. A 70-year-old man presents with a 6-month history of worsening forgetfulness and intellectual decline. He has, however, had frequent episodes of relative lucidness during this period. He tries to chase soldiers whom he thinks he sees in the garden, but his gait has markedly slowed down. His sleeping pattern is now irregular.

2. A 52-year-old woman presents to the emergency department following her first-ever seizure. Her husband said that she had to leave her job because, over a period of 2 months, she rapidly lost the ability to cope with its intellectual demands. A previous cryptic crossword fanatic, she cannot even fill out the simplest tabloid grid. On further questioning, she admits to muscle weakness and difficulty walking.

3. A 72-year-old man who is a lifelong smoker presents with a mild but sudden loss of concentration and problem-solving ability. This has become progressively more severe on three separate occasions without recovery in between.

4. A 54-year-old man has been arrested by the police for stealing furniture and verbally abusing his neighbours. They took him to the hospital because he appeared confused. His family are concerned that he is behaving strangely and is unable to cope with his work and finances. His general demeanour is apathetic.

5. A 69-year-old woman presents after a fall, having been unsteady on her feet for some time. She has severe memory loss, but is relatively well orientated. She has recently developed urinary incontinence. On examination, she has a wide-based gait.

Theme 11: Barriers to communication

Options

A. Cultural differences
B. Distraction
C. Interruption
D. Jargon
E. Language barrier
F. Negative attitude
G. Physical disability
H. Poor listening skills
I. Poor retention
J. Red tape
K. Stereotyping

For each of the following scenarios, select the most appropriate barrier to communication. Each option may be used once, more than once or not at all.

1. A surgeon tells a patient that a 'growth on your bile duct shows features of malignancy'. 'So will it be all right then?', the patient asks.

2. The registrar is obtaining consent from a woman for an upper gastrointestinal endoscopy using a proforma. After explaining the procedure, he asks the patient if she understands and if she has any questions. She says 'I'm afraid I don't have any questions. I don't really remember what you just told me, you see.'

3. A junior doctor is unhappy about the way elective surgical patients are clerked in the hospital. He feels that each ward should clerk their own patients rather than leaving the on-call doctors to do this. Although he would like to bring this up with the surgical managers himself, only the junior doctors' representative is allowed to make suggestions directly to the management.

4. A patient is brought into the emergency department following a fall. Every time he is asked a question, he stares at the doctor's mouth. When he responds, the doctor hears vague mumbles that he cannot interpret.

5. An Asian woman on the ward has a low blood pressure. The male doctor on call comes to assess her, but she screams and shoos him away.

Theme 12: Vasculitis

Options

A. Behçet's disease
B. Churg–Strauss syndrome
C. Giant cell arteritis
D. Kawasaki's disease
E. Microscopic polyangiitis
F. Polyarteritis nodosa
G. Polymyalgia rheumatica
H. Takayasu's arteritis
I. Wegener's disease

For each of the following scenarios, select the most appropriate diagnosis. Each option may be used once, more than once or not at all.

1. A 26-year-old woman presents with a 3-month history of general malaise, fever and weight loss. Over the last week, she has developed an intermittent cramping pain in her right arm. On examination, the upper limbs appear normal, but the radial pulses are not palpable.

2. A 32-year-old man presents with shortness of breath. He feels that it is similar to the asthma that he had as a child. He has also developed hayfever recently, which he has never had before. On examination, a palpable, purple rash is seen on the legs.

3. A 29-year-old man complains of recurrent painful ulceration in his mouth and on his genitals. The ulceration is clearly seen on examination. Swab cultures are taken and found to be negative for herpes simplex virus.

4. A 65-year-old woman presents with a pain in her shoulders. The pain came on suddenly this morning, and now she is barely able to move her arms. She is otherwise well. On examination, shoulder movement is limited by stiffness bilaterally.

5. A 42-year-old man presents with a 2-month history of recurrent nosebleeds. More recently, he has started coughing up blood as well. On examination, there is a deformity in the bridge of his nose.

Theme 13: Complications of liver disease

Options

A. Clotting factor deficiency
B. Hepatic encephalopathy
C. Hepatorenal syndrome
D. Hypoalbuminaemia
E. Hypoglycaemia
F. Lower gastrointestinal bleed
G. Ruptured oesophagus
H. Seizure
I. Spontaneous bacterial peritonitis
J. Thrombocytopenia
K. Upper gastrointestinal bleed

For each of the following scenarios, select the most likely complication. Each option may be used once, more than once or not at all.

1. A 56-year-old man with ascites secondary to alcoholic liver disease presents to the emergency department with severe abdominal pain and fever.

2. A 42-year-old woman with cirrhosis secondary to chronic hepatitis C infection presents to the emergency department with a history of vomiting frank blood and passing offensive, black stools.

3. A 36-year-old man with alcoholic liver disease is noticed to be increasingly confused, clumsy and aggressive after an upper gastrointestinal bleed. He is now sleeping during the day and is awake at night time.

4. A 54-year-old woman with end-stage liver failure secondary to primary biliary cirrhosis is noticed to have a rising serum creatinine and urea, and is passing only small volumes of urine each day.

5. A 19-year-old woman took a significant overdose of paracetamol 2 days ago. She has noticed several large bruises on her limbs and trunk.

Theme 14: Cutaneous lesions 1

Options

A. Cavernous haemangioma
B. Deep capillary naevus
C. Dercum's disease
D. Ganglion
E. Granuloma annulare
F. Kaposi's sarcoma
G. Neurofibroma
H. Pyogenic granuloma
I. Sebaceous cyst
J. Seborrhoeic keratosis
K. Superficial capillary naevus

For each of the following scenarios, select the most appropriate diagnosis. Each option may be used once, more than once or not at all.

1. A 75-year-old man goes to his GP with multiple, dark-brown, flat nodules on his back. These lesions are well demarcated and are rough and greasy to the touch.

2. A 34-year-old woman presents with multiple painful lesions over her body. On examination, each of these lesions is soft and mobile and 2cm in size. She has no other symptoms.

3. A 5-year-old girl was admitted to the emergency department with a seizure. On examination, she has a well-demarcated, purple, flat lesion over her right cheek and forehead. Her parents say that this has been present since birth.

4. An 18-year-old man presents with a lesion on his right wrist. On examination, there is a 2 cm firm lesion on the dorsum of the wrist that is painless and not mobile. There is no neurological deficit in the upper limb.

5. An 18-month-old boy is brought to the GP by his parents with a red lesion on his forehead. This was not present at birth, but has been growing for 3 months. On examination, the lesion is 3 cm, bright red and well defined. There are no other symptoms.

Theme 15: Antimicrobial therapy

Options

A. Amoxicillin
B. Cefotaxime
C. Chloramphenicol
D. Co-amoxiclav
E. Co-trimoxazole
F. Erythromycin
G. Flucloxacillin
H. Metronidazole
I. Vancomycin

For each of the following scenarios, select the most appropriate antibiotic. Each option may be used once, more than once or not at all.

1. This antibiotic is an appropriate first-line drug for treating mild community-acquired pneumonia in a penicillin-allergic patient.

2. This antibiotic should be prescribed with benzylpenicillin to treat cellulitis.

3. This antibiotic can be used for the treatment and prophylaxis of *Pneumocystis* pneumonia.

4. This antibiotic is used to treat uncomplicated bacterial conjunctivitis.

5. This antibiotic should be given in the hospital setting to treat bacterial meningitis.

Practice Paper 1: Answers

Theme 1: Causes of collapse

1. K – Vasovagal syncope

The term 'syncope' describes the sudden loss of consciousness. Presyncope is a feeling of light-headedness. Vasovagal syncope occurs when there is excessive activation of the parasympathetic nervous system in response to certain stimuli, such as heat, fear and stress. The parasympathetic activity causes systemic vasodilatation and bradycardia, which triggers profound hypotension and cerebral hypoperfusion. Collapse is often preceded by a feeling of faintness, nausea, sweating and ringing in the ears. Occasionally, witnesses may describe the patient twitching and a loss of urinary incontinence, which may be confused with seizure activity. Following collapse, cerebral perfusion is restored and recovery is rapid. Situational syncope describes the scenario when vasovagal episodes are triggered by specific actions, such as coughing, urinating or having blood taken.

In all cases of collapse, the patient should be questioned about the presence of chest pain, shortness of breath, urinary incontinence, tongue biting, palpitations, weakness and paraesthesia. A pre-/peri-/post-collapse history is essential, and should be supplemented by a collateral history from a witness when available. Routine investigation should always include ECG, capillary blood glucose, and lying and standing blood pressure.

Syncope, from Greek *syn* = together + *koptein* = to cut off; literally to 'cut short' or 'pause'.

2. M – Wolff–Parkinson–White syndrome

In Wolff–Parkinson–White (WPW) syndrome, there is an abnormal accessory conduction pathway that connects the atria to the ventricles, known as the bundle of Kent. This accessory pathway is able to conduct atrial depolarization to the ventricular myocardium faster than the atrioventricular node. This may trigger dangerous arrhythmias, including supraventricular re-entrant tachycardia, ventricular tachycardia and ventricular fibrillation. Patients may be asymptomatic or suffer from dizziness, palpitations, chest pain, syncope and sudden cardiac death. ECG changes in WPW syndrome include a shortened PR interval, a wide QRS complex and slurred upstroke of the R-wave (the 'delta wave'). Although anti-arrhythmic medications, such as amiodarone and flecainide, can be used as arrhythmia prophylaxis, the treatment of choice for symptomatic WPW syndrome is radio-ablation of the accessory pathway, as this offers a lifetime cure. Drugs that slow atrioventricular conduction (e.g. digoxin and verapamil) should be avoided, as they can promote conduction across the accessory pathway and trigger arrhythmias.

Louis Wolff, American cardiologist (1898–1972).

Sir John Parkinson, English cardiologist (1885–1976).

Paul Dudley White, American cardiologist (1886–1973).

Albert Frank Stanley Kent, British physiologist (1863–1958).

3. B – Cerebrovascular accident

This patient has suffered an embolic cerebral infarct secondary to atrial fibrillation (AF). The inefficient and haphazard atrial contraction that occurs in AF allows blood to stagnate and clot within the atria. Emboli originating from this thrombus may enter the systemic circulation, potentially leading to cerebral, limb or mesenteric infarction. Anticoagulation with warfarin or aspirin is usually indicated to reduce the risk of embolic disease in AF. The decision to anticoagulate must be based on a knowledge of the proposed benefits versus risks of treatment. Warfarin should be avoided in patients at risk of falls and non-compliance.

4. E – First-dose hypotension

First-dose hypotension is a common adverse effect of many antihypertensive medications, but is most commonly associated with angiotensin-converting enzyme (ACE) inhibitor therapy. In order to minimize the risk of first-dose hypotension, patients should be given a low starting dose (e.g. ramipril 1.25 mg) and advised to take the first few doses at night time while in bed. In addition, any diuretic medications should be stopped for the first few days of treatment in order to ensure that the patient is not dehydrated, which may add to the risk of first-dose hypotension and syncope.

5. A – Acute myocardial infarction

Myocardial infarction (MI) typically presents with a history of central crushing chest pain that radiates to the arms and jaw, and is associated with nausea, pallor and sweating. However, in a subgroup of individuals experiencing MI, these symptoms may be absent. In this situation, the patient is said to have had a *silent MI*. Silent MIs account for up to 25% of cases. They are common in elderly people and people with diabetes, and are most likely painless, secondary to autonomic neuropathy. Symptoms that may indicate silent MI include atypical chest pain, epigastric pain, shortness of breath, acute pulmonary oedema, collapse and sudden death. MI should be excluded in all cases of collapse, sudden-onset shortness of breath, acute pulmonary oedema and epigastric pain unless an alternative diagnosis is obvious. Treatment of silent MI is as for any MI.

Theme 2: Nerve lesions of the upper limb

1. L – Upper brachial plexus

Upper brachial plexus injuries, also known as Erb's palsy, involve the C5 and C6 nerve roots (the brachial plexus is made of the roots C5–T1). They are commonly caused by traction injuries, such as motorcycle accidents or birth injuries (due to pulling on the baby's arm). There is flaccid paralysis of the arm abductors, lateral rotators of the shoulder and supinators, so the affected arm hangs limp and is medially rotated, extended at the elbow and pronated, with the hand pointing backwards – the 'waiter's tip' position. Paralysis is accompanied by loss of sensation over the lateral arm and forearm.

Lower brachial plexus injuries, also known as Klumpke's palsy, involve the C8 and T1 nerve roots. They are often caused by breech birth injuries (when the baby's arm remains above its head) and motorcycle accidents. Patients present with a claw hand in all digits (from paralysis of the intrinsic muscles of the hand) and sensory loss along the ulnar border of the forearm and hand.

Wilheim Heinrich Erb, German neurologist (1840–1921).

Augusta Marie Dejerine-Klumpke, French neurologist (1859–1927).

2. F – Long thoracic nerve

The long thoracic nerve of Bell supplies the serratus anterior, a muscle that helps stabilize the scapula. This nerve can be damaged during breast and axillary surgery, radiotherapy and axillary trauma. Lesions of the long thoracic nerve result in winging of the scapula, where the scapula becomes prominent on pushing the arms against resistance.

3. K – Radial nerve

The radial nerve runs in close proximity to the shaft of the humerus in the spiral groove. Common causes of radial nerve palsies include humeral shaft fractures (as in this scenario, in which case patients also suffer bruising to the upper arm), compression of the nerve in the arm with prolonged use of ill-fitting crutches, and elbow dislocations or Monteggia fractures. Damage to the radial nerve is also seen in people who fall asleep with their arm hanging over the back of a chair ('Saturday night palsy').

The radial nerve supplies the extensors to the forearm and wrist, and radial nerve palsy results in an inability to extend the wrist or metacarpophalangeal joints (wrist drop), forearm extensor wasting and a loss of sensation in the anatomical snuffbox. The anatomical snuffbox is the name given to the triangular region on the radial dorsal aspect of the hand at the level of the carpal bones. It is so called as this was the surface used since the 16th century for placing and snorting 'snuff' (powdered tobacco).

4. A – Accessory nerve

The spinal root of the accessory nerve (cranial nerve XI) supplies the trapezius and sternocleidomastoid muscles. It can be damaged during dissections of the neck. Features of accessory nerve palsy include weakness of shoulder shrugging and an inability to turn the head against a force applied by the examiner.

5. C – Axillary nerve

This man presents with an anterior shoulder dislocation. The axillary nerve wraps around the surgical neck of the humerus and is damaged in 5–10%

of anterior dislocations. It can also be affected with fractures of the humeral neck. The axillary nerve supplies the deltoid muscle and gives rise to the lateral cutaneous nerve of the arm (which supplies sensation to the upper, outer arm). Axillary nerve lesions result in anaesthesia of the upper, outer arm (the 'regimental badge patch' area) and paralysis of the deltoid muscle, resulting in limited arm abduction. The arm cannot be abducted, but, if it is passively lifted above 90°, the arm can be held in abduction due to the action of the supraspinatus muscle.

The *posterior interosseous nerve* is a branch of the radial nerve that runs deep in the forearm to supply the wrist and finger extensors except the extensor carpi radialis longus (ECRL) (which is innervated by a proximal branch from the radial nerve). The posterior interosseous nerve can be damaged in forearm fractures, and this damage results in an inability to extend the fingers and a slight wrist drop. The wrist drop is only slight as the ECRL muscle still provides some wrist extension. There is no sensory loss with these nerve lesions. The anterior interosseous nerve is a motor branch of the median nerve in the forearm. Lesions of this nerve are rare and usually arise from deep lacerations to the forearm. The *anterior interosseous nerve* provides motor fibres to flexor pollicis longus, the medial part of flexor digitorum profundus and pronator quadratus. Patients have a weakness in the thumb and index finger characterized by a deformity in the pinch mechanism between the thumb and index fingers.

Compression of the *distal median nerve* can occur in the carpal tunnel as it passes behind the flexor retinaculum. Carpal tunnel syndrome is more common in women, during pregnancy and with certain medical conditions (e.g. rheumatoid arthritis, acromegaly and hypothyroidism). Patients experience tingling and numbness in the radial 3½ digits, which may be followed by wasting of the thenar eminence (supplied by the median nerve). Clinical tests that help confirm carpal tunnel syndrome include Tinel's test (tapping over the median nerve at the wrist reproduces symptoms) and Phalen's test (symptoms are reproduced by holding the wrist palmarflexed for 1 minute). *Proximal median nerve* lesions (i.e. entrapment before the nerve enters the carpal tunnel) manifest as pain in the anterior aspect of the distal upper arm and forearm, with loss of sensation in the radial 3½ digits. Tinel's and Phalen's tests are negative. Proximal median nerve lesions can occur with forearm fractures and elbow dislocation.

The *ulnar nerve* is most commonly damaged behind the elbow (proximal lesions) and at the wrist (distal lesions). The ulnar nerve supplies the small muscles of the hand (except the LOAF muscles: **L**ateral two lumbricals, **O**pponens pollicis, **A**bductor pollicis brevis and **F**lexor pollicis brevis). It also provides sensation to the medial skin of the palm and back of hand, and the medial 1½ digits. Ulnar lesions at the wrist result in sensory loss to the ulnar 1½ digits but not to the hand. This is because the branches of the ulnar nerve that supply the skin of the medial hand (i.e. the palmar cutaneous and dorsal cutaneous branches) originate proximal to the wrist. The digital sensory branch originates in the wrist. Ulnar nerve lesions also result in hand weakness. Chronic lesions of the ulnar nerve result in clawing of the hand. Supracondylar fractures can result in *ulnar nerve lesions at the elbow* (a proximal ulnar nerve lesion). Because the ulnar nerve supplies the flexors to the forearm, lesions of this nerve result in unopposed action of the forearm extensors, with the slight development of a claw hand in the fourth and fifth digits (hyperextension of the metacarpophalangeal joints with flexion of the interphalangeal joints). Proximal ulnar nerve lesions also result in a loss of sensation to the ulnar side of the hand. The clawing that occurs with proximal ulnar nerve lesions is not as marked as that which occurs with distal lesions. This is because the flexor digitorum profundus, which is supplied by the proximal ulnar nerve, is intact in distal lesions, resulting in more flexion of the interphalangeal joints and an exacerbated flexion deformity.

Jules Tinel, French neurologist (1879–1952).

George Phalen, American orthopaedic surgeon (1911–98).

Theme 3: Complications of diabetes mellitus

1. I – Neuropathic ulcer

Neuropathic ulcers are generally small, punched out, well circumscribed and painless. Unless there is coexistent peripheral vascular disease, the foot usually has good peripheral pulses and normal surrounding tissue. The patient usually has generalized sensory neuropathy, often in a 'glove-and-stocking' distribution. In order to prevent the development of neuropathic ulcers, good foot care, including regular podiatry review, must be promoted to all diabetic patients. The complications of neuropathic ulceration include superficial infection, abscess formation and osteomyelitis.

2. B – Autonomic neuropathy

This patient is suffering from postural hypotension. Autonomic neuropathy prevents the patient from compensating for the transient drop of blood pressure on standing, which then leads to cerebral hypoperfusion and collapse. Autonomic neuropathy can also cause erectile dysfunction, gastroparesis, urinary retention and nocturnal diarrhoea. Postural hypotension is usually managed by educating the patient to stand slowly from a sitting/lying position. In severe cases, fludrocortisone, a mineralocorticoid with some glucocorticoid activity, can be prescribed to promote fluid retention and maintain a high intravascular circulating volume.

3. C – Charcot's joint

Also known as neuropathic joint disease, Charcot's joint disease refers to the destruction of weight-bearing joints secondary to sensory neuropathy. The ankles and knees are most commonly affected. Repeated unnoticed trauma and abnormal stresses caused by the absence of pain result in cartilage, ligament, synovium and bone damage, which produces a grossly deformed and unstable, but painless, joint.

Jean-Marie Charcot, French neurologist (1825–93).

4. J – Nephropathy

Diabetic nephropathy is an important cause of morbidity and mortality in the diabetic population, with up to 30% developing chronic renal failure during their lifetime. Diabetic nephropathy has a complex pathophysiology, which can be simplified into three important processes: glomerular involvement, ischaemia and infection. Important contributors to the development of diabetic nephropathy are poor glycaemic control, hypertension and renovascular disease (e.g. renal artery stenosis). The earliest detectable sign of nephropathy is microalbuminuria, i.e. the presence of trace amounts of albumin in the urine that are not detectable using standard dipstick analysis. If untreated, microalbuminuria can progress to intermittent albuminuria and then persistent albuminuria. It is thought that patients with persistent albuminuria are 5–10 years away from end-stage renal failure, even if their creatinine is normal. To reduce the risk of developing end-stage renal failure, all diabetic patients should have their kidney function and urine tested on a regular basis. Good glycaemic and blood pressure control are essential and must be communicated to the patient. Angiotensin-converting enzyme (ACE) inhibitors and angiotensin II receptor antagonists have been shown to reduce the progression of microalbuminuria, and also contribute to blood pressure control.

5. K – Necrobiosis lipoidica

Necrobiosis lipoidica diabeticorum is a rare dermatological complication of diabetes mellitus seen in approximately 1% of patients. It is most often occurs on the anterolateral aspect of the lower limb. The lesion usually begins as a small red nodule that increases in size and flattens over time. Eventually, the lesion becomes depressed, irregular, scaly or waxy, and develops a brownish-yellow discoloration. If the lesion is not ulcerated, topical steroids in association with appropriate dressings can be applied. If ulceration is present, immunosuppressive agents such as ciclosporin can be beneficial. Treatment is often unsuccessful.

Lipoatrophy describes a localized loss of fat tissue, which may occur in people with diabetes at the site of repeated subcutaneous insulin injections. The opposite condition is *lipohypertrophy*, the accumulation of fat at the point of repeated subcutaneous injections. Both of these conditions can be avoided by regularly rotating injection sites.

Theme 4: Diagnosis of respiratory conditions 1

1. N – Small cell lung tumour

Primary lung tumours are associated with smoking, and their incidence is rising. The types of bronchial carcinomas are squamous cell carcinomas (35%), adenocarcinomas (30%), small cell carcinomas (20%) and large cell carcinomas (15%). A Pancoast tumour is a tumour at the apex of the lung that can interfere with the sympathetic chain, resulting in ipsilateral Horner's syndrome. Clinical features include cough, haemoptysis, dyspnoea, stridor, pneumonia and weight loss. Other manifestations of lung tumours include ectopic antidiuretic hormone secretion (small cell, this scenario), ectopic adrenocorticotrophic hormone secretion (small cell), ectopic parathyroid hormone secretion (squamous cell), carcinoid syndrome, gynaecomastia, Eaton–Lambert syndrome, clubbing and hypertrophic pulmonary osteoarthropathy (HPOA). HPOA results in subperiosteal new bone formation in the long bones, with pain and pitting of the anterior shins. Examination in bronchial carcinoma may reveal a monophonic unilateral wheeze (due to fixed bronchial obstruction), a bovine cough (from left recurrent laryngeal nerve palsy), diaphragm paralysis (from phrenic nerve paralysis), pleural effusion and superior vena caval obstruction.

The best investigation for bronchial tumours is bronchoscopy with washings and biopsy. A CT of the thorax should be performed to assess spread. Management is ideally with surgery (although this is not possible in 80% at the time of diagnosis). Contraindications to surgery include spread to contralateral lymph nodes, malignant effusion and metastases. Small cell tumours are best treated with chemotherapy and non-small cell tumours are best treated with radiotherapy. Overall, 80% die within 1 year. Small cell tumours have a worse prognosis, due to early metastases.

Blood-borne lung metastases can occur from various tumours, e.g. renal cell carcinoma. Secondary deposits are often multiple and bilateral, and tend not to cause respiratory symptoms.

2. F – Cystic fibrosis

Cystic fibrosis (CF) is the commonest autosomal recessive condition in white populations in the UK, affecting 1 in 2500 live births. CF is caused by an abnormal gene coding for the cystic fibrosis transmembrane regulator protein (CFTR), located on chromosome 7. CFTR is a cAMP-dependent chloride channel blocker. The most common mutation in CF is the ΔF508 mutation. The poor transport of chloride ions and water across epithelial cells of the respiratory and pancreatic exocrine glands in CF results in an increased viscosity of secretions. The range of presentations is varied, including recurrent chest infections, failure to thrive due to malabsorption and liver disease. In the neonatal period, infants may present with prolonged neonatal jaundice, bowel obstruction (meconium ileus) or rectal prolapse.

The gold standard investigation for CF is the sweat test. The abnormal function of sweat glands results in the excess concentration of sodium chloride (NaCl) in sweat. Sweat is stimulated by pilocarpine iontophoresis, collected on filter paper and analysed.

Normal sweat NaCl concentration = 10–14 mmol/L

Sweat NaCl concentration in CF = 80–125 mmol/L

At least two sweat tests should be performed, as diagnostic errors and false positives are common.

Management options in CF include physiotherapy (for respiratory secretions), antibiotics (for prophylaxis and treatment of lung infections) and pancreatic enzyme supplements (to prevent malabsorption). Complications include diabetes mellitus, hepatic cirrhosis, infertility in males, severe pulmonary hypertension and cor pulmonale, and chronic lung infections (*Pseudomonas aeruginosa* and *Burkholderia cepacia*). Many cases of CF are now being picked up early since the introduction of a national screening programme assessing immunoreactive trypsin (IRT) levels on the Guthrie card at day 8 of life. IRT is a pancreatic enzyme with raised levels in CF.

The boy in this case has bilateral coarse crepitations. Given the history, these are a sign of bronchiectasis. *Bronchiectasis* is an abnormal dilatation of the bronchioles. Causes of bronchiectasis can be congenital (ciliary dyskinesia or CF) or acquired (whooping cough, measles or tuberculosis). Pus accumulates in the dilated bronchi, resulting in a productive cough that is worse in the morning and brought about by changes in posture. Bronchiectasis is associated with clubbing of the fingers. The best investigation to confirm bronchiectasis is CT. Management is by physiotherapy (postural drainage and chest percussion) and prompt antibiotics for respiratory tract infections.

3. H – Mesothelioma

Mesothelioma is a malignant tumour of the pleura (or, less commonly, the peritoneum). Blue asbestos (crocidolite) is the most potent cause. A 20-year lag time between asbestos exposure and development of mesothelioma is typical. Patients present with chest pain and symptoms of pleural effusion. The effusion in mesothelioma tends to be blood stained, but the definitive diagnosis is made by pleural biopsy. There is no curative treatment for mesothelioma, although radiotherapy may slow growth.

4. A – Asbestos-related lung disease

There are three main types of asbestos: chrysotile (white), crocidolite (blue) and amosite (brown). Asbestos is associated with various conditions, and the patient in this scenario has pleural plaques. Pleural plaques are asymptomatic calcified pleural thickenings resembling holly leaves. They are seen on chest X-ray.

Asbestosis is a diffuse fibrosis of the lungs and pleura. It develops in individuals who have been exposed to large amounts of asbestos for years, and affected patients in the UK can claim industrial injury benefit. Clinical features include progressive dyspnoea, clubbing and lower zone inspiratory crepitations. Chest X-ray shows reticulonodular shadowing or honeycombing – features typical of fibrosis. The diagnosis is confirmed by lung biopsy. There is no specific management, and steroids are of no use.

5. B – Asthma

Asthma is a condition of chronic inflammation with airway hyper-reactivity. The pathology includes increased eosinophils, mast cells and immunoglobulin E (IgE) production, with mucus hyperplasia and airway smooth muscle hyperplasia. Asthma affects one in seven children and is associated with a family history of atopy (asthma, allergic rhinitis or eczema). Asthma can be precipitated by pet hairs, smoke, dust mites, pollution, exercise and anxiety. β-Blockers induce bronchoconstriction, and hence are contraindicated. Ten per cent of people with asthma also develop bronchoconstriction with non-steroidal anti-inflammatory drugs (NSAIDs) and aspirin. Features of asthma include wheeze, breathlessness, a cough (which is worse at night) and chest tightness. Peak expiratory flow rates tend to be worse in the mornings. Asthma can be episodic or persistent.

The diagnosis of asthma is made based on a good history and by demonstrating >15% improvement in peak expiratory flow rate (PEFR) with bronchodilator use. Serial PEFR measurements are used to monitor disease and its response to treatment. The chest X-ray in asthma is normal, although during acute attacks the lung fields may be hyperinflated. The routine and emergency management of asthma is covered in 'Management of asthma' (Paper 9 Answers, Theme 13).

Sleep apnoea is a physical condition in which the upper respiratory tract becomes partially occluded during sleep. This can cause transient cessation in breathing, which causes the patient to wake repeatedly during the night, reducing the quality of sleep. Sleep apnoea result in daytime tiredness. It is more common in overweight males who snore. Treatment is by continuous positive airway pressure (CPAP) via a facemask during sleep.

Theme 5: Glomerulonephritis

1. G – Minimal-change glomerulonephritis

Nephrotic syndrome, not to be confused with nephritic syndrome, is characterized by loss of large amounts of protein in the urine due to an excessively leaky glomerular basement membrane. The features of nephrotic syndrome include proteinuria, peripheral oedema, hypoalbuminaemia, hypertension, hyperlipidaemia, hypercoaguability and an increased risk of infection, including spontaneous bacterial peritonitis. In children, the main cause of nephrotic syndrome is minimal-change glomerulonephritis (>90% of cases). Minimal-change disease is thought to be secondary to abnormal T-cell activity that causes a reduction in the synthesis of anion channels within the glomerular basement membrane, thereby making it more permeable. On renal biopsy, the histological appearance is normal. Electron microscopy of the sample may reveal fused and abnormal podocytes. The treatment of minimal-change disease involves steroid therapy, fluid restriction, a low-salt diet, penicillin prophylaxis, angiotensin-converting enzyme inhibitors to reduce proteinuria and statin therapy for hyperlipidaemia. Immunosuppression is occasionally indicated in severe and refractory disease.

Podocyte, from Greek *podos* = foot; so called as these epithelial cells of the kidney have foot-like processes that increase its surface area.

Glomerulus, from Latin *glomerare* = to roll up (describing it as a ball of capillaries).

2. E – Membranous glomerulonephritis

Membranous glomerulonephritis is the most common cause of nephrotic syndrome in adults. In this condition, immune complexes are formed when circulating antibodies bind to basement membrane antigens or antigens deposited in the glomerulus from the circulation. The immune complexes activate an immunological response that involves the complement cascade. This response damages the glomerular basement membrane, making it more permeable. Membranous glomerulonephritis is usually idiopathic (90%), but may be secondary to a number of disease processes, including systemic lupus erythematosus, hepatitis B, systemic infection and drugs. Treatment is largely the same as for nephrotic syndrome in children (see above). The prognosis is variable. Approximately one-third of patients recover spontaneously, one-third will respond to immunosuppression and one-third will develop end-stage renal failure. Up to 5% of patients will develop renal vein thrombosis.

3. C – Goodpasture's syndrome

Goodpasture's syndrome is a rare condition in which autoantibodies are formed against the glomerular basement membrane and the alveolar membrane. The antibodies trigger a type II hypersensitivity reaction that causes renal failure, pulmonary haemorrhage and haemoptysis. The condition is usually diagnosed by the detection of anti-glomerular basement membrane antibody (anti-GBM) in the serum and via renal biopsy. The biopsy often shows focal or diffuse crescentic glomerulonephritis. Immunofluorescence may demonstrate linear deposition of IgG antibodies and complement (C3) on the glomerular basement membrane. Goodpasture's syndrome is usually treated aggressively with plasmapheresis, corticosteroids and immunosuppression.

Ernest William Goodpasture, American pathologist (1886–1960).

4. D – IgA nephropathy

Immunoglobulin A (IgA) nephropathy is probably the most common cause of primary glomerular nephritis worldwide. In this condition, IgA antibodies are deposited within the mesangium and trigger an immune response via activation of the complement cascade. IgA nephropathy may be asymptomatic for many years and discovered only when a random urine dipstick analysis shows microscopic haematuria and proteinuria. Alternatively, it may present with frank haematuria, which usually occurs within 2 days of an upper respiratory tract infection. Renal biopsy is required for diagnosis. Typical changes include mesangium proliferation and expansion of the extracellular matrix. Immunofluorescence shows diffuse IgA deposition throughout the mesangium, with or without evidence of complement, IgG and IgM deposition. Serum IgA is elevated in only about 50% of cases. Treatment involves corticosteroid therapy, immunosuppression and phenytoin, which can cause a reduction in IgA levels. However, in most cases, the condition does not respond to immunomodulation therapy. Up to 30% of patients eventually develop end-stage renal failure.

5. H – Post-streptococcal glomerulonephritis

This form of glomerulonephritis is usually seen 1–2 weeks after an infection caused by a group A β-haemolytic streptococcus, e.g. tonsillitis or cellulitis. The pathophysiology involves immune complex deposition within the glomerular basement membrane. Patients present with acute nephritic syndrome, i.e. fluid retention, peripheral oedema, hypertension, proteinuria and haematuria. The urine is classically dark in colour and is sometimes referred to as 'Pepsi urine'. Investigation usually reveals proteinuria, haematuria, elevated anti-streptolysin O titres and reduced complement (C3). In cases with a clear history and consistent initial investigation results, renal biopsy is often not required. Management is largely supportive with fluid restriction and antihypertensive medications.

Theme 6: Management of hypertension

1. J – Provide lifestyle advice and reassess annually

The recommended target blood pressure for adults is less than 140/85 mmHg (or 130/80 mmHg for those with diabetes). Blood pressure should be viewed as part of the patient's cardiovascular risk factor profile, which also includes variables such as sex, family history, diet, lifestyle, smoking status, lipid profile and the presence of diabetes. The patient in this question has an appropriate blood pressure which requires no active treatment. However, all patients with a systolic blood pressure above 130 mmHg should receive lifestyle advice and be assessed annually.

2. D – Confirm over 4 weeks and treat if persistent

A single blood pressure recording should not be used to decide whether a patient requires treatment, since most antihypertensive agents have side-effects, interactions and contribute to polypharmacy. The British Hypertension Society guidelines (see the reference at the end of the answers to Practice Paper 1, Theme 6) recommend that essential hypertension be confirmed over a period of time prior to initiating treatment. In patients without known cardiovascular risk or end-organ damage, a 4- to 12-week period of assessment should be used to confirm hypertension. Treatment should be initiated only if the blood pressure is persistently over 160/100 mmHg. In contrast, hypertensive patients with significant cardiovascular risk, diabetes or end-organ damage should have the diagnosis confirmed over a 3- to 4-week period. In this high-risk group, the threshold for treatment is lowered so that individuals with blood pressures persistently over 140/90 mmHg are treated sooner. Lifestyle advice should be offered to all patients, and must include the need to stop smoking, reduce salt and saturated fat intake, increase fruit and vegetable intake, and exercise on a regular basis. In addition, patients should be considered for lipid-lowering and antiplatelet therapy in order to reduce their overall cardiac risk.

3. H – Prescribe a single oral antihypertensive agent as an outpatient

According to the British Hypertension Society guidelines, the patient in this question requires pharmacological treatment. Treatment should begin with a single antihypertensive agent. The main classes of drug that are used as first-line agents in the UK are angiotensin-converting enzyme (ACE) inhibitors, β-blockers, calcium channel blockers and diuretics. When deciding which antihypertensive medication to prescribe, the *AB/CD principle* should be employed. In this system, each letter represents a class of drug: A = ACE inhibitors, B = β-blockers, C = calcium channel blockers and D = diuretics.

Non-Afro-Caribbean individuals under 55 years of age should be initially treated with either A or B, i.e. ACE inhibitors or β-blockers, because these drugs are better at reducing renin-dependent hypertension, which is often seen in this cohort of individuals. Afro-Caribbean and older patients (>55 years) should be started on either C or D, i.e. calcium channel blockers or diuretics. If a single agent is ineffective, a second agent from the opposite group should be added, i.e. if A or B does not work, either C or D should be added. For example, a 50-year-old white man whose hypertension was not controlled with an ACE inhibitor should be prescribed either a calcium channel blocker or a thiazide diuretic.

4. B – Admit to hospital for oral antihypertensive medication

This is a case of malignant hypertension, which can be defined as a systolic blood pressure greater than 200 mmHg and/or a diastolic pressure greater than 120 mmHg in association with severe retinopathy (grade III–IV). Patients are often symptomatic and complain of headache, blurred vision and dizziness. This is a serious condition, and if left untreated the mortality rate is approximately 90% after 1 year. In the absence of papilloedema, congestive heart failure and neurological complications such as encephalopathy and seizure, it is usual to treat with oral agents on a general ward. The combination of a β-blocker with a thiazide diuretic (e.g. atenolol with bendroflumethiazide) is the usual first-line treatment.

The aim of treatment is to reduce the blood pressure by approximately 25% over a 4-hour period and then to normal over the following 72 hours. Care must be taken not to drop the blood pressure too quickly, as this may lead to retinal, cerebral and myocardial infarction due to the failure of autoregulatory perfusion mechanisms. Once the acute stage of the episode is over, the patient should be investigated for end-organ damage such as retinopathy, nephropathy and neuropathy. In addition, a cause for secondary hypertension such as phaeochromocytoma, Cushing's syndrome and renal artery stenosis should be excluded before a diagnosis of essential hypertension can be made. Follow-up of these patients is essential.

5. A – Admit to high-dependency unit for monitoring and intravenous antihypertensive medication

This patient is suffering from severe malignant hypertension with papilloedema and encephalopathy. This condition warrants urgent treatment and monitoring to prevent serious complications such as haemorrhagic stroke, blindness, renal failure, aortic dissection and death. All patients with features of severe disease require admission to the high-dependency or intensive therapy unit. Intravenous sodium nitroprusside and furosemide are the first-line treatments of hypertensive encephalopathy, and should be used to reduce blood pressure by approximately 25% over 1–2 hours and then to normal levels over the following 72 hours. Intravenous β-blockers (e.g. labetalol) and long-acting calcium channel blockers may be considered as second-line agents if first-line medications are not adequate. As previously mentioned, the blood pressure should not be dropped too quickly.

Guidelines for management of hypertension

For more information, see:

Williams B, Poulter NR, Brown MJ et al. British Hypertension Society guidelines for hypertension management 2004 (BHS-IV): summary. *BMJ* 2004; **328**: 634–40.

Theme 7: Interpretation of cerebrospinal fluid results

1. A – *Cryptococcus neoformans* (fungal)

2. E – Mumps (viral)

3. D – Multiple sclerosis

4. G – *Neisseria meningitidis* (bacterial)

5. F – *Mycobacterium tuberculosis* (tuberculous)

The cerebrospinal fluid (CSF) abnormalities found in bacterial, viral, tuberculous and fungal meningitis are summarized in the following table. Make sure that you learn these.

	Normal	*Bacterial*	*Viral*	*Tuberculous*	*Fungal*
Pressure	50–180 mmH$_2$O	Normal/↑	Normal	Normal/↑	Normal
Colour	Clear	Cloudy	Clear	Clear/cloudy	Clear
Red cells	0–4/mm^3	Normal	Normal	Normal	Normal
White cells	0–4/mm^3	>1000 neutrophils	<1000 lymphocytes	>1000 lymphocytes	0–50 lymphocytes
Glucose	>60% blood	↓	Normal	↓	↓
Protein	<0.45 g/L	↑	Normal/↑	↑	↑
Microbiology	Sterile	+ve stain	Sterile/virus	+ve stain	+ve stain

Different stains need to be used to pick up different pathogens. Bacteria are stained with Gram stain (*N. meningitidis* is a Gram-negative diplococcus, streptococci are Gram-positive). *M. tuberculosis* stains with Ziehl–Neelsen stain. India ink stains *C. neoformans*. In addition to the above findings, the presence of oligoclonal bands of immunoglobulin in the CSF is strongly indicative of multiple sclerosis. In subarachnoid haemorrhage, xanthochromia may be seen in the CSF. Xanthochromia is a yellow colour caused by the presence of erythrocyte breakdown products.

Theme 8: Thyroid disease

1. A – De Quervain's thyroiditis

De Quervain's thyroiditis describes inflammation of the thyroid gland, which is usually secondary to a self-limiting viral infection. The patient often complains of neck swelling (goitre), tenderness, fever and flu-like symptoms. Blood tests will usually reveal a high C-reactive protein (CRP) level and a high erythrocyte sedimentation rate (ESR). Thyroid function tests will initially show a high thyroxine (T_4) level in association with suppressed thyroid-stimulating hormone (TSH). Following the acute phase, the patient will often enter a hypothyroid state before becoming euthyroid after 4–6 months. De Quervain's thyroiditis requires no specific treatment, but non-steroidal anti-inflammatories can be given for pain.

Fritz de Quervain, Swiss surgeon (1868–1940).

2. B – Graves' disease

Graves' disease is the most common cause of hyperthyroidism. It is an autoimmune disease in which circulating IgG immunoglobulins stimulate the TSH receptors of the thyroid gland, causing the release of T_4 into the circulation. Graves' disease is the only cause of thyroid eye disease. Autoantibodies are also directed against retro-orbital structures, causing proptosis, ophthalmoplegia and periorbital oedema. Common symptoms of hyperthyroidism include heat intolerance, weight loss, anxiety, diarrhoea, tremor and palpitations. Thyroid function tests are likely to show a high T_4 level and a reduced TSH level. The patient may also have a normocytic anaemia, deranged liver function tests and a high ESR. Hyperthyroidism can be treated in a variety of ways. β-Blockers improve the symptoms of hyperthyroidism, but have no effect on the underlying disease. Carbimazole reduces T_4 synthesis, and can either be titrated against the patient's thyroid function until they are euthyroid or be given at higher doses to completely suppress endogenous T_4 synthesis, which is then supplemented with exogenous T_4. The latter method is known as the 'block-and-replace' regimen and has the advantage of allowing better control of T_4 levels. Carbimazole should be withdrawn after 18 months of treatment, although 50% of patients will relapse and require further treatment.

Robert James Graves, Irish physician (1797–1853).

3. F – Hypothyroidism secondary to lithium therapy

Lithium, a drug used to treat bipolar disorder (manic depression), is one of a number of medications known to affect the thyroid gland. Lithium can cause goitre formation and inhibit T_4 and triiodothyronine (T_3) secretion from the thyroid gland. Therefore, prior to starting lithium, every patient should receive a neck examination and have their thyroid function checked. The majority of patients taking lithium become subclinically hypothyroid (i.e. are asymptomatic, with a normal T_4 level and a high TSH). Unless the patient is acutely unwell, it is usual practice to continue the lithium and start the patient on T_4 replacement. After commencing therapy, thyroid function should be tested every 6 months.

4. C – Hashimoto's thyroiditis

Hashimoto's thyroiditis is an autoimmune disease in which the thyroid gland becomes infiltrated by plasma cells and lymphocytes. This leads to the development of goitre and thyroid dysfunction. At presentation, the majority of patients are euthyroid, a significant proportion are hypothyroid and a minority are hyperthyroid. However, up to 50% will eventually become hypothyroid, as in this case. Serology often reveals the presence of autoantibodies to thyroid peroxidase and thyroglobulin. Treatment is with T_4 if the patient is hypothyroid.

Hashimoto Hakaru, Japanese physician (1881–1934).

5. G – Sick euthyroid syndrome

Sick euthyroid syndrome describes abnormal thyroid function in the presence of systemic disease. There are many different subtypes of sick euthyroidism, but, as a general rule, the T_3 and T_4 levels are low, with TSH levels falling in more severe disease (i.e. everything is low). As the patient recovers from the underlying disease, the thyroid function usually returns to normal.

Theme 9: Transfusion reactions

1. K – Slow the transfusion and prescribe paracetamol

The development of low-grade pyrexia in the absence of other symptoms is indicative of a non-haemolytic febrile transfusion reaction. It is relatively common and is caused by anti-leucocyte antibodies in the patient's serum reacting to leucocytes in the transfused blood. The condition is treated by slowing the infusion rate and prescribing paracetamol. Close monitoring should follow a non-haemolytic febrile reaction, as it may very occasionally proceed to anaphylaxis. In order to reduce the risk of non-haemolytic febrile reactions, all blood products in the UK are leucocyte depleted.

2. N – Stop the transfusion and inform the blood bank. Take blood for full blood count, clotting screen and Coombs' testing, and begin fluid resuscitation

This man is having an acute haemolytic reaction due to ABO incompatibility. This potentially fatal condition is usually caused by human error and can be avoided by following strict transfusion protocols. Within minutes of beginning the transfusion, the patient becomes febrile and experiences chest, abdominal and loin pain. The patient is at risk of developing disseminated intravascular coagulation (DIC) and acute renal failure. If an acute haemolytic reaction is suspected, the transfusion should be stopped immediately, and the remaining blood and giving set should be sent to the blood bank together with a sample of the patient's own blood to test for incompatibility. Blood should also be taken from the patient for full blood count, urea and electrolytes, clotting studies and direct Coombs' testing.

The initial management is ABC. Fluid resuscitation is necessary to treat renal failure and should begin straight away. If there is evidence of DIC, the patient will require cryoprecipitate or fresh frozen plasma. The patient should be transferred to the high-dependency or intensive care unit for further treatment and monitoring. The mortality rate of acute haemolytic reaction following transfusion is around 10%.

3. M – Stop the transfusion and exclude a haemolytic reaction. Send blood cultures and prescribe broad-spectrum antibiotics

This patient had developed sepsis secondary to bacterial contamination of the blood product. Contamination can occur at any stage of the product's life. Before diagnosing sepsis secondary to bacterial contamination, it is important to first exclude a haemolytic reaction, as the conditions are often indistinguishable in the early stages (a haemolytic reaction is less likely in this scenario, as the symptoms take 40 minutes to develop and the pyrexia is very high). Blood cultures should be taken and broad-spectrum antibiotics started immediately. Antibiotics can later be amended based on bacterial sensitivities when these become available.

4. J – Slow the transfusion and prescribe furosemide

Any intravenous infusion, including blood, has the potential to cause fluid overload resulting in peripheral and pulmonary oedema. Certain groups of patients, including elderly people and individuals with ischaemic heart disease, are particularly at risk. In order to prevent this complication, the blood should be infused slowly and furosemide prescribed between units.

5. F – Prescribe intravenous calcium gluconate, intravenous insulin and glucose

Massive blood transfusion is defined as the patient receiving 150% of their circulating blood volume, or having had their whole circulating volume replaced by donor blood within a 24-hour period. Complications of massive blood transfusion include hypothermia, thrombocytopenia, hypocalcaemia, deranged clotting and hyperkalaemia. This patient is hyperkalaemic, judging from the typical ECG changes of a widened QRS complex and tall, tented T-waves. Calcium gluconate should be given immediately, as it protects the myocardium from the arrhythmogenic actions of potassium. Intravenous insulin and glucose should then be prescribed to drive potassium into the intracellular compartment. Cardiac monitoring should be started when available.

Guidelines for transfusion

Further information on blood transfusion is available at:
www.transfusionguidelines.org.uk.

Theme 10: Dementia 1

Dementia is defined as a progressive, irreversible decline in cognitive function *without* impaired consciousness. It can affect all aspects of higher brain function: concentration, memory, language, personality and emotional control.

Dementia, from Latin *de* = away + *mens* = mind.

1. F – Lewy body dementia

Lewy body dementia is the second most common dementia after Alzheimer's disease. Characteristic features of Lewy body dementia include day-to-day fluctuating levels of cognitive functioning, visual hallucinations, sleep disturbance, transient loss of consciousness, recurrent falls and parkinsonian features (tremor, hypokinesia, rigidity and postural instability). Although people with Lewy body dementia are prone to hallucination, antipsychotics should be avoided, as they precipitate severe parkinsonism in 60%. Lewy bodies are abnormalities of the cytoplasm found within neurons, containing various proteins and granular material. They are found in the cerebral cortex in patients with Lewy body dementia, and are also found in patients with Parkinson's disease.

Frederick Lewy, German neurologist (1885–1950).

2. B – Creutzfeldt–Jakob disease

Creutzfeldt–Jakob disease (CJD) is a rapidly progressive dementia caused by prions (infectious agents composed only of protein). The prion proteins can be transmitted by neurosurgical instruments and human-derived pituitary hormones. Features of CJD include rapid cognitive impairment, which may be preceded by anxiety and depression. Eventually, physical features become prominent, including muscle disturbance (rigidity, tremor, wasting, spasticity, fasciculations, cyclonic jerks and choreoathetoid movements). Convulsions may also occur. The EEG is characteristic (showing stereotypical sharp wave complexes). Death occurs within 6–8 months.

New variant CJD (nvCJD) occurs secondary to ingestion of bovine spongiform encephalopathy (BSE)-infected beef. It is more common in younger adults. The features are as for CJD, but decline is slower, with death occurring within 18 months. There are no typical EEG changes in nvCJD, although there is a characteristic feature on MRI (symmetrical hyperintensity in the posterior nucleus of the thalamus – the pulvinar sign).

Other prion diseases include kuru (in Papa New Guinea, transmitted by cannibalistic consumption of human neural tissue) and Gerstmann–Straussler syndrome (an autosomal dominant mutation of the prion protein gene on chromosome 20).

Hans Gerhard Creutzfeldt, German neuropathologist (1885–1964).

Alfons Maria Jakob, German neurologist (1884–1931).

3. J – Vascular dementia

Vascular dementia is an ischaemic disorder characterized by multiple small cerebral infarcts in the cortex and white matter. When >100 mL of infarcts have occurred, dementia becomes clinically apparent. Vascular dementia begins in the 60s with a stepwise deterioration of cognitive function. Other features include focal neurology, fits and nocturnal confusion. Risk factors for vascular dementia are as for any atherosclerotic disease (male sex, smoking, hypertension, diabetes and hypercholesterolaemia). Death in vascular dementia often occurs within 5 years, due to ishaemic heart disease or stroke.

4. I – Pick's disease

Pick's disease is a form of frontotemporal dementia (it can only be differentiated from other forms postmortem, so 'frontotemporal dementia' is the preferred term). Clinical features include disinhibition, inattention, antisocial behaviour and personality changes. Later on, apathy, akinesia and withdrawal may predominate. Memory loss and disorientation only occur late. Postmortem examination shows atrophy of the frontal and temporal lobes (knife blade atrophy) and Pick's bodies (cytoplasmic inclusion bodies of tau protein) in the substantia nigra. In advanced cases, the atrophy may be seen on MRI.

Arnold Pick, Czechoslovakian neurologist and psychiatrist (1852–1924).

5. G – Normal-pressure hydrocephalus

Normal-pressure hydrocephalus is characterized by the triad of dementia (mainly memory problems), gait disturbance and urinary incontinence. It is caused by an increased volume of CSF, but with only a slightly raised pressure (as the ventricles dilate to compensate). There is an underlying obstruction in the subarachnoid space that prevents CSF from being reabsorbed but allows it to flow from the ventricular system into the subarachnoid space. Diagnosis is by lumbar puncture (to demonstrate a normal CSF opening pressure) followed by head CT/MRI (showing enlarged ventricles). Treatment is with ventriculoperitoneal shunting.

Theme 11: Barriers to communication

This is an example of a question for which you may not specifically revise but can crop up in examinations. It is easy to feel frustrated at being presented with such questions in summative examinations, but on the whole they are straightforward, so be grateful for the easy marks!

1. D – Jargon

2. I – Poor retention

3. J – Red tape

4. G – Physical disability (deafness)

5. A – Cultural differences

Theme 12: Vasculitis

1. H – Takayasu's arteritis

Vasculitis is an inflammation of the blood vessels. Takayasu's arteritis (also known as 'pulseless disease') is a rare granulomatous inflammation of the aorta and its major branches. This results in poor blood flow to the peripheries and a lack of distal pulses. It is commonest in Japanese women. Patients present with systemic illness (malaise, fever and weight loss) and arm claudication. A third of patients suffer visual disturbance. Examination reveals absent pulses and arterial bruits. Diagnosis is by angiography, which demonstrates the inflamed constricted major vessels. Treatment is with steroids, but surgery may be required to bypass significantly stenosed or obliterated vessels.

Mikito Takayasu, Japanese ophthalmologist (1860–1938).

2. B – Churg–Strauss syndrome

Churg–Strauss syndrome is a rare systemic vasculitis that is associated with eosinophilia and asthma. The disease may be triphasic, with a prodromal period (rhinitis and allergies), eosinophilia (asthma or eosinophilic gastroenteritis) and finally a systemic vasculitis. Churg–Strauss syndrome is associated with perinuclear antineutrophil cytoplasmic antibodies (pANCAs). Treatment is with steroids.

Jacob Churg, American pathologist (b1910).

Lotte Strauss, American pathologist (1913–85).

3. A – Behçet's disease

Behçet's disease (pronounced 'beh-chet') is a chronic vasculitis most common in Turkey and the eastern Mediterranean. There is a strong association with HLA-B5 and disease is more severe in males. Behçet's disease is characterized by an occlusive vasculitis and venulitis. The diagnosis is based on the clinical features, which include recurrent oral and genital ulceration, recurrent iritis, skin lesions, and thrombophlebitis. The pathergy reaction (where red papules >2 mm develop after 48 hours at sites of needle pricks) is pathognomonic of Behçet's disease.

Pathergy, from Greek *pathos* = suffering.

Hulusi Behçet, Turkish dermatologist (1889–1948).

4. G – Polymyalgia rheumatica

Polymyalgia rheumatica is not a vasculitis but is found in 50% of people with temporal arteritis (below). It is commonest in females over 50 years. Patients present with abrupt-onset proximal muscle pain (shoulder and hips) and stiffness *without* weakness. (The lack of weakness helps distinguish polymyalgia rheumatica from polymyositis.) Symptoms are worse in the morning. Treatment is with corticosteroids, and the response is prompt and dramatic.

Giant cell arteritis (temporal arteritis) is an inflammatory vasculitis of the cranial branches arising from the aorta. It is most common in the over-50s and is twice as frequent in females. Clinical features include general malaise, temporal headache, scalp tenderness and jaw claudication. Eventually, visual disturbance or visual loss can occur due to ischaemic optic neuritis caused by arteritis of the posterior ciliary artery and branches of the ophthalmic arteries. On examination, an enlarged, tender, non-pulsatile temporal artery is seen on the affected side. Temporal artery biopsy is the definitive investigation (showing patchy granulomatous inflammation), but skip lesions may be present and investigation should not delay treatment. Management is with prednisolone.

5. I – Wegener's disease

Wegener's disease is a granulomatous necrotizing vasculitis characterized by a classic triad of involvement: upper airway pathology (epistaxis, saddle nose deformity, rhinitis, deafness and proptosis), respiratory disease (pulmonary nodules and pulmonary haemorrhage) and renal disease (glomerulonephritis). It is associated with cytoplasmic antineutrophil cytoplasmic antibodies (cANCAs) in 90% of cases. Treatment is with steroids and immunosuppressants.

Friedrich Wegener, German pathologist (1907–90).

Polyarteritis nodosa is a necrotizing vasculitis of small and medium-sized vessels associated with microaneurysm formation. It is more frequent in areas endemic for hepatitis B infection, and the hepatitis B surface antigen is present in 30% of cases. Clinical features can involve any organ, and include constitutional symptoms, abdominal pain, joint pain, mononeuritis multiplex and skin lesions. ANCAs are positive in less than 10% of cases. The diagnosis of polyarteritis nodosa is confirmed using histology and a renal angiography demonstrating microaneurysm formation.

Microscopic polyangiitis is a necrotizing focal segmental glomerulonephritis that tends to affect the small arteries of the kidney. Features are usually renal, with haematuria and proteinuria, although other organs can be involved. ANCAs are positive in most cases (cANCAs or pANCAs).

Kawasaki's disease is an acute febrile systemic vasculitis affecting children. It is most common in Japanese boys. The diagnosis is made clinically as follows: patients must have a fever for 5 or more days *plus* four of the following:

- cervical lymphadenopathy
- oral mucosal erythema (red lips, strawberry tongue)
- conjunctivitis without exudates
- rash
- extremity changes such as oedema and desquamation (peeling).

There may also be thrombocytosis. Treatment is with anti-inflammatories and intravenous immunoglobulins. The main complication of Kawasaki's disease is the development of coronary aneurysms (which can result in heart attack and sudden death), and patients conventionally undergo coronary angiography after recovery to rule this out.

Tomisaku Kawasaki, Japanese paediatrician (described the condition in 1967).

Theme 13: Complications of liver disease

1. I – Spontaneous bacterial peritonitis

Patients with ascites are at risk of developing spontaneous bacterial peritonitis (SBP), which usually presents with severe generalized abdominal pain, worsening ascites, vomiting, fever and rigors. The most common causative organisms are Gram-negative bacilli such as *Escherichia coli* and *Klebsiella* spp., which enter the systemic circulation from the intestinal lumen and colonize the ascitic fluid. SBP can lead to rapid decompensation of liver disease causing hepatic encephalopathy and death. The diagnosis of SBP is confirmed by paracentesis, which involves taking a sample of ascitic fluid from the abdomen using a needle. The aspirated ascitic fluid is analysed for white cell count, glucose and protein. In addition, the fluid should be sent to microbiology for culture and Gram staining. If the white cell count is greater than 250 cells/mm^3, the patient requires intravenous antibiotics (e.g. cefotaxime or ceftriaxone). Some patients also require human albumin solution to restore their intravascular fluid volume. Patients who have had a previous episode of SBP, and those who are considered to be at high risk of developing SBP, should be considered for prophylactic oral antibiotics (e.g. norfloxacin or ciprofloxacin).

2. K – Upper gastrointestinal bleed

Patients with cirrhosis are at risk of upper gastrointestinal bleeding secondary to the formation of oesophageal varices. The disruption of the hepatic architecture in cirrhosis can lead to a build-up of pressure within the portal vein, causing portal hypertension. The high pressure within the portal vein forces blood into collateral veins such as the submucosal oesophageal, rectal and umbilical veins. The diversion of high-pressure blood into the collateral veins causes them to become tortuous, friable, dilated and prone to bleeding (i.e. varicose). Oesophageal varices can rupture and bleed treacherously, causing haematemesis, melaena, hypotension, collapse and death. The treatment of variceal bleeds usually involves therapeutic endoscopy, during which the varices are banded or sclerosed to alleviate the haemorrhage and prevent recurrence. If haemostasis is required urgently, or the bleeding is not responding to first-line treatments, haemostasis can be temporarily achieved using balloon tamponade. The Sengstaken–Blakemore tube, which is often used for this purpose, has one balloon that lies within the stomach, compressing the veins at the gastro-oesophageal junction, and a second balloon that lies within the oesophagus, compressing the superficial oesophageal veins. This method of haemostasis is invasive and has complications, including oesophageal rupture. Primary and secondary prophylactic measures are available to reduce the risk of variceal bleeding and re-bleeding. These include elective endoscopic variceal banding/sclerotherapy and treatment with propranolol, a non-selective β-blocker that reduces portal venous pressure.

3. B – Hepatic encephalopathy

This patient is exhibiting the classic features of hepatic encephalopathy. Hepatic encephalopathy is a potentially reversible neuropsychiatric disease that occurs in patients with significant hepatocellular disease and/or portal hypertension. In health, the toxic metabolites that are formed from the metabolism of protein in the intestinal lumen by commensal bacteria enter the portal vein and are transported to the liver for detoxification. In patients with significant hepatocellular disease and portal hypertension, the toxic metabolites are not filtered by the liver and enter the systemic circulation unprocessed. The circulating toxic metabolites, (e.g. ammonia) cross the blood–brain barrier and accumulate, causing hepatic encephalopathy.

The clinical features of hepatic encephalopathy include a reversed sleep pattern, asterixis, constructional apraxia, agitation, reduced consciousness, coma and death. Common precipitants of hepatic encephalopathy include a high-protein diet, upper gastrointestinal bleeding, hypokalaemia, alcohol ingestion, benzodiazepines and diuretics. The treatment of hepatic encephalopathy involves correcting the underlying cause and initiating supportive measures such as a low-protein diet and nursing the patient in a light room with access to a clock and familiar faces. Lactulose, an osmotic laxative, is used to clear the intestine of the commensal bacteria that metabolize protein into ammonia. In some situations, antibiotics are indicated, but their use should be discussed with senior colleagues. Patients with known portal hypertension and oesophageal varices can have prophylactic treatment in the form of β-blockers, regular endoscopic sclerotherapy/banding or portosystemic shunting.

4. C – Hepatorenal syndrome

Hepatorenal syndrome is seen in up to 20% of patients with cirrhosis and portal hypertension. In hepatorenal syndrome, the patient develops acute renal failure despite having histologically normal kidneys. It is thought to arise secondary to the release of vasoactive substances that cause dilatation of the splanchnic vasculature and constriction of the renal cortical vasculature. This combination of events reduces the glomerular filtration rate. The treatment of hepatorenal syndrome involves restoring the intravascular volume with human albumin solution and reversing the splanchnic dilatation with potent arterial vasoconstrictors such as terlipressin. Severe and refractory disease may require liver transplantation for cure.

5. A – Clotting factor deficiency

This patient has taken a significant overdose of paracetamol, resulting in hepatocellular necrosis and liver failure. Clotting factors are synthesized in the liver, and measurement of clotting is a sensitive method of assessing liver function. In cases of significant hepatocellular damage, the production of clotting factors is impaired, resulting in a propensity to bleed, which may present as bruising or haemorrhage. The clotting profile is usually measured in terms of the prothrombin time (PT), which is converted into the international normalized ratio (INR). In cases of significant bleeding with a raised INR, the patient should be treated with intravenous vitamin K and blood products that contain clotting factors, such as fresh frozen plasma and cryoprecipitate.

Theme 14: Cutaneous lesions 1

1. J – Seborrhoeic keratosis

Seborrhoeic keratoses (or basal cell papillomas) are common pigmented benign tumours of basal keratinocytes that often occur in large numbers on the face and trunk of elderly people. They are dark, rough and greasy, and have a 'stuck-on' appearance with a well-defined edge. These lesions have no malignant potential, but may be removed by excision, cautery or cryotherapy if the patient wishes.

2. C – Dercum's disease

These woman's lesions are lipomas – soft, mobile lesions composed of fatty tissue that are usually painless. However, the presence of multiple painful lipomas is known as Dercum's disease (or adiposis dolora). This occurs most commonly in obese middle-aged women, and may be accompanied by headaches, amenorrhoea and reduced sweating. Simple lipomas can be removed by excision for cosmetic reasons.

Francis Xavier Dercum, American neurologist (1856–1931).

3. B – Deep capillary naevus

A deep capillary naevus (or port-wine stain) is a malformation of the capillaries in the deep and superficial dermis. These are congenital malformations that can occur anywhere in the body but are most often found unilaterally on the face. Occasionally, a port-wine stain is associated with seizures, learning difficulties and eye abnormalities (glaucoma and optic atrophy) due to underlying cranial malformations. This is known as Sturge–Weber syndrome and is usually associated with a port-wine stain in the distribution of the ophthalmic or maxillary division of the trigeminal nerve. (Trigeminal, from Latin *tri* = three + *gemini* = twins; which together means 'triplets'. The trigeminal nerve has three divisions.)

Superficial capillary naevi (also known as salmon patches) are small, flat, pink patches of skin with poorly defined borders. They are commonly found on the forehead ('angel's kiss') or on the nape of the neck ('stork mark'). Most superficial naevi disappear in the first year of life.

William Allen Sturge, English physician (1850–1919).

Frederick Parkes Weber, English physician (1863–1962).

4. D – Ganglion

A ganglion is a benign, tense, cystic swelling, often at the back of the wrist, that occurs due to degeneration of the fibrous tissue surrounding the joints. Ganglia are most common in young women. Ganglia are usually painless and asymptomatic, although they may occasionally press on adjacent nerves (ulnar and median nerves). Asymptomatic ganglia do not require treatment, and many spontaneously resolve. Lasting cure is by excision (aspiration is simpler, but 50% will recur). The traditional method of curing ganglia by striking them with a large Bible is no longer recommended.

5. A – Cavernous haemangioma

A cavernous haemangioma (or strawberry naevus) is a condition that appears in the first months of life as a bright-red lesion on the face or trunk that grows rapidly. Occasionally, these lesions bleed or ulcerate. Cavernous haemangiomas eventually regress and disappear spontaneously, so intervention is required only if lesions persist beyond a few years of age. Cavernous haemangiomas may rarely be associated with thrombocytopenia and haemolytic anaemia secondary to trapping and destruction of platelets and erythrocytes within the lesions. This is known as Kasabach–Merritt syndrome.

Haig Kasabach, American paediatrician (1898–1943).

Katherine Merritt, American paediatrician (1886–1986).

Theme 15: Antimicrobial therapy

1. F – Erythromycin

The majority of community-acquired pneumonias are caused by *Streptococcus pneumoniae, Haemophilus influenzae* and *Mycoplasma pneumoniae*. Amoxicillin is the first-line antibiotic and can be given orally in mild-to-moderate infections. If the patient is allergic to penicillin, the first-line antibiotic of choice is erythromycin, which can also be given orally.

2. G – Flucloxacillin

Cellulitis is usually caused by a streptococcal infection. It tends to present with systemic illness in association with a well-demarcated area of raised erythematous skin that may be blistered. If the patient is unwell or septic, they will require intravenous antibiotics. The first-line agents are benzylpenicillin and flucloxacillin, which cover streptococci and staphylococci respectively. If the patient is fit enough for oral therapy, they are prescribed flucloxacillin and phenoxymethylpenicillin, since benzylpenicillin is available only as an intravenous preparation.

3. E – Co-trimoxazole

Pneumocystis jiroveci (previously *Pneumocystis carinii*) is a fungus that can cause life-threatening pneumonia in immunocompromised individuals, such as patients with HIV. Co-trimoxazole is a combination of trimethoprim and sulfamethoxazole that is often used as the first-line treatment. Intravenous therapy is indicated in acute infection. Co-trimoxazole is also used as a primary prophylactic agent in susceptible individuals, e.g. an HIV patient with a low CD4 count.

4. C – Chloramphenicol

Bacterial conjunctivitis is a common cause of red eye, and is often seen in children who present with conjunctival injection and a mucopurulent discharge that causes the eyelids to stick together. The majority of bacterial conjunctival infections clear up spontaneously, but antibiotics are often prescribed to reduce the course of the illness and the risk of complications. Topical chloramphenicol is the first-line antibiotic of choice. The main complication of chloramphenicol therapy is aplastic anaemia, but this is extremely unlikely to occur with topical treatment (although a number of cases have been reported in the literature).

5. B – Cefotaxime

It is essential to begin treating suspected bacterial meningitis immediately. A third-generation cephalosporin (e.g. cefotaxime) is usually the first-line antibiotic in the treatment of bacterial meningitis. If the patient is seen in the community, a one-off dose of intramuscular benzylpenicillin can be given while transfer to a hospital is being arranged. Treatment can be altered in relation to the patient's clinical status and microbiological sensitivities when these become available.

Practice Paper 2: Questions

Theme 1: Bleeding disorders

Options

A. Acquired haemophilia
B. Antibiotic side-effect
C. Complication of warfarin therapy
D. Congenital haemophilia
E. Disseminated intravascular coagulation
F. Global reduction in clotting factor synthesis
G. Heparin overdose
H. Hereditary haemorrhagic telangiectasia
I. Hypofibrinogenaemia
J. Pancytopenia
K. Thrombocytopenia
L. Von Willebrand's disease

For each of the following scenarios, select the most likely underlying bleeding disorder. Each option may be used once, more than once or not at all.

1. A 14-year-old boy being treated for meningococcal meningitis begins to bruise easily and bleed from his central line site and peripheral cannula. A full blood count shows a haemoglobin concentration of 9 g/dL, a platelet count of 90×10^9/L and a white blood cell count of 16×10^9/L. Coagulation studies reveal a prolonged PT and APTT, raised D-dimers and reduced fibrinogen levels.

2. A 15-month-old boy is brought to the emergency department with a grossly swollen right knee. His parents claim that he has had several episodes of bleeding into his joints and muscles over the previous 6 months. A clotting screen was requested and showed a significantly prolonged APTT with a normal PT and bleeding time. The full blood count showed a mild microcytic anaemia.

3. A 45-year-old woman complains of excessive bruising. She is known to have chronic hepatitis C infection. Her PT and APTT are slightly prolonged. The bleeding time is normal.

4. A 75-year-old man presents to the emergency department following a minor head injury. On arrival, he is alert and orientated, but is later found in bed unresponsive, with a Glasgow Coma Scale score of 3. Fifteen minutes after an emergency set of blood tests has been sent, the laboratory calls to inform the duty doctor that the patient's INR is above 8. When his wife arrives, she mentions that he is on some medication for an irregular heart beat and has recently started a course of antibiotics for a chest infection.

5. A 13-year-old boy is brought to the emergency department with a nosebleed. His adoptive mother says that he has several episodes a month. On examination, he has a number of spidery, red lesions on his lips, tongue and fingers. A full blood count and clotting screen are both within normal limits.

Theme 2: Chronic heart failure

Options

A. Angiotensin II receptor antagonist
B. Angiotensin-converting enzyme inhibitors
C. Amlodipine
D. β-Blockers
E. Brain-type natriuretic peptide
F. Digoxin
G. Lipid profile
H. Loop diuretics
I. Myoglobin
J. Potassium-sparing diuretics
K. Spironolactone
L. Thiazide diuretics
M. Thyroid function tests
N. Transoesophageal echocardiography
O. Transthoracic Doppler echocardiography
P. Troponin I

In the following scenarios, we follow Mrs X through her chronic heart failure. For each scenario, select the most appropriate step in her investigation or management. Each option may be used once, more than once or not at all.

1. Mrs X is an 80-year-old woman with a history of ischaemic heart disease. She presents to the emergency department with a 3-month history of worsening shortness of breath associated with swollen ankles. Her ECG demonstrates no abnormality, but you suspect that she has heart failure. What simple blood test could you do to effectively rule out heart failure in this patient?

2. The blood test that you performed on Mrs X suggests that she may have heart failure. Which investigation should be requested if chronic heart failure is suspected?

3. Mrs X is now on the ward. Your investigations demonstrate that she indeed has heart failure. Which class of drug is recommended as first line in the treatment of chronic heart failure and may help to remodel the left ventricle?

4. Two days after her admission, Mrs X is still complaining of shortness of breath. Which class of diuretic is used as a first-line symptomatic treatment when managing chronic heart failure?

5. Six months after her original diagnosis, Mrs X visits her GP because she still gets very short of breath, especially when she lies down. Her current medications include enalapril, atenolol, zopiclone, aspirin and furosemide. What additional treatment should the doctor prescribe her?

Theme 3: Motor weakness 1

Options

A. Bell's palsy
B. Guillain–Barré syndrome
C. Hypokalaemia
D. Lambert–Eaton syndrome
E. Mononeuritis multiplex
F. Motor neuron disease
G. Multiple sclerosis
H. Muscular dystrophy
I. Myasthenia gravis
J. Poliomyelitis
K. Spinal cord compression
L. Spinal muscular atrophy

For each of the following scenarios, select the most likely cause of motor weakness. Each option may be used once, more than once or not at all.

1. A 41-year-old man presents with a 2-week history of bloody diarrhoea and lower limb weakness. He denies any other symptoms. On examination, there is bilateral weakness in the distal limbs, with absent deep tendon reflexes and diminished sensation. There is no abnormality in the upper limbs or cranial nerves.

2. A 29-year-old woman presents to the emergency department with pain in her left ear. When she looked in the mirror, she noticed that the left side of her face was drooping. These symptoms occurred 2 days ago, but have not improved. On examination, the left side of her face is weak and she is not able to smile or frown adequately. Sensation to the face is unaffected.

3. A 34-year-old woman attends the GP with a 2-week history of intermittent double vision. She also feels generally weaker, particularly after playing tennis. She demonstrates this by opening and closing her hand repeatedly and showing how the motion gets gradually slower. On examination, her eyes appear partially closed. There is no sensory deficit and reflexes are present.

4. A 58-year-old man presents with a 2-month history of progressive weakness in his lower limbs, resulting in walking difficulties. On examination, his lower limbs are markedly wasted, although the reflexes are brisk. There is no sensory deficit.

5. A 62-year-old man presents to the emergency department with weight loss, weakness and a cough productive of blood-stained sputum. He feels weak in his limbs, but the weakness improves with repeated muscle use. On examination, there is no sensory deficit.

Theme 4: Skin manifestations of systemic disease 1

Options

A. Acanthosis nigricans
B. Alopecia
C. Diabetic dermopathy
D. Eruptive xanthomas
E. Erythema ab igne
F. Hyperhidrosis
G. Necrobiosis lipoidica diabeticorum
H. Paget's disease
I. Pretibial myxoedema
J. Thrombophlebitis migrans
K. Tylosis
L. Xanthelasma

For each of the following scenarios, select the most appropriate diagnosis. Each option may be used once, more than once or not at all.

1. A 45-year-old woman presents to the GP complaining of a new rash. The skin under her arms and on the back of her neck is dark and velvety in texture. She has diabetes mellitus, but is otherwise well.

2. A 45-year-old woman presents to the GP complaining of a new rash. There are multiple, light-brown, depressed lesions on her shins, each around 2 cm in size. She has diabetes mellitus, but is otherwise well.

3. A 45-year-old woman presents to the GP complaining of a new rash. There are raised, erythematous, firm plaques on the front of both of her shins. She has recently started treatment for an overactive thyroid, but is otherwise well.

4. A 45-year-old woman presents to the GP complaining of a new rash. There is a dark-brown, lacy rash over the front of both of her shins. She has recently started treatment for an underactive thyroid, but is otherwise well.

5. A 45-year-old woman presents to the GP complaining of a new rash. There are small yellow deposits in the skin around her eyes. She has hypothyroidism, but is otherwise well.

Theme 5: Acute ECG interpretation

Options

A. 3rd-degree heart block
B. Atrial fibrillation
C. Atrial flutter
D. Bifid P-waves
E. Delta wave
F. J-waves
G. Sinus arrhythmia
H. Sinus tachycardia
I. Tented T-waves
J. U-waves

For each of the following scenarios, select the most likely ECG finding. Each option may be used once, more than once or not at all.

1. A 34-year-old woman has been suffering from profuse diarrhoea and vomiting for 4 days. She is now complaining of extreme muscle weakness and muscle cramps.

2. A 55-year-old man known to be in end-stage renal failure presents to the emergency department feeling generally unwell and experiencing palpitations. He admits to missing his last haemodialysis appointment as he went away on holiday.

3. A 40-year-old woman presents with left-sided chest pain that is worse on breathing in. She is also experiencing shortness of breath on exertion and has coughed up a small amount of frank blood. She is otherwise well, with no significant past medical history. Her only regular medication is the oral contraceptive pill.

4. An 85-year-old man with dementia is brought to the emergency department by the ambulance after escaping from his care home during the night. He was found wandering on the local moors by a farmer in the early hours of the morning. He is shivering and confused. His core temperature is 31°C.

5. A 32-year-old man is involved in a road traffic collision. He has no obvious injuries.

Theme 6: Hepatitis B serology

Options

A. α-Fetoprotein
B. Alanine aminotransferase
C. Hepatitis B core antibody (HBcAb)
D. Hepatitis B core antigen (HBcAg)
E. Hepatitis B e antigen (HBeAg)
F. Hepatitis B surface antibody (HBsAb)
G. Hepatitis B surface antigen (HBsAg)
H. Hepatitis B RNA titre

For each of the following descriptions, select the most appropriate serological marker. Each option may be used once, more than once or not at all.

1. This serological marker is used to measure immunity following hepatitis B immunization.
2. This serological marker is the first to indicate acute hepatitis B infection.
3. This serological marker would indicate chronic hepatitis B infection if detected 6 months after the original infection.
4. This serological marker indicates high infectivity in a chronic hepatitis B carrier.
5. This serological marker, if high, would indicate low infectivity in a chronic hepatitis B carrier.

Theme 7: Headache 1

Options

A. Cluster headache
B. Coitus-induced headache
C. Giant cell arteritis
D. Ice-cream headache
E. Idiopathic intracranial hypertension
F. Meningitis
G. Migraine
H. Sagittal sinus thrombosis
I. Sinusitis
J. Space-occupying lesion
K. Subarachnoid haemorrhage
L. Tension headache
M. Trigeminal neuralgia

For each of the following scenarios, select the most appropriate cause of headache. Each option may be used once, more than once or not at all.

1. A 32-year-old man presents to the emergency department with a sudden-onset severe occipital headache. It started an hour ago and is accompanied by vomiting. He has a history of polycystic kidney disease. On examination, he has a stiff neck.

2. A 45-year-old man presents to the GP with a 3-week history of severe headaches. The headaches have occurred at the same time each day – about 2 a.m. – and last around 30 minutes. Headaches are accompanied by lacrimation and redness of the right eye.

3. A 62-year-old woman presents with intermittent scalp pain. She says that the pain is specifically on the left side at the front and is worse when touching the area. She has no medical history. She is very tender over the affected area. Examination is otherwise unremarkable.

4. An 18-year-old woman presents with a 6-month history of intermittent headaches. She describes these as throbbing and on the left side. The headaches are accompanied by vomiting and she occasionally sees flashing lights in her visual field.

5. A 24-year-old woman presents to the GP with a 4-month history of headaches. These are intermittent and are frequently accompanied by blurring of vision. She is otherwise well. Fundoscopy shows bilateral papilloedema.

Theme 8: Complications of the treatment of thyroid disease

Options

A. Agranulocytosis
B. Angina
C. Bilateral recurrent laryngeal nerve injury
D. Bronchoconstriction
E. Hyperthyroid storm
F. Hypocalcaemia
G. Hypothyroidism
H. Laryngeal oedema
I. Malignancy
J. Unilateral recurrent laryngeal nerve injury

For each of the following scenarios, select the most appropriate complication. Each option may be used once, more than once or not at all.

1. A 34-year-old woman who is being treated for hyperthyroidism with carbimazole becomes generally unwell with fever, rigors and a sore throat. In the emergency department, her full blood count shows a haemoglobin of 13.6 g/dL, a white cell count of 1.0×10^9/L and a neutrophil count of 0.2×10^9/L.

2. A 56-year-old woman complains of a hoarse voice and dry cough following a thyroidectomy. She is otherwise well.

3. A 45-year-old woman presents to the GP with weight gain and lethargy 9 months after having radioactive iodine therapy for hyperthyroidism.

4. A 67-year-old man with secondary hypothyroidism was recently started on a daily dose of thyroxine (100 μg). He presents to the emergency department with central chest pain that started when he was gardening but resolved when he rested.

5. A 57-year-old woman becomes short of breath while in the recovery room following a subtotal thyroidectomy. Her observations show respiratory rate 28/min, heart rate 120 beats/min and blood pressure 140/96 mmHg. She has obvious stridor and falling oxygen saturations.

Theme 9: Common drug doses

Options

A. 1 g four times daily
B. 1 mg of 1:1000 solution i.m.
C. 1 mg of 1:1000 solution i.v.
D. 1 mg of 1:10000 solution i.m.
E. 1 mg of 1:10000 solution i.v.
F. 10 mg three times daily
G. 200 mg once daily
H. 200 mg twice daily
I. 4 mg three times daily
J. 40 mg once daily
K. 400 mg three times daily
L. 50 mg three times daily

For each of the following scenarios, select the most appropriate dose of the required drug. Each option may be used once, more than once or not at all.

1. A 26-year-old woman presents to her GP with dysuria, urinary frequency and suprapubic pain. The urine dipstick is positive for nitrites and leucocytes. She is diagnosed with a urinary tract infection and started on trimethoprim.

2. A patient on your ward spikes a temperature of 38°C. The nurses ask you to prescribe paracetamol.

3. You are called to see a 45-year-old woman who is complaining of nausea and vomiting. You wish to prescribe an antiemetic. She reports being allergic to cyclizine, so you prescribe metoclopramide.

4. A 25-year-old man presents to the emergency department with an acute exacerbation of asthma. You decide to prescribe an oral dose of prednisolone after stabilizing his breathing.

5. A 26-year-old woman is admitted to the emergency department with anaphylactic shock after being stung by a bee. She is has facial swelling and stridor and is hypotensive. You decide that she requires adrenaline.

Theme 10: Urinary tract infections

Options

A. Acute bacterial prostatitis
B. Acute pyelonephritis
C. Bacterial epididymo-orchitis
D. Balanitis
E. Chronic prostatitis
F. Chronic pyelonephritis
G. *Escherichia coli* cystitis
H. Mumps epididymo-orchitis
I. *Proteus mirabilis* urinary tract infection
J. Renal tuberculosis
K. Testicular torsion
L. Testicular trauma
M. Urinary tract obstruction

For each of the following scenarios, select the most appropriate diagnosis. Each option may be used once, more than once or not at all.

1. A 45-year-old woman presents to her GP with lower abdominal pain, frequency of urination and pain on passing urine. She describes her urine as dark and offensive. The urine dipstick shows leucocytes, nitrites and blood.

2. A 34-year-old woman has had frequent episodes of lower abdominal pain, urinary frequency and nocturia over the past few years. On all these occasions, the urine dipstick showed nitrites, blood and leucocytes. Today, she developed sudden-onset, severe right-sided loin pain and macroscopic haematuria. An X-ray on admission to hospital confirmed the presence of a ureteric calculus.

3. A 75-year-old man presents to his GP feeling generally unwell and feverish. He also describes a vague lower back and perineal pain. He has a history of benign prostatic hyperplasia.

4. A 15-year-old boy with a past medical history of ureteric reflux presents to the emergency department complaining of lethargy, fever, vomiting, left loin pain and pain on urination. Examination reveals tenderness in the left loin.

5. An 18-year-old man presents to the emergency department with an acutely painful left testicle. This was preceded by 5 days of purulent urethral discharge. On examination, the left testicle is swollen and exquisitely tender. The patient's temperature is 38.3°C.

Theme 11: Diabetic emergencies

Options

A. Decrease insulin dose temporarily
B. Increase insulin dose temporarily
C. Intravenous bicarbonate
D. Intravenous glucose
E. Intravenous glucagon
F. Intravenous insulin with fluid resuscitation
G. Oral glucose
H. Rectal diazepam
I. Subcutaneous insulin with fluid resuscitation
J. Urgent referral to an endocrinologist

For each of the following scenarios, select the most appropriate management plan. Each option may be used once, more than once or not at all.

1. A 13-year-old boy is brought to the emergency department by his mother. He has been complaining of severe abdominal pain and thirst, and has been passing large volumes of urine. He is clinically dehydrated. Investigations show a plasma glucose concentration of 20 mmol/L, a potassium of 5.2 mmol/L, a sodium of 148 mmol/L, a urea of 13.4 mmol/L and a creatinine of 60 µmol/L. A blood gas shows a pH of 7.15, a Pco_2 of 2.3 kPa, a Po_2 of 13 kPa and a base excess of –7.

2. A 68-year-old man is admitted to the emergency department with reduced consciousness. He has recently complained to his wife about passing large amounts of urine and excessive thirst. Investigation show a plasma blood glucose of 31.0 mmol/L, a potassium of 3.8 mmol/L, a sodium of 150 mmol/L, a urea of 16 mmol/L and a creatinine of 68 µmol/L.

3. A 19-year-old woman with type 1 diabetes enters her GP's surgery in a confused state. She appears anxious, pale and sweaty. The practice nurse manages to settle the patient and takes a capillary blood glucose reading, which gives a result of 2.0 mmol/L.

4. A 22-year-old woman who has been newly diagnosed with type 1 diabetes begins to fit in the outpatient waiting room. She appears pale and clammy. After securing her airway and starting intravenous fluids, the nurse requests a capillary blood glucose, which shows a level of <1.0 mmol/L.

5. The mother of a 14-year-old type 1 diabetic boy phones the GP's surgery asking for advice. Her son has a chest infection and is not eating. She is worried about his blood sugar levels.

Theme 12: Dermatomes 1

Options

A. C1
B. C2
C. C4
D. C6
E. C7
F. C8
G. T4
H. T6
I. T10
J. L1
K. L3
L. L5
M. S1
N. S3
O. S5
P. Trigeminal nerve

For each of the following descriptions, select the most appropriate dermatome. Each option may be used once, more than once or not at all.

1. This dermatome supplies the nipple line.
2. This dermatome supplies the thumb.
3. This dermatome supplies the back of the head.
4. This dermatome supplies the perianal area.
5. This dermatome supplies the umbilicus.

Theme 13: Shortness of breath

Options

A. Acute coryza
B. Asbestosis
C. Aspergillosis
D. Bronchiectasis
E. Chronic obstructive pulmonary disease
F. Cryptogenic fibrosing alveolitis
G. Extrinsic allergic alveolitis
H. Pneumoconiosis
I. Sarcoidosis
J. Tuberculosis

For each of the following scenarios, select the most appropriate cause of shortness of breath. Each option may be used once, more than once or not at all.

1. A 54-year-old man presents to the GP with worsening shortness of breath and a cough productive of bloody sputum. He has lost a stone in weight over the last month. A chest X-ray shows consolidation at the left apex.

2. A 42-year-old woman presents to the GP with a 6-month history of worsening shortness of breath associated with a dry cough. A chest X-ray shows bilateral hilar lymphadenopathy.

3. A 56-year-old man presents to the GP with a 6-month history of worsening shortness of breath. Examination reveals bilateral end-inspiratory crackles and clubbing. A chest X-ray shows reticulo-nodular shadowing, especially in the lower zones.

4. A 47-year-old man presents to the GP with a 4-month history of worsening shortness of breath. Examination reveals bilateral end-inspiratory crackles. A chest X-ray shows reticulonodular shadowing, especially in the upper zones.

5. A 38-year-old man presents with an episode of massive haemoptysis. He says that he has had two similar episodes in the last month. He often feels short of breath, but has recently finished a course of treatment for pulmonary tuberculosis. Examination is unremarkable. A chest X-ray shows a cavitating lesion with an opaque mass within it.

Theme 14: Sexually transmitted infections 1

Options

A. Bacterial vaginosis
B. Cervical cancer
C. Chancroid
D. Chlamydia infection
E. Epstein–Barr virus
F. Genital candidiasis
G. Genital herpes
H. Genital warts
I. Gonorrhoea
J. Granuloma inguinale (donovanosis)
K. HIV
L. Lymphogranuloma venereum
M. Molluscum contagiosum
N. Phthiriasis
O. Reiter's syndrome
P. Scabies
Q. Syphilis
R. Trichomoniasis

For each of the following scenarios, select the most appropriate diagnosis. Each option may be used once, more than once or not at all.

1. A 32-year-old man has developed multiple painful ulcers on his penis, with an associated phimosis. On examination, there is inguinal lymph node enlargement and a discharging sinus. A culture demonstrates *Haemophilus ducreyi*.

2. A 21-year-old female student presents with abdominal pain in the right upper quadrant. She has had multiple casual sexual partners with whom she used no barrier protection. When questioned further, she admits to having a burning sensation on passing urine.

3. A 32-year-old woman attends the GP with a grey–white vaginal discharge, which she says has a 'fishy' odour.

4. A 29-year-old woman attends the GP complaining of feeling generally unwell. She says that she is tired and mildly feverish, with headaches and an itchy diffuse skin rash. She also complains of pains in her joints. She noticed a painless ulcer on her labia that healed about 5 weeks previously. She was last sexually active 4 months ago.

5. A 48-year-old woman who works in a nursing home is complaining of itching on her fingers and wrists, especially at night. Her partner developed a similar pattern of itching 3 weeks later, which has now spread to his penis.

Theme 15: Diagnosis of joint pain 1

Options

A. Ankylosing spondylitis
B. Enteropathic arthritis
C. Golfer's elbow
D. Gout
E. Osteoarthritis
F. Pseudogout
G. Psoriatic arthritis
H. Reiter's syndrome
I. Rheumatoid arthritis
J. Septic arthritis
K. Still's disease
L. Tennis elbow

For each of the following scenarios, select the most likely diagnosis. Each option may be used once, more than once or not at all.

1. A 75-year-old woman presents with sudden-onset pain in her right knee. On examination, the knee is swollen, red and painful. She has a temperature of 36.8°C. An X-ray of the knee shows a bright line on the surface of the meniscus

2. A 56-year-old woman presents with pain in her hands and swelling of the fingers. The pain is mainly in the distal interphalangeal joints. On examination, the nails of the hands are pitted and appear to be lifted off the skin at the distal edges.

3. A 15-year-old girl presents with difficulty walking on her left leg because of pain. On examination, her left ankle is hot, swollen and tender. She has a temperature of 38.6°C.

4. A 30-year-old man presents with a 2-day history of left knee pain and a burning sensation on passing urine. On examination, his temperature is 37.2°C and you notice that his eyes are red.

5. A 63-year-old man presents with a 2-year history of worsening pain in his knees. The pain is worse when he walks. He is otherwise well. On examination, there is no apparent deformity, but crepitus is elicited bilaterally.

Practice Paper 2: Answers

Theme 1: Bleeding disorders

1. E – Disseminated intravascular coagulation

Disseminated intravascular coagulation (DIC) is an acquired consumptive coagulopathy that is usually seen in association with severe systemic disease. The pathophysiological process is secondary to the release into the circulation of prothrombotic factors that trigger widespread and inappropriate activation of the clotting cascade. Both the intrinsic and extrinsic pathways are activated, resulting in conversion of fibrinogen into fibrin. This process creates multiple thrombi, which clog up the microcirculation, causing end-organ ischaemia, intravascular haemolysis and thrombocytopenia secondary to platelet destruction. DIC results in rapid consumption of clotting factors, platelets and fibrinogen, placing the patient at risk of paradoxical bleeding. Clotting studies reveal prolonged prothrombin time (PT) and activated partial thromboplastin time (APTT) due to a global clotting factor deficiency. The bleeding time is usually normal unless the platelet count is independently extremely low. Clinical features include extensive bruising, purpura, oozing from cannulation sites and multi-organ failure secondary to end-organ ischaemia. Treatment involves correcting the underlying cause and replacing lost blood products with platelets, fresh frozen plasma and cryoprecipitate.

2. D – Congenital haemophilia

Haemophilia A is an X-linked recessive disorder of coagulation in which the patient cannot synthesize clotting factor VIII due to a gene mutation. Haemophilia B (also known as Christmas disease) is caused by an inability to synthesize factor IX and is clinically indistinguishable from the much more common haemophilia A. Although usually familial, a significant proportion of cases are caused by sporadic mutations. Factors VIII and IX are essential in the extrinsic clotting cascade, meaning that patients with haemophilia have a prolonged APTT. The intrinsic pathway does not require factors VIII or IX, and is therefore unaffected by haemophilia – shown by a normal PT. The bleeding time is also normal. Symptoms usually begin when the patient becomes mobile, i.e. when they begin to crawl or walk. Patients with haemophilia typically suffer painful recurrent bleeds into the joints and soft tissues (haemarthrosis), which may eventually lead to crippling arthropathy and neuropathy.

Treatment of haemophilia A is with factor VIII concentrate either as a regular infusion or when actively bleeding. Patients receiving regular infusions have higher factor VIII levels and a better quality of life, but are at higher risk of developing antibodies to the extrinsic factor VIII, which reduces its efficiency. Patients who receive factor VIII only when bleeding are less likely to form antibodies, but are at increased risk of bleeding. Patients with mild disease may be treated with desmopressin (DDVAP), which releases factor VIII from internal stores. Factor VIII concentrate should be given prior to invasive procedures such as tooth extraction and surgery. Haemophilia B is treated with factor IX concentrate. It should be noted that many patients with haemophilia who received blood products prior to the initiation of blood screening programmes have contracted bloodborne viruses such as HIV and hepatitis C.

Stephen Christmas, the first person described to have factor IX deficiency (1947–93). He eventually died from AIDS, transmitted via a transfusion. The original case report of Christmas disease was reported in the Christmas edition of the *British Medical Journal* in 1952.

3. F – Global reduction in clotting factor synthesis

All clotting factors are synthesized in the liver. Therefore, patients with liver disease such as alcoholic cirrhosis and hepatitis are prone to quantitative and qualitative clotting factor deficiency and deranged coagulation. In reality, the process is much more complex than a simple factor deficiency, and is likely to involve a combination of vitamin K deficiency, thrombocytopenia, splenomegaly and marrow suppression. Vitamin K is an essential cofactor in the carboxylation of clotting factors II, VII, IX and X, and a deficiency of vitamin K results in a hypocoagulable state similar to that produced by taking warfarin. The treatment of clotting abnormalities in liver disease and hypovitaminosis K is with oral vitamin K supplements, unless the patient is actively bleeding, in which case cryoprecipitate and fresh frozen plasma are required to replace the deficient factors.

4. C – Complication of warfarin therapy

This patient has suffered an intracranial bleed secondary to minor trauma. The history suggests that he is taking warfarin for atrial fibrillation. Warfarin is a common anticoagulant that works by inhibiting an essential step in the synthesis of vitamin K-dependent clotting factors (II, VII, IX and X). Anticoagulation is measured using the PT which is converted into the international normalized ratio (INR) using the following formula:

$$\text{INR} = (\text{measured PT}/\text{normal PT})^{\text{ISI}}$$

where ISI (the international sensitivity index) is a constant that represents how the particular manufactured batch of tissue factor used in the laboratory compares with an internationally standardized sample. It is usual for patients on warfarin to have a target INR of 2–4.5, depending on the condition being treated. Warfarin therapy is complicated, and some patients develop an inappropriately high INR, which places them at increased risk of bleeding. The most common causes for developing an inappropriately high INR are dosing errors, accidental overdose and drug interaction. Drugs that are known to potentiate the action of warfarin include antibiotics, thyroxine, alcohol, antidepressants, aspirin, amiodarone and quinine. In this case, it is likely that the antibiotics prescribed for the chest infection increased the action of warfarin, causing a significant rise in INR, which placed the patient at risk of a major bleed from minor trauma. The treatment of an inappropriately high INR depends on the specific circumstances. A moderately high INR with no bleeding can usually be corrected by omitting a dose of warfarin. In situations when the INR is significantly raised without bleeding, the warfarin should be omitted and an oral dose of vitamin K prescribed. A high INR associated with active bleeding warrants a dose of oral or intravenous vitamin K plus the administration of a prothrombin complex concentrate such as Beriplex that contains the deficient factors II, VII, IX and X.

When a prothrombin complex concentrate is not available, fresh frozen plasma may be used as an alternative.

5. H – Hereditary haemorrhagic telangiectasia

Hereditary haemorrhagic telangiectasia (also known as Osler–Weber–Rendu syndrome) is a rare autosomal dominant disease in which the patient develops multiple telangiectasias on the skin, lips and mucosal surfaces. Arteriovenous malformations may also be found in the soft tissues, brain, liver and lungs. These lesions are friable and prone to bleeding. The most common symptom is recurrent and severe epistaxis. Patients with gastrointestinal lesions can suffer acute or chronic gastrointestinal bleeding. Problematic telangiectasias on the skin, nose and gastrointestinal tract may be treated by laser therapy. Larger arteriovenous malformations can be treated with embolization or surgery. Oral iron supplementation is often required to treat iron-deficiency anaemia that develops secondary to chronic blood loss

Theme 2: Chronic heart failure

Heart failure, where the heart cannot maintain an adequate output, affects 10% of 80-year-olds. The most common causes of left heart failure are ischaemic heart disease, hypertension, valvular disease and high-output states (e.g. anaemia and thyrotoxicosis). The most common causes of right heart failure are left heart failure and chronic lung disease (cor pulmonale).

The features of heart failure stem from pulmonary oedema (leading to dyspnoea, orthopnoea and paroxysmal nocturnal dyspnoea), poor renal perfusion (leading to oliguria and uraemia) and low cardiac output (leading to fatigue, poor exercise tolerance, cold peripheries and hypotension). Other features include weight loss (cardiac cachexia) and arrhythmias (sudden death due to ventricular fibrillation occurs in 50% with heart failure).

1. E – Brain-type natriuretic peptide

Brain-type natriuretic peptide (BNP) is a serum marker for impaired left ventricular function that is rarely raised in individuals with normal cardiac function. It is secreted from the ventricles in response to pressure overload, and acts to reduces systemic vascular resistance and cardiac preload while promoting natriuresis (the excretion of large amounts of sodium in the urine). BNP should be used alongside ECG to identify patients who require further imaging and assessment. Patients with a normal ECG and negative BNP are unlikely to have heart failure. In addition to its diagnostic role, BNP may have a prognostic value, as higher serum levels are associated with more severe disease. Other investigations that are useful in the initial assessment of cardiac failure include full blood count, urea and electrolytes, thyroid function tests and chest X-ray.

Natriuresis, from Latin *natrium* = sodium + Greek *ourein* = to urinate.

2. O – Transthoracic Doppler echocardiography

Transthoracic Doppler echocardiography is indicated for patients with features of chronic heart failure in association with either a raised serum BNP or ECG evidence of left ventricular hypertrophy. Echocardiography is a non-invasive investigation that is able to assess ventricular function, visualize the heart valves and detect any other cardiac lesions that may be contributing to heart failure. If the results of transthoracic Doppler echocardiography are inconclusive, alternative, more detailed investigations such as transoesophageal echocardiography, radionuclide angiography and cardiac MRI are available.

3. B – Angiotensin-converting enzyme inhibitors

General measures that can be implemented to manage heart failure include having a low-salt diet and taking regular exercise. Patients are also advised to stop smoking and reduce their alcohol intake.

Angiotensin-converting enzyme (ACE) inhibitors prevent the production of angiotensin II and aldosterone, thereby preventing sodium/water retention and sympathetically mediated vasoconstriction. Overall, therefore, they reduce preload and afterload on the heart. ACE inhibitors have been shown to improve symptoms and prognosis in all degrees of heart failure. They are the first-line treatment in all patients unless contraindicated. Side-effects include first-dose hypotension, renal impairment, hyperkalaemia and an intractable cough (which occurs secondary to a build-up of bradykinin in the lungs). ACE inhibitors must not be prescribed to patients with bilateral renal stenosis, as they may precipitate acute renal failure. Prior to starting an ACE inhibitor, and at regular intervals thereafter, the patient should have their renal function measured, with particular attention being paid to the serum potassium level. ACE inhibitors should be avoided in patients with hyperkalaemia and should never be prescribed in conjunction with potassium supplements. In patients who suffer from an intolerable cough, an angiotensin II receptor antagonist may be used as an alternative. Examples include valsartan and losartan.

4. H – Loop diuretics

Loop diuretics, such as furosemide and bumetanide, inhibit sodium and chloride reabsorption at the ascending loop of Henle and are the first-line diuretics used in the treatment of symptomatic heart failure. The lowest dose that controls symptoms should be used. Side-effects of loop diuretics include hypokalaemia, hyponatraemia and hypotension. If symptoms are not controlled with high doses of a loop diuretic, a thiazide diuretic such as bendroflumethiazide may be added. Thiazides inhibit sodium and chloride reabsorption in the distal collecting tubule. Side-effects include hypokalaemia and hyperuricaemia, which can precipitate acute gout.

Friedrich Gustav Jacob Henle, German physician and anatomist (1809–85).

5. K – Spironolactone

Spironolactone is an aldosterone antagonist; therefore it causes increased sodium secretion and reduced potassium excretion. Because it does not cause hypokalaemia (unlike the thiazide and loop diuretics), spironolactone is known as a potassium-sparing diuretic. Amiloride is another example of such a drug. Spironolactone is indicated in patients with severe symptomatic disease that is not controlled by optimal medical therapy to improve symptoms and mortality. Since this medication reduces potassium excretion by the kidneys, it should not be given to patients with a potassium level over 5.0 mmol/L or to patients taking potassium supplements. Patients should have their serum potassium measured prior to prescription and at regular intervals thereafter in order to detect hyperkalaemia. Other well-known side-effects of spironolactone include hyponatraemia, gynaecomastia and menstrual disturbance.

β-Blockers, such as atenolol, are also used in the treatment of heart failure. These drugs counteract the adverse effects of enhanced sympathetic stimulation (i.e. reduce afterload). β-Blockers have been shown to decrease hospitalization and improve mortality in heart failure. Digoxin is used to manage heart failure in patients with atrial fibrillation.

Theme 3: Motor weakness 1

Muscle weakness is graded using the Medical Research Council (MRC) system as follows:

Grade 5: normal power
Grade 4: active movements against gravity and resistance
Grade 3: active movements against gravity
Grade 2: active movement with gravity eliminated
Grade 1: flicker of contraction
Grade 0: no contraction.

1. B – Guillain–Barré syndrome

Guillain–Barré syndrome (also known as post-infective demyelination polyneuropathy) is an immune-mediated demyelination of the spinal roots or peripheral nerves. It often develops weeks after a respiratory or diarrhoeal infection, especially with *Campylobacter jejuni*. Patients present with rapidly progressive muscle weakness, which ascends from the lower to the upper limbs, with loss of deep tendon reflexes. Distal paraesthesia, limb pain and facial/bulbar weakness may also develop. Twenty per cent of cases develop respiratory weakness requiring ventilator support, so it is important to measure serial peak flows in all patients. An unusual variant (described by Miller Fisher) is characterized by ophthalmoplegia, ataxia and areflexia. Management of Guillain–Barré syndrome is supportive. Around 80% recover fully, 4% die and 16% are left with residual disability.

Georges Guillain, French neurologist (1876–1961).

Jean Alexander Barré, French neurologist (1880–1967).

2. A – Bell's palsy

Bell's palsy is a lower motor neuron lesion of the facial nerve (cranial nerve VII), often within the facial canal. The cause is often unknown, but may be latent herpes simplex infection. Symptoms develop over a few hours and include loss of movement over one side of the face (without sensory loss), pain around the ear, hyperacusis and loss of salivation/tear secretion. Although there is no specific treatment, prednisolone and antivirals may speed recovery. Most cases of Bell's palsy recover spontaneously, although aberrant innervations may occur during recovery, giving rise to unwanted facial movements (e.g. tear secretion during salivation – known as crocodile tear syndrome).

Sir Charles Bell, Scottish surgeon (1774–1842).

3. I – Myasthenia gravis

Myasthenia gravis is characterized by an inability to sustain a maintained or repeated contraction of striated muscle (fatigability). It is caused by autoimmune destruction of postsynaptic acetylcholine receptors (AChRs) in the neuromuscular junction. It is more common in women between 20 and 40 years of age. The first symptom may be diplopia or ptosis, and the cardinal feature is fatigability. Symptoms are worse after exercise and at the end of the day. Occasionally, a sudden weakness can occur (myasthenic or cholinergic crisis). Diagnosis of myasthenia gravis is by the Tensilon test: intravenous edrophonium bromide (a short-acting anticholinergic) is administered and, if the weakness transiently improves, myasthenia is confirmed. Anti-AChR antibodies are found in 80%. All patients with myasthenia gravis should have a CT scan to rule out thymoma. Management is with anticholinergics (e.g. pyridostigmine). An overdose of anticholinergics can cause a cholinergic crisis (leading to muscle fasciculation, paralysis, pallor, sweating, excessive salivation and small pupils). This may be distinguished from a myasthenia crisis (severe weakness due to exacerbation of myasthenia) by injection of edrophonium.

A large proportion of cases of myasthenia gravis are associated with either a thymoma or thymic hyperplasia. It is also associated with other autoimmune conditions.

4. F – Motor neuron disease

Motor neuron disease (MND) is a progressive degeneration of motor neurons within the spinal cord, motor cortex and cranial nerve nuclei. Some cases are autosomal dominant (5%), while others are caused by viral infection, trauma and toxins. MND affects 1 in 20 000 and is most common in males over the age of 50. Clinically, there is a combination of upper and lower motor neuron signs (limb weakness, fasciculations, spasticity and exaggerated reflexes) with no sensory involvement or intellectual impairment. The presence of brisk reflexes in wasted fasciculating limbs is typical. Symptoms of MND begin in one area and spread relentlessly. There are different patterns of involvement of MND – these include progressive muscular atrophy (weakness of distal limb muscles first), progressive bulbar palsy (early involvement of tongue and pharyngeal muscles, with dysarthria and dysphagia) and amyotrophic lateral sclerosis (combination of distal and proximal muscle wasting and spasticity). Management is supportive, although riluzole can prolong life expectancy.

5. D – Lambert–Eaton syndrome

Lambert–Eaton syndrome is caused by impaired neurotransmitter release due to autoantibodies to presynaptic voltage-gated calcium channels. Patients suffer muscle weakness and autonomic dysfunction (dry mouth, blurred vision and impotence). The cardinal sign is an absence of tendon reflexes and weakness that returns immediately after sustained contraction of the relevant muscle. Lambert–Eaton syndrome is associated with an underlying malignancy, often of the lung. Diagnosis is by electrophysiology. Management is with 3,4-diaminopyridine, which blocks neural potassium channels, allowing the affected calcium channels to stay open for longer.

Edward Howard Lambert, American neurophysiologist (b1915).

Lealdes McKendree Eaton, American neurologist (1905–58).

Theme 4: Skin manifestations of systemic disease 1

1. A – Acanthosis nigricans

The presence of a black, velvety overgrowth in the axillae, neck and groin is typical of acanthosis nigricans. This rash is associated with insulin resistance (diabetes), Cushing's syndrome, acromegaly, polycystic ovarian syndrome, lymphomas and adenocarcinomas of the gastrointestinal tract.

Other cutaneous features of internal malignancy include *Paget's disease* (scaly, eczematous rash on the nipple – breast cancer), *thrombophlebitis migrans* (recurrent thrombophlebitis in different parts of the body – pancreatic cancer), *tylosis* (hyperkeratosis of the palm and soles – oesophageal cancer), *dermatomyositis* (purple rash on eyelids and scaly pink rash on knuckles – lung and breast cancer) and *necrolytic migratory erythema* (blistering erythematous rash of buttocks, groin and legs – glucagonoma).

Acanthosis nigricans, from Latin *acanthosis* = thorn + *neger* = black.

2. C – Diabetic dermopathy

Diabetic dermopathy describes the presence of depressed pigmented scars in the shin. It is associated with diabetic microangiopathy.

Other skin features of diabetes include *necrobiosis lipoidica diabeticorum* (shiny, atrophic, yellowish-red plaques on the shins), *cheiroarthropathy* (a scleroderma-like thickening of the skin of the hands), *granuloma annulare* (small, papular lesions arranged in a ring and found on the back of the hands or feet) and acanthosis nigricans.

3. I – Pretibial myxoedema

Pretibial myxoedema is the presence of raised erythematous plaques due to mucopolysaccharide deposition in the dermis over the shins and dorsa of the feet. It is seen in hyperthyroidism. Other skin features of hyperthyroidism are alopecia, palmar erythema and hyperhidrosis (excess sweating).

4. E – Erythema ab igne

Erythema ab igne is a brown lacy rash seen on skin that has been exposed to heat for long periods of time. It classically develops in hypothyroid patients who are cold and spend a lot of time in front of the fire. Excessive hot water bottle use can also result in the rash.

Other cutaneous features of hypothyroidism include alopecia (especially loss of the outer third of the eyebrows), dry coarse hair, puffy yellow skin, periorbital oedema, xanthomas and a malar flush on an otherwise pale face ('strawberries and cream' appearance).

Ab igne, from Latin *ab* = from + *ignis* = fire.

5. L – Xanthelasma

Xanthelasma are yellowish plaques around the eyelid, and may be due to hyperlipidaemia.

Both primary and secondary hyperlipidaemia can produce a variety of xanthomatous deposits. These include:

- eruptive xanthomas: red–yellow papules on shoulders and buttocks
- tendinous xanthomas: subcutaneous nodules on hand, foot or Achilles' tendon
- palmar xanthomas: yellow–orange macules in palmar creases
- tuberous xanthomas: yellow–orange nodules on knees and elbows.

Xanthelasma, from Greek *xanthos* = yellow, *elasma* = flat plate.

Theme 5: Acute ECG interpretation

1. J – U-waves

The 4-day history of diarrhoea and vomiting followed by the development of severe muscle weakness and cramps suggests hypokalaemia secondary to excessive gastrointestinal potassium loss. Other causes of reduced total body potassium include diuretic use, Conn's syndrome, excessive sweating and burns. Potassium can also be redistributed from the extracellular compartment into the intracellular compartment, resulting in a reduction in bioavailable potassium despite there being normal total body potassium levels. Causes of potassium redistribution include β_2-antagonist use (e.g. salbutamol), excess insulin administration and alkalosis. The clinical features of hypokalaemia become evident with serum potassium levels less than 2.5 mmol/L. These include lethargy, polyuria, profound muscle weakness, muscle cramps, palpitations and arrhythmia. ECG changes in hypokalaemia include U-wave formation (upward deflections following the T-waves), flattened T-waves, ST-segment depression, and atrial and ventricular arrhythmias. Treatment of hypokalaemia involves correcting the underlying cause and replacing the lost potassium. Patients with potassium levels above 2.5 mmol/L can usually be managed with oral potassium supplements. Symptomatic patients and those with potassium levels under 2.5 mmol/L should receive intravenous potassium supplementation at a rate no higher than 20 mmol/h at a concentration no higher than 40 mmol/

L, unless a central line, monitoring and expertise are available. Hypokalaemia in association with hypomagnesaemia is often refractory to treatment and will require correction of serum magnesium levels in addition to potassium supplementation.

2. I – Tented T-waves

Patients receiving haemodialysis are usually in end-stage renal failure. Haemodialysis is used to remove metabolic toxins such as urea and potassium from the bloodstream. In addition, if the patient is fluid overloaded, haemodialysis can be used to remove excess fluid (ultrafiltration). In this scenario, the missed dialysis session has led to an accumulation of potassium, resulting in palpitations. ECG findings in hyperkalaemia include tall tented T-waves, P-wave flattening, PR prolongation, a widened QRS complex, and arrhythmias such as ventricular tachycardia and ventricular fibrillation.

3. H – Sinus tachycardia

This patient has many clinical features of pulmonary embolism (shortness of breath, pleuritic chest pain and haemoptysis). The most common ECG findings in pulmonary embolism are sinus tachycardia, right bundle-branch block and right axis deviation. The S1, Q3, T3 combination (large S-waves in lead 1, Q-waves in lead III and inverted T-waves in lead III) is a characteristic ECG finding in pulmonary embolism, but is rarely seen.

4. F – J-waves

This patient is hypothermic secondary to prolonged environmental exposure. Severe hypothermia can lead to coagulopathy, bradycardia, heart failure, arrhythmia and death. The ECG in severely affected patients may show an upward deflection following the R-wave of the QRS complex (J-wave). Patients with hypothermia should be re-warmed slowly at a rate no greater than 0.5°C/h, as rapid re-warming can cause vasodilatation, hypotension and circulatory collapse. Methods of re-warming include removal of wet clothing, supplying warmed humidified oxygen, applying a bear hugger device and infusing warm saline intravenously. More invasive methods of re-warming include peritoneal, pleural and bladder lavage with warmed fluid. Due to the risk of arrhythmia, hypothermic patients should be managed on a cardiac and blood pressure monitor.

5. H – Sinus tachycardia

Patients in the emergency department are likely to be highly anxious and may be suffering from acutely painful conditions. The physiological response to pain and anxiety can induce sinus tachycardia and autonomic symptoms such as sweating. It is important to exclude other potential causes of sinus tachycardia, such as hypovolaemic shock, before making a diagnosis of pain- or anxiety-induced tachycardia. If there is no evidence of a serious underlying cause, the patient should be reassured and offered analgesia (and reassessed later).

Theme 6: Hepatitis B serology

1. F – Hepatitis B surface antibody (HBsAb)

Hepatitis B virus (HBV) is a DNA virus that is mainly transmitted via blood products and sexual activity. Certain individuals, such as those who work in healthcare, are required to be vaccinated against HBV. The vaccine contains the hepatitis B surface antigen (HBsAg), against which the immune system produces HBsAb. It is HBsAb that is measured after vaccination to evaluate the response to the vaccine. Some individuals have a poor response to the vaccine and require higher doses of vaccine or booster shots. HBsAb is also found in patients who have had hepatitis in the past. In this situation, patients will also have developed antibodies to the hepatitis B core antigen (HBcAg), which are not present in patients who have been immunized.

2. G – Hepatitis B surface antigen (HBsAg)

HBsAg can usually be detected within 4 weeks of infection and is the earliest marker of HBV infection. It is not found in patients vaccinated against HBV.

3. G – Hepatitis B surface antigen (HBsAg)

If HBsAg is still detected in the serum 6 months after an acute HBV infection, the patient has become a chronic carrier of the virus. The risk of developing chronic HBV infection is related to age at the time of infection. The majority of infected neonates develop chronic infection, whereas only 5–10% of adults do so. Patients with chronic hepatitis B are at risk of developing cirrhosis, liver failure and hepatocellular carcinoma. The treatment of chronic hepatitis B can involve interferon-α, peginterferon-α2a, lamivudine and (in some patients) eventual liver transplantation.

4. E – Hepatitis B e antigen (HBeAg)

HBeAg can be present in both acute and chronic hepatitis B and indicates a high level of infectivity. The presence of HBeAg in chronic hepatitis B suggests that the patient is infective and has an aggressive disease requiring treatment. In addition to establishing infectivity, measurement of HBeAg can be used to assess the efficacy of treatment, with falling levels indicating success. It should be noted that there are some mutant strains of HBV found in Asia and the Middle East that do not produce HBeAg. HBV DNA levels can also be used to assess disease activity, with high levels indicating active disease and infectivity.

5. C – Hepatitis B core antibody (HBcAb)

HBcAb can be present in acute and chronic infection. They are formed against the HBcAg, which is found only within the liver and therefore cannot be detected using serology. In acute infection, it is the second marker to be detected, after HBsAb, and is usually seen after 4 weeks of infection. In chronic disease, the presence of high titres of HBcAb, in the absence of HBeAg, indicates low infectivity and disease activity. This serological picture is associated with a better prognosis, with fewer individuals progressing to cirrhosis and hepatocellular carcinoma.

Theme 7: Headache 1

1. K – Subarachnoid haemorrhage

Subarachnoid haemorrhage (SAH) presents with a severe, sudden-onset ('thunder clap') occipital pain that is often accompanied by vomiting. Other features include irritability, photophobia, neck stiffness (meningism) and reduced consciousness. All patients with a history of 'first-ever worst-ever' headache should have a CT scan to rule out SAH (an SAH shows fresh blood within the ventricles, which appears white on an unenhanced scan). It is important to remember that the CT scan is negative in 15% of SAHs, so a lumbar puncture should be performed after 12 hours to look for evidence of blood or xanthochromia (yellow-tinted cerebrospinal fluid due to the presence of erythrocyte breakdown products). Cerebral artery vasospasm is a complication of SAH that can result in ischaemic brain injury and brain damage. Administration of nimodipine (a calcium channel blocker) reduces the risk of this complication. SAH is usually caused by an aneurysm in a cerebral artery (especially in the circle of Willis). Such aneurysms are more common in people with polycystic kidney disease and collagen defects (e.g. Ehlers–Danlos syndrome). Most cases occur in the under-65s.

2. A – Cluster headache

Patients with cluster headache present with unilateral, severe periorbital pain accompanied by conjunctival injection, lacrimation and nasal congestion. The headaches last between 30 and 90 minutes. Cluster headaches develop at around the same time each day, often in the early hours, and may be relieved by pacing around outside. Cluster headaches may occur repeatedly for weeks, followed by respite for months, before another cluster occurs. They are much more common in men and are associated with heavy smoking and alcohol consumption. Acute attacks of cluster headache may be relieved by inhalation of 100% oxygen. Prophylactic therapies are available and include the calcium channel blocker verapamil and ergotamine.

3. M – Trigeminal neuralgia

Trigeminal neuralgia describes sharp, stabbing pains in the second and third divisions of the trigeminal nerve. The pain is severe, brief and repetitive, often causing the patient to flinch. (This feature gives rise to the French name for the condition 'tic douloureux' – painful twitch). The pain may often have triggers, such as touching or eating. Trigeminal neuralgia is most common in older women, and the condition has a tendency to improve and relapse. The underlying cause may be compression of the trigeminal nerve rootlets at their entry into the brain stem by aberrant loops of cerebellar arteries. Management options include carbamazepine, phenytoin or gabapentin, which can improve the neuropathic pain.

4. G – Migraine

Migraine may be caused by vasodilatation of the extracranial arteries. The triad of classic migraine includes paroxysmal headache, nausea/vomiting and auras (often visual). People without an aura are said to have common migraine. Features include severe, unilateral, throbbing headache with photophobia and vomiting. During the headache, patients prefer to lie in a dark room and sleep.

Headaches may be preceded by a prodrome (aura and irritability). Auras most commonly take the form of fortification spectra (shimmering, zigzag lines that appear across the visual field), but some people experience tingling, numbness, and even transient aphasia. True weakness during a migraine is rare.

Migraine is most common in females with a genetic predisposition, and may be exacerbated by contraceptive pill use, red wine, chocolate and cheese. Management options include avoidance of precipitating factors. Acute attacks are treated with analgesia and antiemesis. Codeine preparations should be avoided, as they may worsen migraine in the long term. Severe attacks are treated with serotonin agonists (e.g. sumatriptan), which act by vasoconstricting the extracranial arteries. Prophylactic options include propranolol, pizotifen (serotonin antagonist) and amitriptyline.

5. E – Idiopathic intracranial hypertension

This woman is likely to have idiopathic intracranial hypertension (previously known as benign intracranial hypertension). Idiopathic intracranial hypertension is characterized by a raised intracranial pressure in the absence of space-occupying lesions, ventricular dilatation or impaired consciousness. It usually occurs in younger, obese women and can be precipitated by drugs (contraceptive pill, tetracyclines or steroid withdrawal). Features include a history of intermittent headaches, transient diplopia and blurring, and papilloedema. The CT scan is normal and a lumbar puncture may confirm a raised opening pressure. Management options include weight loss, removal of offending triggers, acetazolamide (a carbonic anhydrase inhibitor that decreases production of cerebrospinal fluid) and repeated lumbar puncture. If untreated, idiopathic intracranial hypertension can lead to blindness.

Theme 8: Complications of the treatment of thyroid disease

1. A – Agranulocytosis

Agranulocytosis is a complication of carbimazole therapy. In agranulocytosis, the concentrations of neutrophils, basophils and eosinophils (the granulocytes) fall dramatically, predisposing the patient to infection and overwhelming sepsis. All patients taking carbimazole should be advised to seek medical attention if they develop a fever or sore throat or become generally unwell. On presentation, the patient should have a full external examination, a full blood count, blood cultures, urine cultures, wound swabs and a chest X-ray. Patients with agranulocytosis are initially prescribed broad-spectrum intravenous antibiotics (e.g. piperacillin and gentamicin), which are altered according to bacterial sensitivities.

2. J – Unilateral recurrent laryngeal nerve palsy

The recurrent laryngeal nerve can be damaged during thyroidectomy via a number of mechanisms, including transection, infarction, diathermy burns and accidental ligation. Unilateral recurrent laryngeal nerve injury usually presents in the days following surgery with a hoarse voice and dyspnoea. In some cases, the symptoms will disappear after a few months. For those who do not recover, a number of surgical interventions are available. In total thyroidectomy, both laryngeal nerves can be damaged. This is a potentially life-threatening complication, since both vocal cords are paralysed, resulting in upper airway obstruction at extubation. If this is the case, the patient should be re-intubated and have their neck explored to assess the extent of any damage. If extubation continues to fail, the patient will require a tracheostomy. In the long term, surgical correction may allow the airway to be maintained without tracheostomy, but the voice will not recover.

3. G – Hypothyroidism

Radioiodine therapy is used to treat hyperthyroidism that is not responsive to standard therapy (e.g. carbimazole). It involves oral administration of a solution containing radioactive iodine (^{131}I), which is absorbed from the gastrointestinal tract. Once in the bloodstream, it is transported to the thyroid gland, where it is stored. While in storage, the radioactive iodine damages the cells of the thyroid gland, preventing them from secreting thyroxine. Radioactive iodine therapy is regarded as a safe treatment, but it is contraindicated in pregnant women and women who are breast-feeding. The treatment can take several months to work, and some individuals will require a second treatment. A common side-effect of this treatment is the development of hypothyroidism. If this occurs, the patient should be started on thyroxine replacement therapy.

4. B – Angina

Thyroxine should be started with caution in elderly individuals and in those with a history of cardiovascular disease. If started at too high a dose, it can cause angina, heart failure and arrhythmia. In otherwise healthy individuals, it is usual to start with 100 μg daily, which should be adjusted based upon thyroid function tests, taken at least 6 weeks after starting treatment. In elderly people and those with cardiovascular disease, an initial dose of 25 μg or lower should be used.

5. H – Laryngeal oedema

The development of post-thyroidectomy laryngeal oedema is a rare but potentially life-threatening complication of this procedure. It is usually due to the development of a postoperative haematoma that obstructs venous and lymphatic drainage of the larynx, leading to laryngopharyngeal oedema. This condition usually presents 2–6 hours following surgery. The patient is likely to complain of dyspnoea, stridor, facial swelling and neck pain. Laryngeal oedema can cause a rapid deterioration in the patient's clinical status secondary to upper airway obstruction. If postoperative laryngeal oedema is suspected, the patient should be intubated immediately and taken to theatre for wound exploration and closure. If the patient is haemodynamically unstable, the wound must be decompressed on the ward by removing the cutaneous stitches and dividing the underlying muscle.

Theme 9: Common drug doses

1. H – 200 mg twice daily

Trimethoprim is often the first-line antibiotic of choice when treating uncomplicated urinary tract infections in a young woman. The length of the antibiotic course varies, but is usually between 3 and 5 days. Other antibiotics used to treat simple urinary tract infections include amoxicillin, cefradine and nitrofurantoin.

2. A – 1 g four times daily

In hospital, paracetamol is used as much for its antipyretic actions as it is for its analgesic properties. The adult dose of paracetamol is 1 g taken every 4–6 hours, with a maximum daily dose of 4 g. Paracetamol can be given orally, rectally or intravenously.

3. F – 10 mg three times daily

Metoclopramide is a dopamine receptor antagonist with prokinetic properties. It is usually used for its antiemetic properties, but may also be used to promote gastric motility in conditions such as diabetic gastroparesis. The usual dose is 10 mg three times daily.

4. J – 40 mg once daily

Prednisolone is a corticosteroid used in the treatment of many acute and chronic illnesses, including asthma, giant cell arteritis, inflammatory bowel disease and nephrotic syndrome. Prednisolone is often prescribed as part of the management of acute and severe asthma once the patient is stable, as an initial 40 mg dose. The prednisone should be continued for at least 5 days or until the patient has fully recovered from the acute exacerbation. If the patient is unable to swallow, an intravenous dose of hydrocortisone 100 mg can be given followed by 100 mg every 6 hours until the patient has recovered.

5. B – 1 mg of 1:1000 solution IM

Anaphylaxis is a life-threatening condition that can lead to death within minutes if not treated correctly. The presence of stridor and upper airway oedema warrants the urgent administration of adrenaline. Adrenaline is available in a 1:1000 solution and a 1:10 000 solution. Therefore, to achieve the maximum single dose of 1 mg, 1 mL of 1:1000 solution or 10 mL of 1:10 000 solution is required. When treating anaphylaxis, the intramuscular route is preferred, meaning that the more concentrated 1:1000 solution can be given. However, the 1:1000 solution should never be given as an intravenous dose, and in cardiac arrest the 1:10 000 solution is usually given as a 1 mg (10 mL) bolus.

Theme 10: Urinary tract infections

1. G – *Escherichia coli* cystitis

Cystitis usually presents with dysuria, frequency of urine, suprapubic discomfort and fever. Cystitis is much more common in women than in men due to the shorter urethra in women. *Escherichia coli*, usually found in the bowel, is the most common pathogen responsible for uncomplicated cystitis in the UK. Cystitis can be confirmed by the presence of leucocytes, nitrites and blood in the urine. A midstream urine (MSU) sample should be sent to microbiology for microscopy, culture and sensitivity. A positive culture is when more than 10^5 of a single organism are grown per millilitre of urine. The growth of mixed bacterial species usually indicates contamination of the sample. Antibiotic treatment should be guided by local patterns of bacterial resistance and MSU sensitivity results. Uncomplicated cystitis is usually treated with a 3- to 5-day course of trimethoprim. Other antibiotics that are used to treat cystitis include amoxicillin, ciprofloxacin, cefradine and nitrofurantoin. Patients who are susceptible to recurrent urinary tract infection can be prescribed prophylactic antibiotics (e.g. 100 mg of trimethoprim once nightly). Patients should be advised to drink lots of fluids and avoid dehydration. Urinary tract infections in men and children require further investigation

2. I – *Proteus mirabilis* urinary tract infection

Proteus mirabilis is a Gram-negative anaerobic pathogen that can cause urinary tract infection. In addition, *P. mirabilis* infection causes the urine to become more alkaline, which predisposes to the development of urinary calculi. *P. mirabilis* infection is more common in patients with structural abnormalities of their urinary tract and in patients with long-term catheters.

3. A – Acute bacterial prostatitis

Acute bacterial prostatitis is a relatively uncommon condition. The patient presents systemically unwell with lethargy, fever, perineal pain and lower back pain. In severe cases, there may be acute urinary retention, urethral discharge or anal discharge. Bacteria can reach the prostate via the urinary tract or from the bloodstream and lymphatic system. On digital rectal examination, the prostate is usually inflamed and painful to palpation. Common pathogens include *E. coli* and *Streptococcus faecalis*. Treatment is with intravenous or oral antibiotics (e.g. ciprofloxacin for 4–6 weeks) and bed rest. If acute bacterial prostatitis is missed or not treated appropriately in the acute stage, the patient may develop a more chronic form of the disease

4. B – Acute pyelonephritis

Acute pyelonephritis describes renal infection and inflammation. This condition is usually secondary to an ascending urinary tract infection, but may also be seen following instrumentation of the urogenital tract or haematological transfer of infection from the bloodstream to the kidney. Certain conditions, such as urinary reflux, anatomical abnormalities and urinary stasis secondary to urinary tract obstruction, predispose to the development of pyelonephritis. Patients present with a history of malaise, fever, rigors, vomiting, dysuria, haematuria and loin pain. *E. coli* and *Enterobacter faecalis* are the most common pathogens causing acute pyelonephritis. Investigation of acute pyelonephritis requires urine dipstick analysis, urine cultures, blood cultures, serum inflammatory markers, and serum urea and electrolytes. An abdominal X-ray and renal tract ultrasound should be performed to identify any calculi and rule out an obstruction respectively. The treatment of pyelonephritis requires intravenous antibiotics (e.g. cefuroxime ± gentamicin for up to 14 days). Alterations to antibiotics should be made on the basis of culture and sensitivity results.

5. C – Bacterial epididymo-orchitis

Epididymo-orchitis, literally meaning inflammation of the epididymis and testicle, can be caused by a number of pathogens. It may occur secondary to cystitis, chlamydial/gonococcal urethritis or prostatitis and following urethral instrumentation. Less commonly, the mumps virus is responsible. Patients present with an acute scrotum (an acutely painful and swollen testicle) with discoloration of the scrotal skin. There may also be a history of unprotected sex and urethral discharge, although it often presents anew. In young men presenting with an acute scrotum, it is essential to exclude testicular torsion before diagnosing epididymo-orchitis. Further investigation of suspected epididymo-orchitis should include a full blood count, blood cultures, urine culture and urethral swabs for sexually transmitted infection. The treatment of epididymo-orchitis is with oral antibiotics (e.g. ciprofloxacin for 4–6 weeks), scrotal support, analgesia and bed rest. If a sexually transmitted infection is confirmed, the patient should be given advice on how to access the genitourinary medicine (GUM) clinic for further advice, testing, and partner tracking and notification.

Theme 11: Diabetic emergencies

1. F – Intravenous insulin with fluid resuscitation

This patient has diabetic ketoacidosis (DKA), a condition that can occur in those with known or previously undiagnosed type 1 diabetes. Since the pathogenesis of DKA requires an absolute deficiency of endogenous insulin, it is almost exclusively seen in type 1 diabetes. DKA is usually triggered by an underlying illness (e.g. a chest infection) during which the patient's insulin requirements increase. The lack of insulin and the presence of counter-regulatory hormones such as glucagon mean that plasma glucose levels rise significantly. This glucose enters the renal tubules, causing an osmotic diuresis and profound dehydration. Although DKA is accompanied by a high urinary potassium loss, patients can have a paradoxically high serum potassium level. This is because the potassium ions move from the intracellular compartment into the extracellular compartment in exchange for hydrogen ions in an attempt to correct the acidosis. A catabolic state ensues during which there is excessive production of free fatty acids from the metabolism of adipose stores. The free fatty acids are metabolized in the liver into β-hydroxybutyrate and acetoacetate (ketone bodies), which are metabolic acids. In DKA, the production of ketone bodies surpasses their uptake, resulting in a metabolic acidosis. This is shown on blood gas analysis at a pH <7.35 in association with a low CO_2, a low bicarbonate, a low base excess and a high anion gap.

DKA is managed with aggressive fluid therapy and insulin. An intravenous insulin sliding scale should be started straight away. A suggested fluid resuscitation regimen is a litre of 0.9% saline immediately followed by a litre over 1 hour, a litre over 2 hours, a litre over 4 hours and then a litre over 6 hours. The first bag of saline should not contain potassium unless the serum potassium concentration is known beforehand, in order to avoid hyperkalaemia. Potassium should be added to subsequent bags and titrated against the serum potassium concentration. Blood glucose should be measured hourly and, if it falls below 12 mmol/L, the intravenous fluid should be changed to 5% glucose. Adjuncts to treatment include intravenous antibiotics if infection is suspected, urinary catheterization if the urine output is poor, and subcutaneous heparin if the patient is immobile for a prolonged period of time. Once the patient is stabilized, they should have blood and urine cultures and a chest X-ray, and have any suspicious lesions swabbed. When the fluid balance and plasma glucose are stable, the patient can be transferred to subcutaneous insulin therapy.

2. F – Intravenous insulin with fluid resuscitation

This patient has entered a hyperosmolar non-ketotic state (HONK). HONK is seen in people with type 2 diabetes, including previously undiagnosed patients. The event is usually triggered by an underlying illness, the ingestion of a high sugar load or the use of medications that cause a rise in plasma glucose (e.g. steroids). Patients usually present in a confused state, with a history of polyuria and polydipsia. The patient has a high plasma glucose, which can be in excess of 30 mmol/L. In HONK, the circulating insulin is sufficient to prevent ketogenesis but insufficient to allow the peripheral uptake and metabolism of glucose. Therefore the patient does not become acidotic. The hyperglycaemia causes an osmotic diuresis that rapidly dehydrates the patient and produces an extremely high plasma osmolality.

HONK is treated with a combination of intravenous fluid resuscitation and intravenous insulin. Care must be taken not to reduce the glucose levels or sodium concentration too rapidly, as the resultant osmotic shifts can result in fatal cerebral oedema. The insulin should therefore be started at a low rate (e.g. 3 units/h) and only isotonic (0.9%) saline should be prescribed. HONK also places the patient at high risk of thromboembolic events such as deep vein thrombosis, pulmonary embolism and stroke; therefore all patients should receive prophylactic heparin. The mortality rate of HONK approaches 30%, which is likely to be a reflection of the advanced age of many of the patients and the presence of underlying illness.

3. G – Oral glucose

This patient has mild- to -moderate hypoglycaemia. Symptoms of hypoglycaemia usually appear when the glucose level drops below 3 mmol/L. Common symptoms include drowsiness, sweating, hunger, palpitations, anxiety and personality changes. Patients with longstanding diabetes can become unaware of hypoglycaemia and become profoundly hypoglycaemic before symptoms develop. In mild-to-moderate hypoglycaemia, the treatment of choice is with oral glucose in the form of either sugary drinks/food or a glucose gel (e.g. GlucoGel – formerly known as Hypostop Gel), which is applied to, and directly absorbed from, the buccal membrane. Hypoglycaemia is also seen in a number of non-diabetic conditions, which can be remembered using ExPLAIN:

Exogenous agents (e.g. insulin, oral hypoglycaemic agents, alcohol)
Pituitary insufficiency (ACTH deficiency)
Liver failure
Addison's disease (due to glucocorticoid deficiency)
Insulinoma
Neoplasms

4. D – Intravenous glucose

This patient's profound hypoglycaemia has triggered a seizure. In patients with diabetes, hypoglycaemia is usually secondary to insulin or oral hypoglycaemic medications. Patients experiencing hypoglycaemic seizures are often pale and extremely clammy, and may have exhibited bizarre behaviour beforehand. The treatment of choice depends upon the situation. If the patient has venous access, 50 mL of 50% glucose is given intravenously, followed by a large saline flush. If the patient does not have venous access, 1 mg intramuscular glucagon is given to mobilize hepatic glucose stores. Recovery is usually prompt. Once the seizure has stopped, the patient should be placed on a glucose drip, be encouraged to drink sugary drinks and have regular capillary blood glucose levels recorded. Patients in the community who are prone to hypoglycaemia can be given glucagon to be administered by a responsible person in case of severe hypoglycaemia.

5. B – Increase insulin dose temporarily

Although this case does not represent a true diabetic emergency, the patient is at risk of deteriorating. As discussed above in Case 1, in the presence of illness, the patient's insulin requirements increase even if they are not eating. If the insulin dose is lowered or remains the same, the patient may become ketoacidotic. The patient in this scenario should therefore be advised to increase his insulin dose temporarily and seek medical attention. Regular capillary blood glucose measurement is essential until an improvement is seen.

Theme 12: Dermatomes 1

1. G – T4

2. D – C6

3. B – C2

4. O – S5

5. I – T10

A dermatome is an area of skin that is supplied by a pair of spinal nerve roots. Each dermatome is named after the nerve root that supplies it. They are useful in clinical examination to delineate the site of neurological damage, but can be used only as a guide, as there may be considerable overlap between dermatomes. Useful locations to test the dermatomes are as follows:

C2	back of the head, occipital protuberance
C3	neck
C4	acromioclavicular joint
C5	anterolateral shoulder
C6	thumb
C7	middle finger
C8	little finger
T1	medial arm
T2	apex of the axilla
T4	nipple line
T6	xiphoid process
T10	umbilicus
T12/L1	inguinal ligament
L2	medial thigh
L3	medial knee
L4	big toe
L5	dorsum of foot
S1	lateral foot
S2	popliteal fossa
S3	ischial tuberosity
S4/S5	perianal area

There is no C1 dermatome. The face is supplied by the three branches of the trigeminal nerve (cranial nerve V).

Dermatome, from Greek *derma* = skin + *tomos* = cut.

Theme 13: Shortness of breath

1. J – Tuberculosis

Tuberculosis (TB) is the most common infection in the world, with a greater risk in developing countries, HIV infection and malnutrition. It is caused by the Gram-positive organism *Mycobacterium tuberculosis*, although some cases are caused by *M. bovis* and *M. africanum*. Primary TB infection occurs through droplet infection and leads to the development of the primary lung lesion (a focus of TB organisms surrounded by macrophages, known as the Ghon focus). This may be associated with enlarged hilar lymph nodes (Ghon complex), but is often asymptomatic. The pathology of TB is caseating granulomas. Ninety per cent of primary lesions heal spontaneously, although a severe, disseminated infection occurs in 10% (miliary TB – seen as 1–2 mm fine lesions through the lung fields on X-ray). Re-infection or reactivation of TB results in post-primary disease. Post-primary pulmonary TB presents with a subacute illness with cough, haemoptysis, dyspnoea, fever, night sweats and anorexia. A chest X-ray shows lesions in the upper lobes. Features of extrapulmonary TB include painless lymphadenopathy, constrictive pericarditis, ascites, spinal disease, septic arthritis and kidney infection.

The diagnosis of TB can be made by sputum staining (using Ziehl–Neelsen stain) and culture (on Lowenstein–Jensen media; this can take up to 6 weeks). The bacille Calmette–Guérin (BCG) vaccine is made of attenuated *M. bovis* and provides some protection. Skin tuberculin testing can be used to screen for TB. There are two types: the Heaf test (a multipuncture method that is read after 5 days and is positive if there is ring-shaped induration) and the Mantoux test (an intradermal tuberculin injection that is read at 3 days and is positive when induration is >5 mm). False negatives to tuberculin screening are seen with severe TB, HIV, malnutrition, malignancy and sarcoidosis, and in people taking immunosuppressants.

Drug treatment of TB is with 6 months of antituberculous therapy (e.g. rifampicin, isoniazid, pyrazinamide and ethambutol for 4 months followed by just rifampicin and isoniazid for 2 months). Ethambutol can be omitted if drug resistance is unlikely (e.g. in white, HIV-negative patients). Twelve months of treatment is given for central nervous system disease. Multidrug-resistant TB (MDRTB) is defined as TB infection that is resistant to rifampicin and isoniazid. MRDTB is treated with five drugs for 24 months (including, for example, clarithromycin and streptomycin). Drugs are given as a single daily dose before breakfast. The side-effects of the commonly used antituberculous drugs are as follows:

- rifampicin: orange urine, purple tears, hepatitis, induces liver enzymes
- isoniazid: hepatitis, peripheral neuropathy
- pyrazinamide: hepatitis, photosensitivity, gout
- ethambutol: optic neuritis
- streptomycin: ototoxic, nephrotoxic.

Anton Ghon, Austrian pathologist (1866–1936).

Miliary, from Latin *miliarius* = grain seeds.

2. I – Sarcoidosis

Sarcoidosis is a multisystem disease characterized by the production of non-caseating granulomas. It is most common in West Indians and Scandinavians. The lungs are affected in 90% of cases, presenting with dyspnoea and a dry cough. Other features include erythema nodosum (painful, purple, tender lesions on the shins), lupus pernio (sarcoidosis lesions on the skin), arthralgia and lymphadenopathy. Sarcoid tissue can activate vitamin D and cause hypercalcaemia. Chest X-ray shows bilateral hilar lymphadenopathy. Serum calcium and angiotensin-converting enzyme (ACE) levels are elevated and the tuberculin test is negative. The diagnosis of sarcoidosis is confirmed by biopsy and histology (showing non-caseating granulomas). The Kveim–Siltzbach test – where a sample of splenic tissue is injected into the skin in order to try to produce granulation tissue – is no longer done. Sarcoidosis is staged according to chest X-ray findings as follows:

Stage 1: bilateral hilar lymphadenopathy
Stage 2: bilateral hilar lymphadenopathy and lung involvement
Stage 3: lung involvement only
Stage 4: lung fibrosis.

Treatment is with steroids and immunosuppressants.

Morton Ansgar Kveim, Norwegian pathologist (1892–1966).

Louis Siltzbach, American physician (1906–80).

3. F – Cryptogenic fibrosing alveolitis

Cryptogenic fibrosing alveolitis (CFA) is a fibrosing alveolitis that is not associated with another disease. It is most common in older male smokers. CFA presents with exertional dyspnoea and a dry cough. Examination may reveal clubbing and bilateral end-inspiratory crepitations, especially at the lower zones. As disease progresses, central cyanosis and cor pulmonale develop. Chest X-ray demonstrates diffuse pulmonary opacities, or honeycombing in advanced disease. Pulmonary function tests show a restrictive defect (with a reduced vital capacity and reduced forced expiratory volume). The diagnosis is confirmed with high-resolution CT. Treatment is with prednisolone and azathioprine, although CFA tends to respond poorly. Death usually occurs within 5 years of diagnosis.

Cryptogenic, from Greek *kryptos* = secret + Latin *genus* = origin.

4. G – Extrinsic allergic alveolitis

Extrinsic allergic alveolitis is caused by the inhalation of organic dusts, resulting in an immune complex-mediated reaction with the formation of granulomas within the lung (and eventual lung fibrosis). Patients present with fever, muscle aches, cough, dyspnoea (no wheeze) and headaches. Examination reveals widespread end-inspiratory crepitations. Chest X-ray demonstrates micronodular shadowing, especially in the upper zones. Lung function tests confirm a restrictive defect. The diagnosis of extrinsic allergic alveolitis is made by demonstrating typical clinical and radiological features along with identifying the underlying allergen. Treatment is with prednisolone and requires avoidance of the precipitating allergen. Examples of allergens that cause extrinsic allergic alveolitis include:

- farmer's lung: *Aspergillus fumigatus* in mouldy hay
- bird fancier's lung: avium serum proteins found in bird droppings and feathers
- malt worker's lung: *A. clavatus* in mouldy maltings.

5. C – Aspergillosis

Aspergillosis is caused by the fungus *Aspergillus fumigatus*. It is associated with atopic asthma, extrinsic allergic alveolitis and the development of aspergillomas. Aspergillomas occur when spores of *Aspergillus* lodge in pulmonary tissue, usually in lung that has been previously damaged (e.g. by TB or bronchiectasis). Patients may present with recurrent severe haemoptysis. A chest X-ray demonstrates a tumour-like opacity (the fungal ball) within a cavity. The diagnosis is confirmed by finding fungal hyphae on sputum microscopy, and treatment is by surgical removal (antifungals do not work).

Pneumoconiosis is a diffuse lung fibrosis caused by chronic inorganic dust exposure. Coal pneumoconiosis follows chronic coal dust inhalation. There are two types: simple pneumoconiosis (disease does not progress once the miner leaves the industry) and progressive massive fibrosis (disease progresses). Affected patients have a cough productive of black sputum (melanoptysis). *Silica* is the most fibrogenic dust, resulting in progressive lung fibrosis even when exposure has finished. Patients with silicosis characteristically have egg-shell calcification of the hilar nodes.

Theme 14: Sexually transmitted infections 1

Anyone who presents with a sexually transmitted infection (STI) is at risk of carrying further infections.

1. C – Chancroid

Chancroid is caused by the Gram-negative bacterium *Haemophilus ducreyi*, and is found mostly in tropical countries. It is an ulcerative condition of the genitalia that develops within a week of exposure. Lesions begin as a small papule, which eventually ulcerates to form single or multiple, painful, superficial ulcers. Inflammation may lead to phimosis. Enlargement and suppuration of inguinal lymph nodes may occur, leading to a unilocular abscess (bubo) that can rupture to form a discharging sinus. Treatment is with appropriate antibiotics (e.g. erythromycin).

2. D – Chlamydia infection

The right upper quadrant pain with non-specific urethritis in a girl with this history suggests chlamydial infection. Chlamydia infection is caused by the oculogenital serovars D–K of *Chlamydia trachomatis.* Infection tends to be asymptomatic, although there can be increased vaginal discharge, dysuria and urinary frequency. Ascending infection can cause salpingitis and, if it enters the abdominal cavity, perihepatitis (Fitz-Hugh–Curtis syndrome), which leads to right upper quadrant pain and tenderness. Chlamydia infection is a major cause of infertility and increases the possibility of a future ectopic pregnancy. In males, symptoms include mucopurulent discharge and dysuria, although it is asymptomatic in 25%. Epididymo-orchitis is a complication. Diagnosis of chlamydial infection is by urine antigen detection or vaginal swab culture. Treatment is with doxycycline.

Acute pelvic inflammatory disease is characterized by pelvic pain, pyrexia, cervical excitation, adnexal tenderness and a raised white cell count. It is most often caused by chlamydia infection and gonorrhoea.

Chlamydia, from Greek *chlamys* = cloak (as chlamydia is often 'cloaked', i.e. asymptomatic).

Thomas Fitz-Hugh Jr, American physician (1894–1963).

Arthur Curtis, American gynaecologist (1881–1955).

3. A – Bacterial vaginosis

Bacterial vaginosis (BV) is not a sexually transmitted infection but rather an imbalance of the polymicrobial vaginal flora. There is often a preponderance of mixed anaerobic flora (e.g. *Gardnerella vaginalis* and *Mycoplasma hominis*). It is often asymptomatic, but can cause a creamy-grey discharge with a fishy odour. There is no itching. The diagnosis of BV is by the Amsel criteria (at least three of the following): homogeneous discharge, clue cells on microscopy, pH of vaginal fluid >4.5, and release of a fishy odour on addition of 10% potassium hydroxide to the discharge. Clue cells are epithelial cells with bacteria adherent to the surface. BV can be treated with antibiotics (e.g. metronidazole), but there is a high rate of recurrence.

4. Q – Syphilis (specifically secondary syphilis)

This woman has had a painless ulcer followed by systemic symptoms (fever, malaise, headache and skin rash). This history is indicative of secondary syphilis. For more information about syphilis, see 'Sexually transmitted infections 2' (Paper 9 Answers, Theme 4).

5. P – Scabies

Scabies is caused by *Sarcoptes scabiei,* a mite that burrows into the skin, where the female lays her eggs. Scabies is often a sexually transmitted infection, but can be spread throughout households. Patients develop an intense itch, which is worse at night. This is caused by an allergic response to the eggs. The burrows made by the mite tend to be symmetrical and affect finger webs, sides of digits, flexor surfaces of the wrists and the penis. Secondary infection of affected areas can occur. Immunocompromised and institutionalized patients can develop a more severe infestation, with thick hyperkeratotic crusting on affected areas. This is known as Norwegian scabies (first described in Norway in 1848 – it was originally thought to be a distant variant of leprosy). Management of scabies is by application of topical pesticides (e.g. malathion and permethrin).

Scabies, from Latin *scabere* = to scratch.

Genital herpes is caused by the DNA-containing herpes simplex virus (HSV) types 1 and 2. The infection remains prevalent due to asymptomatic virus shedding. Clinical features of primary infection include dysuria with painful, itchy ulcers and occasionally urethral or vaginal discharge. Patients may also complain of constitutional symptoms (fever, headache, malaise and myalgia). Lesions are papular, vesicular or pustular; these crust and heal within 4 weeks. Examination may reveal inguinal lymphadenitis. HSV remains dormant in dorsal root ganglia, and reactivation occurs in 75% of cases. Recurrent attacks tend to be milder, shorter and not associated with systemic features. Diagnosis is by viral swabs. Severe infections can be managed with aciclovir.

Genital warts are most commonly caused by human papillomavirus (HPV) types 6b and 11. Incubation is normally about 3 months, but warts may take up to 2 years to develop. When large warts coalesce, the appearance is known as condylomata acuminata. Genital warts increase in size during pregnancy, and wart-induced obstruction of labour may be an indication for caesarean section. Management options for genital warts include excision, cautery and caustic agents (podophyllin and imiquimod).

Condylomata acuminata, from Latin *condylomata* = knuckles + *acuminatum* = pointed.

Theme 15: Diagnosis of joint pain 1

1. F – Pseudogout

Calcium pyrophosphate deposition disease is caused by the deposition of calcium pyrophosphate dihydrate crystals in the joints. The crystals deposit along the cartilages, producing a linear chondrocalcinosis that is best seen on the meniscus on X-ray. Shedding of crystals into the joint precipitates an acute synovitis known as pseudogout. Patients present with acute-onset pain, swelling and redness in the affected joint. Pseudogout is most common in elderly women and usually affects the knee or wrist. The diagnosis is made by joint aspiration, demonstrating the weakly positively birefringent brick-shaped crystals of calcium pyrophosphate. The joint fluid should always be sent for culture to exclude a septic arthritis. The treatment of pseudogout is with non-steroidal anti-inflammatory drugs (NSAIDs). The chondrocalcinosis itself cannot be treated.

2. G – Psoriatic arthritis

Psoriatic arthritis affects 5% of patients with psoriasis, but it may precede the onset of skin symptoms. It is more common in psoriasis patients who have nail disease (e.g. onycholysis and nail pitting). Psoriatic arthritis is characterized by distal interphalangeal joint involvement and dactylitis (sausage-shaped swelling of the fingers from inflammation). Arthritis mutilans is a severe form of psoriatic arthritis where there is destruction of the small bones of the hand, resulting in shortening of the fingers. The shortened fingers can be passively extended to their original length (telescoping). An X-ray of the hand in arthritis mutilans demonstrates central joint erosions in the interphalangeal joints, resulting in a 'pencil in cup' appearance. Although the hand may look significantly deformed, functional ability is well preserved.

Dactylitis, from Greek *daktylos* = finger.

3. J – Septic arthritis

Septic arthritis should always be considered with the presentation of a hot, swollen, tender joint with a restricted range of movement in the unwell patient. Septic arthritis is an infection within the synovial joint, most often caused by *Staphylococcus aureus* infection. It is most common in the hip and knee. Risk factors for developing septic arthritis include being very old, very young, intravenous drug use, diabetes and having pre-existing joint complaints. X-ray is normal in the early stages, but ultrasound and joint aspiration should be done to culture organisms. Management of septic arthritis is with surgical washout of the joint and intravenous antibiotics (e.g. flucloxacillin and benzylpenicillin) until the patient is clinically well, followed by a few weeks of oral antibiotics. Complications of septic arthritis include joint destruction (leading to arthritis), spread of infection to the bone (osteomyelitis) and ankylosis (bony fusion across the joint).

4. H – Reiter's syndrome

The triad of arthritis, urethritis and iritis is indicative of Reiter's syndrome. For more information on this condition, see 'Sexually transmitted infections 2' (Paper 9 Answers, Theme 4).

5. E – Osteoarthritis

Osteoarthritis is a non-inflammatory disorder of the synovial joints characterized by wear and tear of the articular surfaces. It is the most common joint disease, affecting 70% of the over-70s. Risk factors for osteoarthritis are obesity, female sex, hypermobility, trauma and repetitive use. It most commonly affects the distal interphalangeal joints (Heberden's nodes), proximal interphalangeal joints (Bouchard's nodes) and the base of the thumb, hips, knees and spine. Patients complain of joint pain that is worse with movement and relieved by rest, stiffness, joint instability and deformity. On examination, bony swellings, joint effusions and crepitus may be seen. Joint X-rays can show four characteristic features in osteoarthritis: narrowing of the joint space (due to cartilage loss), subchondral sclerosis, cyst formation and osteophytes (bony swellings). Heberden's and Bouchard's nodes are examples of osteophytes, and the Baker's cyst of the knee is an example of joint effusions. Management options in osteoarthritis include weight loss, physiotherapy, NSAIDs, intra-articular steroid injections, arthrodesis and joint replacement.

William Heberden, English physician (1710–1801).

Charles-Joseph Bouchard, French pathologist (1837–1915).

Tennis elbow is inflammation at the insertion of the tendon into the lateral epicondyle of the elbow. This often occurs in response to repetitive strain of the tendon. There is pain over the lateral epicondyle that radiates down the forearm and is exacerbated by wrist extension. Management options are rest, NSAIDs and steroid injection. Severe cases are treated by surgery, where the tendon of the forearm extensors is stripped from the lateral epicondyle and replaced. *Golfer's elbow* describes a similar condition but on the medial epicondyle, with pain that is worse on wrist flexion.

Practice Paper 3: Questions

Theme 1: Motor weakness 2

Options

A. Ataxia telangiectasia
B. Charcot–Marie–Tooth disease
C. Guillain–Barré syndrome
D. Hypokalaemia
E. Lambert–Eaton syndrome
F. Mononeuritis multiplex
G. Motor neuron disease
H. Multiple sclerosis
I. Muscular dystrophy
J. Myasthenia gravis
K. Poliomyelitis
L. Spinal cord compression
M. Spinal muscular atrophy

For each of the following scenarios, select the most likely cause of motor weakness. Each option may be used once, more than once or not at all.

1. A 32-year-old woman presents to the GP with a sudden pain behind her right eye associated with blurred vision. Last month, she experienced sudden loss of use of her left arm, but this resolved spontaneously within 48 hours. On examination, there was no limb weakness or sensory loss.

2. A 6-month-old baby boy is brought to see the doctor by his mother. She is worried that he is becoming increasing floppy and can no longer lift his head. He is also finding it difficult to bottle-feed. On examination, although the baby lies flat and does not move much, he is obviously alert.

3. A 6-year-old boy is brought in by his mother as he has had progressive difficulty walking over the last few months. He especially finds it difficult to stand up after he has been playing on the floor. On examination, his calves appear large. There is no sensory deficit.

4. A 47-year-old woman presents with difficulty writing and walking. Over the last week, she has had numbness and weakness of the first three digits of the right hand. She is on insulin for type 2 diabetes mellitus. On examination, there is a left-sided foot drop.

5. A 20-year-old man attends his GP with worsening difficulty walking and a tendency to fall over. This clumsiness has caused him to twist his knee and tear his left anterior cruciate ligament. On examination, there is weakness in both his lower limbs and a loss of sensation below the knees. The muscles of the feet are wasted, and this has resulted in a high-arching deformity.

Theme 2: Diabetic eye disease

Options

A. Background retinopathy
B. Cataract
C. Glaucoma
D. Hypertensive retinopathy
E. Macular degeneration
F. Macular oedema
G. Pre-proliferative retinopathy
H. Proliferative retinopathy
I. Retinal detachment
J. Vitreous haemorrhage

For each of the following scenarios, select the most appropriate description of diabetic eye disease. Each option may be used once, more than once or not at all.

1. A 50-year-old man with type 2 diabetes is found to have retinal microaneurysms, haemorrhages and hard exudates on fundoscopy. He claims to have no visual impairment.

2. A 67-year-old woman with a long history of poorly controlled type 2 diabetes is having problems with her sight. Examination reveals reduced visual acuity. Fundoscopy demonstrates evidence of background retinopathy but no other pathology.

3. A 47-year-old man with type 1 diabetes presents to the emergency department with a sudden deterioration in the vision of his left eye associated with flashes and objects floating across his visual field. He describes the visual loss as a curtain moving across his visual field.

4. A 35-year-old patient with type 1 diabetes is found to have microaneurysms, hard exudates and cotton-wool spots on fundoscopy.

5. A 40-year-old patient with type 1 diabetes is found to have new vessel formation around the optic disc on fundoscopy.

Theme 3: Complications of acute myocardial infarction

Options

A. First-degree heart block
B. Acute mitral valve regurgitation
C. Acute pericarditis
D. Atrial ectopic beats
E. Atrial fibrillation
F. Cardiac tamponade
G. Complete (third-degree) heart block
H. Dressler's syndrome
I. Pulmonary embolism
J. Subacute left ventricular failure
K. Ventricular aneurysm
L. Ventricular ectopic beats
M. Ventricular tachycardia
N. Ventricular wall rupture

For each of the following scenarios, select the most likely complication. Each option may be used once, more than once or not at all.

1. You are asked to see a 68-year-old woman who had an anterior myocardial infarction 2 days ago. She has become acutely short of breath and is coughing up pink frothy sputum. On examination, her jugular venous pressure is raised and she has a systolic murmur. On auscultation, you can hear bilateral crackles at the lung bases.

2. A 58-year-old man complains of central chest pain, fever and lethargy 4 weeks after suffering a myocardial infarction. The chest pain is worse on inspiration, is stabbing in nature, and is relieved by ibuprofen and sitting forward.

3. You are asked to review a 72-year-old woman who had a myocardial infarction 12 hours ago. Her heart rate is 40 beats/min and her blood pressure is 90/60 mmHg. The ECG shows abnormally wide QRS complexes occurring at a rate of 40 beats/min and P-waves occurring at a rate of 90 beats/min. There is no relationship between the P-waves and QRS complexes.

4. A 66-year-old man, known to have had an anterior myocardial infarction 2 days previously, collapses. On examination, you notice that he has a raised jugular venous pressure that rises with inspiration. Auscultation seems normal. His blood pressure is 80/50 mmHg and his heart rate is 100 beats/min. The ECG shows sinus tachycardia with small QRS complexes.

5. A 60-year-old man who had a myocardial infarction 4 weeks ago presents to his GP complaining of increasing shortness of breath since discharge. It is worse at night time on lying flat, and he occasionally wakes up acutely short of breath in the early hours of the morning.

Theme 4: Cutaneous lesions 2

Options

A. Cellulitis
B. Erysipelas
C. Ganglion
D. Granuloma annulare
E. Impetigo
F. Kaposi's sarcoma
G. Necrotizing fasciitis
H. Neurofibroma
I. Pyogenic granuloma
J. Sebaceous cyst
K. Seborrhoeic keratosis

For each of the following scenarios, select the most appropriate diagnosis. Each option may be used once, more than once or not at all.

1. A 37-year-old woman goes to the primary-care diabetes follow-up clinic. She has a lesion on the back of her hand that has appeared recently. It does not cause any problems, but she was curious. On examination, the lesion is made up of reddish bumps arranged in a ring.

2. A 12-year-old girl has developed multiple lumps on her arms and trunk. One examination, the lesion feels firm and rubbery and the patient reports some tingling on palpation.

3. A 57-year-old man is in hospital being treated for severe pneumonia. He develops an area of erythema around his intravenous cannula site. On examination, the area is swollen and warm, with some superficial blistering. The patient has a temperature of 38.5°C and feels unwell.

4. A 37-year-old woman presents with a bright-red nodule on the end of her index finger that bleeds easily. This lesion has grown rapidly in the last week and is now 1 cm in diameter.

5. A 42-year-old man had a renal transplant last year for end-stage renal failure. He presents to his GP with multiple painless purple lesions that have gradually appeared over the last few weeks. These lesions are found all over his body.

Theme 5: Dizziness

Options

A. Benign paroxysmal positional vertigo
B. Drug-induced ototoxicity
C. Hyperventilation
D. Labyrinthitis
E. Ménière's disease
F. Multiple sclerosis
G. Ramsay Hunt syndrome
H. Posterior circulation stroke
I. Trauma

For each of the following scenarios, select the most appropriate underlying cause. Each option may be used once, more than once or not at all.

1. A 45-year-old woman presents with a 6-month history of intermittent ringing in her ears and dizziness. She had also noticed a gradual worsening in the hearing of her right ear. Examination is unremarkable.

2. A 56-year-old man presents to the GP with a 3-day history of intermittent dizziness. The dizziness only comes on when he turns his head to the left. He has no hearing problems.

3. A 35-year-old man is in hospital being treated for pyelonephritis. One day on the ward round, he complains that he cannot hear that well and that he is intermittently dizzy. He has never had any problems like this before. On examination, there is marked sensorineural deafness bilaterally.

4. A 48-year-old woman attends the emergency department with pain and a rash on her left ear. This is associated with dizziness, vertigo and weakness of the left side of her face.

5. A 58-year-old man woke up in the night with sudden-onset severe dizziness and nausea. He got up, but found it difficult to walk down the stairs because of the dizziness. The symptoms were no worse in any particular position and there was no hearing loss.

Theme 6: Diagnosis of joint pain 2

Options

A. Ankylosing spondylitis
B. Enteropathic arthritis
C. Golfer's elbow
D. Gout
E. Osteoarthritis
F. Pseudogout
G. Psoriatic arthritis
H. Reiter's syndrome
I. Rheumatoid arthritis
J. Septic arthritis
K. Still's disease
L. Tennis elbow

For each of the following scenarios, select the most likely diagnosis. Each option may be used once, more than once or not at all.

1. A 64-year-old man presents with sudden-onset severe pain in his left great toe that occurred at rest. He is otherwise well. On examination, the small joint of the toe is swollen, red and tender. The patient is unable to move the joint for the pain.

2. A 36-year-old man presents with a 4-month history of worsening lower back pain and stiffness. The pain is worse in the morning, but gets better throughout the day. Examination is unremarkable.

3. A 12-year-old boy presents with painful joints. He recently had a bout of gastroenteritis, which he blames on a 'dodgy donor kebab'. His stools were loose and contained blood. He says that his stools have contained blood for at least a month prior to the bout of gastroenteritis. On examination, both knee joints are tender and hot.

4. A 43-year-old woman presents with a 2-month history of pain in her hands. She finds the small joints in both her hands extremely painful and stiff, especially in the morning. On examination, the small joints of the hand are tender and appear swollen.

5. A 3-year-old girl presents with a 2-week history of pain in her joints and muscles. She feels very unwell and is difficult to settle. On examination, she has a raised temperature.

Theme 7: Complications of drug therapy

Options

A. Agranulocytosis
B. Bronchospasm
C. Dry cough
D. Dry mouth
E. Nausea and vomiting
F. Peripheral oedema
G. Oculogyric crisis
H. Reye's syndrome
I. Vomiting after alcohol

For each of the following drugs, select the most characteristic side-effect. Each option may be used once, more than once or not at all.

1. Metoclopramide used to treat nausea in a 15-year-old girl.

2. Aspirin used to treat a 5-year-old boy with fever.

3. Morphine used to treat a 28-year-old man with severe abdominal pain.

4. Metronidazole used to treat a 32-year-old woman with intra-abdominal sepsis

5. Propranolol used to treat anxiety in a 21-year-old woman with asthma.

Theme 8: Interpretation of liver function tests

Options

A. Acute liver failure
B. Biliary tract obstruction
C. Gilbert's syndrome
D. Haemolytic anaemia
E. Hepatocellular carcinoma
F. Hepatocellular inflammation
G. Paracetamol overdose
H. Short-term alcohol abuse

For each of the following scenarios, select the most likely diagnosis. Each option may be used once, more than once or not at all.

1. An 18-year-old man has routine blood tests taken as part of a medical trial. A mildly raised bilirubin level was incidentally discovered. The man is asymptomatic and is usually fit and well.

2. A 45-year-old woman presents to the emergency department with severe right upper quadrant abdominal pain. She is found to have significantly raised alkaline phosphatase and bilirubin levels. ALT and AST are only mildly raised.

3. A 19-year-old man is shown to have a raised γ-glutamyltranspeptidase level after he is admitted to the emergency department following an alcohol binge. Liver function tests, full blood count, and urea and electrolytes are all normal.

4. A 56-year-old man presents to the GP with abdominal pain and jaundice. His liver function tests are globally deranged. ALT and AST levels are significantly raised, and there is a mild rise in bilirubin and alkaline phosphatase.

5. A 45-year-old man presents to the emergency department with confusion, lethargy and jaundice. His stools and urine are a normal colour. Blood tests show a raised unconjugated bilirubin, a raised lactate dehydrogenase, a raised ALT and a haemoglobin of 8.1 g/dL. Alkaline phosphatase, ALT and AST levels are normal.

Theme 9: Diagnosis of respiratory conditions 2

Options

A. Acute coryza
B. Asthma
C. Bronchiectasis
D. Chronic obstructive pulmonary disease
E. Closed non-tension pneumothorax
F. Cryptogenic fibrosing alveolitis
G. Cystic fibrosis
H. Extrinsic allergic alveolitis
I. Open non-tension pneumothorax
J. Pneumoconiosis
K. Pneumonia
L. Pulmonary embolism
M. Sleep apnoea
N. Tension pneumothorax

For each of the following scenarios, select the most appropriate diagnosis. Each option may be used once, more than once or not at all.

1. A 67-year-old man has a 3-day history of worsening shortness of breath. He can normally walk 100 m but now can barely get to the front door. Although he says he normally coughs up small amounts of clear sputum, he is now expectorating large amounts of greeny-yellow sputum. Auscultation reveals widespread wheeze.

2. A 32-year-old man is stabbed in the right side of his chest. He struggles to the hospital. On arrival, he is in some respiratory distress. On examination, there is decreased air entry and hyper-resonance to percussion on the right side. The trachea is not deviated. The doctor notes the presence of a 'sucking' wound in the right chest.

3. A 26-year-old man presents with a 2-day history of feeling generally unwell and short of breath. Today, he started coughing up thick green sputum that had flecks of dry blood in. He complains of a sharp pain over the right side of his chest, which is worse on breathing in. Auscultation reveals bronchial breathing at the right base.

4. A 48-year-old woman presents with sudden-onset shortness of breath and a sharp pain on the right side of her chest. She was previously well. On examination, there is no wheeze or crackles and no areas of hyper-resonance.

5. A 21-year-old woman is involved in a road traffic accident. When the paramedics arrive, she has a heart rate of 122 beats/min, a respiratory rate of 32/min and a blood pressure of 86/42 mmHg. On examination, there are absent breath sounds and hyper-resonance to percussion on the left side. The trachea is deviated to the right.

Theme 10: Renal investigations

A. Angiography
B. Cystoscopy
C. DMSA scan
D. End-stream urine sample for microscopy, culture and sensitivity
E. Kidney–ureter–bladder X-ray
F. Micturating cystourethrogram
G. Midstream urine sample for microscopy, culture and sensitivity
H. MRI
I. Renal biopsy
J. Renal tract ultrasound scan
K. Three early morning urine samples for microscopy, culture and Ziehl–Neelsen staining
L. Water deprivation test

For each of the following scenarios, select the most appropriate investigation. Each option may be used once, more than once or not at all.

1. A 34-year-old woman presents to her GP with a 2-day history of pain on urinating, frequency of urination and the production of offensive urine. A urine dipstick shows that the sample is positive for nitrites and leucocytes and contains 1+ blood and 1+ protein.

2. A 25-year-old man presents to the emergency department complaining of severe loin pain and vomiting. He has had three episodes of this pain today, each lasting 10 minutes. On examination, he is pale, sweaty and tender in his right loin. A urine dipstick shows 3+ blood, 1+ protein, no nitrites and no leucocytes.

3. A 16-year-old boy with a transplanted kidney is shown to have worsening renal function over the previous 2 weeks. He is complaining of pain around the transplanted kidney. He has had no significant complications since his transplant 4 months ago. An ultrasound scan of his transplanted kidney showed no significant abnormalities.

4. A 2-year-old boy is seen by a paediatrician as he is experiencing recurrent urinary tract infections and is failing to thrive. There is a strong family history of vesico-ureteric reflux.

5. A 27-year-old man from India presents to his GP with an 8-week history of weight loss, night sweats, loin pain and pain on passing urine. A urine dipstick shows blood and leucocytes. A urine sample sent off a week earlier has been reported as 'no growth'.

Theme 11: Study design

Options

A. Case–control study
B. Case report
C. Case series
D. Cohort study
E. Meta-analysis
F. Non-systematic review
G. Randomized controlled trial
H. Systematic review

For each of the following descriptions of a study, select the most appropriate design. Each option may be used once, more than once or not at all.

1. Over the last year, you have seen eight patients with congenital absence of the left ear associated with a green rash on the trunk and a long QT interval on ECG. You wish to write this up for publication.

2. You are interested in finding out what is known about the use of doxycyline in treating multiple sclerosis, and write a good-quality paper for publication. A database search has found 12 studies addressing this question, and you aim to use them all.

3. You have a hunch that crayons can increase the risk of children developing autism. To test your theory, you follow up two groups of children for 10 years – a group that uses crayons and a group that does not – and compare the incidence of autism between the groups.

4. Your project supervisor wants you to look at whether regular music therapy is more likely to improve outcome in moderate depression compared with fluoxetine. He suggests that you randomize patients with a new diagnosis of depression to receive either one of the two therapies and follow them up for a year before finally comparing the outcomes.

5. Several studies have been published looking at the association between aortic aneurysm rupture and head size. While you would love to study this yourself, your department will not provide you with a grant. Instead, you decide to statistically analyse the available literature as a whole to come up with a more definite conclusion.

Theme 12: Management of neurological conditions 1

Options

A. Amphetamines
B. Aspirin
C. Carbamazepine
D. Chlordiazepoxide
E. Donepezil
F. Levodopa
G. Lorazepam
H. Metronidazole
I. Penicillin
J. Reassurance
K. Rifampicin and isoniazid

For each of the following scenarios, select the most appropriate management. Each option may be used once, more than once or not at all.

1. A 22-year-old woman has developed what she calls 'sleeping attacks'. These can come on at any time of day and last around 10 minutes. She is worried that they are interfering with her job in the stock market.

2. A 54-year-old woman attends the GP with a persistent headache. She also has multiple painless ulcers over her body. On examination, you notice that her pupils are small and unequal in size. The light reflex is absent.

3. A 74-year-old woman presents to the GP with a 12-month progressive decline in her memory function. Her husband says that she now gets lost trying to find the bathroom at home. She has previously been fit and well, and physical examination is unremarkable. She scores 23/30 on a Mini-Mental State Examination.

4. A 42-year-old man has a 2-month history of worsening headache, photophobia, neck stiffness, cough and malaise. Last week, he also developed weakness in his right arm.

5. A 63-year-old man was admitted for an elective cholecystectomy. On the second postoperative day, he complains of sweating and tremor. He is confused, anxious and tachycardic, and appears to be responding to visual hallucinations.

Theme 13: Anaemia

Options

A. α-Thalassaemia
B. β-Thalassaemia major
C. β-Thalassaemia trait
D. Anaemia of chronic disease
E. Autoimmune haemolytic anaemia
F. Glucose-6-phosphate dehydrogenase deficiency
G. Hereditary spherocytosis
H. Iron-deficiency anaemia secondary to gastrointestinal bleeding
I. Iron-deficiency anaemia secondary to iron malabsorption
J. Iron-deficiency anaemia secondary to menorrhagia
K. Megaloblastic macrocytic anaemia secondary to vitamin B_{12} deficiency
L. Megaloblastic macrocytic anaemia secondary to folate deficiency
M. Megaloblastic microcytic anaemia secondary to vitamin B_{12} deficiency
N. Normal variant
O. Sickle cell anaemia

For each of the following scenarios, select the most likely cause of anaemia. Each option may be used once, more than once or not at all.

Reference ranges: haemoglobin (Hb) (male) 13.5–17.7 g/dL, Hb (female) 11.5–16.5 g/dL, mean cell volume (MCV) 80–96 fL.

1. A 68-year-old woman who is being investigated for altered bowel habit is found to have an Hb of 8.3 g/dL, an MCV of 67 fL, a low ferritin level and a raised total iron-binding capacity.

2. A 24-year-old woman with active Crohn's disease is shown to have an Hb of 9.5 g/dL, an MCV of 101 fL and a normal ferritin level. A peripheral blood film shows a number of hypersegmented neutrophils.

3. A 55-year-old woman with a long history of rheumatoid arthritis is shown to have an Hb of 10.5 g/dL, an MCV of 80 fL and a raised ferritin level. Her arthritis is treated only symptomatically with paracetamol.

4. A previously well 8-month-old baby boy becomes generally unwell. His health visitor notices that he is failing to thrive. Investigation shows a microcytic, hypochromic anaemia in association with high levels of HbF and HbA_2.

5. A 56-year-old man presents to the emergency department feeling generally unwell and complaining of palpitations and breathlessness. He is clearly jaundiced on examination. Apart from hypertension, there is no significant medical history. The full blood count reveals an Hb of 7.4 g/dL, an MCV of 95 fL and a normal ferritin level. The peripheral blood film shows a larger than expected number of reticulocytes. Coombs' test is later shown to be positive.

Theme 14: Diagnosis of thyroid disease 1

Options

A. Anaplastic carcinoma
B. De Quervain's thyroiditis
C. Follicular carcinoma
D. Graves' disease
E. Hashimoto's thyroiditis
F. Haemorrhage into a cyst
G. Medullary carcinoma
H. Papillary carcinoma
I. Riedel's thyroiditis
J. Struma ovarii
K. Toxic multinodular goitre

For each of the following scenarios, select the most appropriate diagnosis. Each option may be used once, more than once or not at all.

1. A 25-year-old woman presents to the clinic with a slowly enlarging lump on the left side of her neck. She denies any other symptoms. On examination, there is a 2 cm, smooth, regular, firm lump that moves up with swallowing, but not with tongue protrusion. Lymph nodes are palpable in the left side of the neck.

2. A 54-year-old man presents to the clinic with a midline neck mass that has been increasing in size over a few months. On examination, the thyroid gland is enlarged, firm and irregular, although the patient does not complain of any pain. No cervical nodes are palpable. A core biopsy is taken, and the histology report denies the presence of malignancy.

3. A 42-year-old woman presents to her GP with a large goitre that she admits to having had for a long time. More recently, she has been suffering with constipation, lethargy and weight gain. On examination, her pulse is 64 beats/min and regular. She has a diffusely enlarged, smooth, firm goitre. No lymph nodes are palpable.

4. A 46-year-old woman presents to the emergency department with palpitations. She is clearly nervous and describes having multiple paroxysms of fast palpitations over the preceding fortnight. On examination, you find an enlarged, lumpy thyroid gland, which is not fixed to the overlying skin.

5. An 84-year-old woman presents with a lump in her neck that was first noticed last month and has since been growing rapidly. On further questioning, she admits to having problems swallowing her food. On examination, there is a 5 cm, irregular, hard mass on the left side, which is fixed to the overlying skin.

Theme 15: Secondary hypertension

Options

A. Acromegaly
B. Adult polycystic disease
C. Aortic dissection
D. Berry aneurysm
E. Coarctation of the aorta
F. Conn's syndrome
G. Cushing's disease
H. Non-steroidal anti-inflammatory drug use
I. Oral contraception
J. Phaeochromocytoma
K. Pre-eclampsia
L. Stress at work
M. White coat syndrome

For each of the following scenarios, select the most likely cause of hypertension. Each option may be used once, more than once or not at all.

1. A 30-year-old man presents to the emergency department with headache and muscle weakness. He also complains of increased thirst and urine production. Apart from a blood pressure of 190/95 mmHg, examination was normal. Initial bloods tests demonstrated a serum potassium of 2.2 mmol/L, a serum sodium of 150 mmol/L, a serum urea of 4.3 mmol/L and a creatinine of 69 μmol/L.

2. A previously fit and well 35-year-old female doctor presents to her GP with a history of 'panic attacks', during which she feels extremely anxious and experiences palpitations, chest tightness and headaches. While in the surgery, she experiences a similar episode, becoming flushed and anxious. Her heart rate was 120 beats/min and her blood pressure reached 185/80 mmHg.

3. A 27-year-old woman with known Turner's syndrome presents to her GP with recurrent nose bleeds. On examination, her blood pressure is 190/95 mmHg. Auscultation reveals a mid-late systolic murmur best heard in between the shoulder blades.

4. A 45-year-old man was found to have a persistently raised blood pressure by his GP. On examination, a vague mass could be felt on the left side of the abdomen. He mentioned that his father died at 26 years of age following a 'brain haemorrhage'.

5. A 55-year-old woman is noted to have an elevated blood pressure on three separate occasions by her GP. She has a recent history of persisting acne and hirsutism, for which a dermatology referral has been made. Marked bruising is observed on examination.

Practice Paper 3: Answers

Theme 1: Motor weakness 2

1. H – Multiple sclerosis

Multiple sclerosis (MS) is an autoimmune destruction of the myelin-producing oligodendrocytes. The myelin loss in the central nervous system (CNS) results in slowed nerve conduction. The incidence is highest in temperate climates and in middle-aged women. Symptoms that suggest CNS demyelination include optic neuritis, unilateral dorsal column loss, a coarse tremor, trigeminal neuralgia in the under-50s, recurrent facial nerve palsy, sixth cranial nerve palsy and Lhermitte's phenomenon (tingling in the spine or limbs in neck flexion). A diagnosis of MS requires all of the following:

- age <60 years
- deficit in two or more anatomically distinct sites
- abnormalities apparent on examination
- one of the following patterns:
  - o two episodes lasting >24 hours and >1 month apart or
  - o slow progression over 6 months
- no other explanation for the symptoms.

Eighty per cent of cases of MS have the relapsing and remitting type, 15% have a primary progressive course and 5% have fulminating disease with early death. The best investigation to demonstrate demyelination is MRI. Electrophoresis of cerebrospinal fluid shows oligoclonal bands of IgG immunoglobulin. High-dose steroids can shorten acute relapses of MS, but do not affect long-term outcome. Immunosuppressants and interferons reduce the number of relapses and improve outcome. Complications of MS include spasticity, ataxia, neuropathic pain and bladder dysfunction.

2. M – Spinal muscular atrophy

Spinal muscular atrophy describes a group of genetic disorders affecting spinal and cranial motor neurons. There is degeneration of anterior horn cells, resulting in progressive proximal and distal weakness, wasting, and fasciculation (usually symmetrical). An example is Werdnig–Hoffmann disease: autosomal recessive severe muscle weakness, with death occurring by 12 months. Spinal muscular atrophy is the second most common cause of neuromuscular disease in the UK.

3. I – Muscular dystrophy

Muscular dystrophy describes a group of inherited disorders with progressive degeneration of groups of muscles without involvement of the nervous system. It is characterized by symmetrical wasting and weakness, with no fasciculations or sensory loss. The most common muscular dystrophy is the Duchenne type, an X-linked recessive deficiency of the protein dystrophin, which is required to maintain the integrity of muscle cell walls. Duchenne muscular dystrophy begins in childhood and affects the proximal arms and legs. There is pseudohypertrophy of the calves (due to replacement of muscle by fibrosis and fat), a waddling gait and difficultly standing (children may 'climb' up their legs to help stand up – Gower's sign). Death by respiratory failure or cardiomyopathy occurs in the early 20s. A diagnosis of muscular dystrophy is confirmed by electromyography and biopsy. Creatine kinase may also be elevated. Management of muscular dystrophy is supportive.

Other forms of muscular dystrophy include Becker muscular dystrophy (X-linked recessive, with features similar to Duchenne muscular dystrophy but less severe, and with death occurring by the early 40s), myotonic dystrophy (autosomal dominant, weakness of temporal, facial, sternomastoid and distal limb muscles), fascioscapulohumeral dystrophy (autosomal dominant, affecting facial and shoulder girdle muscles) and limb girdle dystrophy (autosomal recessive, affecting pelvic and shoulder girdles). Additional features of myotonic dystrophy include myotonia (slow relaxation of muscles), frontal balding, cataracts, ptosis and gonadal atrophy.

Guillaume Benjamin Amand Duchenne, French neurologist (1806–75).

4. F – Mononeuritis multiplex

Mononeuritis multiplex is a form of peripheral neuropathy where there is damage to at least two anatomically distinct peripheral or spinal nerves. There may be a variety of underlying pathologies, such as ischaemia or inflammation of the nerves. Common causes of mononeuritis multiplex include diabetes mellitus, polyarteritis nodosa, rheumatoid arthritis and systemic lupus erythematosus.

5. B – Charcot–Marie–Tooth disease

Charcot–Marie–Tooth disease (also known as hereditary motor and sensory neuropathy) is characterized by symmetrical, distal, slowly progressive muscle wasting, and is often autosomal dominant. Symptoms often begin in early adulthood, and include foot drop (peroneal nerve damage), claw toes, pes cavus (high-arched feet), areflexia and distal sensory loss. Wasting of the distal leg muscles gives rise to an 'inverted bottle' appearance. Weakness of the upper limbs occurs later in the disease. Diagnosis is by nerve biopsy, which shows an 'onion bulb formation' due to repeated cycles of nerve demyelination followed by attempted remyelination. Disease is chronic, and death usually occurs by 40 years.

Jean-Marie Charcot, French neurologist (1825–93).

Pierre Marie, French neurologist (1853–1940).

Howard Henry Tooth, English physician (1856–1925).

Theme 2: Diabetic eye disease

The classification of diabetic retinopathy is as follows:

- background: microaneurysms, blot haemorrhages, hard exudates
- maculopathy: hard exudates involving the macula
- pre-proliferative: retinal haemorrhages, cotton-wool spots
- proliferative: neovascularization, fibrosis.

1. A – Background retinopathy

Diabetic eye disease is a serious microvascular complication of diabetes, and is the leading cause of blindness in the under-60 age group in the developed world. Background retinopathy is asymptomatic and is usually detected during the screening of diabetic patients. The pathological processes leading to retinopathy relate to increased retinal arterial blood flow secondary to hyperglycaemia, which results in the formation of microaneurysms, increased capillary permeability and retinal ischaemia. The pathognomonic changes of background retinopathy are blot haemorrhages, capillary microaneurysms (dots) and hard exudates, which appear as yellow plaques and contain lipid deposits. If a patient is shown to have background retinopathy, they must receive annual fundoscopy or diabetic photography to assess disease progression. If there is concern that disease is progressing, the patient should be reviewed again after 3 months. Each patient must undergo a holistic review of their glycaemic control, blood pressure, lipid profile and lifestyle. If the glycaemic control, hypertension and hyperlipidaemia are not corrected, the background retinopathy can progress to pre-proliferative and proliferative retinopathy, which is associated with a significant risk of blindness, vitreous haemorrhage and retinal detachment.

2. F – Macular oedema

Diabetic maculopathy is most commonly seen in older patients with type 2 diabetes and is the leading cause of blindness in this group. Macular oedema cannot be seen on fundoscopy, but must always be suspected if the patient complains of deteriorating vision or if there is objective evidence of deteriorating visual acuity (i.e. using a Snellen chart). In addition to macular oedema, the macula can be affected by retinopathy, including the presence of haemorrhages, exudates and neovascularization. If maculopathy is suspected, the patient should be referred to an ophthalmologist for assessment and possible retinal photocoagulation therapy.

Hermann Snellen, Dutch ophthalmologist (1834–1908).

3. I – Retinal detachment

Retinal detachment occurs when the outer pigment epithelium detaches from the inner retina, which contains the neurons. In patients with proliferative retinopathy, the retina detaches as a result of traction caused by the formation and deposition of fibrous bands. Patients complain of visual floaters, reduced visual acuity and visual field loss (often described as a curtain passing across their visual field). If the macula becomes detached, which usually occurs when the upper half of the retina detaches, the patient will suffer permanent damage to their central vision. On fundoscopy, the retina often appears grey and lifeless and bulges forward. If retinal detachment is suspected, the patient should be referred for urgent ophthalmological review.

4. G – Pre-proliferative retinopathy

Pre-proliferative retinopathy represents disease progression from background retinopathy. In addition to blot haemorrhages, capillary microaneurysms and hard exudates, there is evidence of retinal ischaemia in the form of soft exudates (cotton-wool spots) and venous bleeding. Soft exudates are seen as whitish-grey indistinct lesions on the retina. Pre-proliferative retinopathy requires a non-urgent referral to an ophthalmologist and a review of diabetic control and management.

5. H – Proliferative retinopathy

This patient has new vessel formation (neovascularization) in the retina, which is pathognomonic of proliferative retinopathy. This is a serious condition, and requires urgent referral to an ophthalmologist. Fundoscopy demonstrates new vessel formation, blot haemorrhages, capillary microaneurysms (dots), hard exudates and soft exudates. The new vessels are thin-walled, tortuous and prone to rupture (resulting in retinal and vitreous haemorrhage). The treatment of proliferative retinopathy is with retinal photocoagulation therapy, which has been shown to reduce the progression to blindness, especially in patients with disc involvement.

Theme 3: Complications of acute myocardial infarction

1. B – Acute mitral valve regurgitation

Acute mitral regurgitation is usually seen 2–10 days after an inferior myocardial infarction (MI) and is often fatal. It is usually secondary to rupture of a papillary muscle or the chordae tendineae. It presents with symptoms and signs of acute left ventricular failure, including shortness of breath and the production of pink frothy sputum. On auscultation, there is a loud pansystolic murmur best herd at the apex that radiates into the axilla. The patient is usually haemodynamically compromised, with severe hypotension, low oxygen saturation and poor urine output. If the patient survives the initial period, a surgical opinion should be sought regarding possible repair/valve replacement.

2. H – Dressler's syndrome

Dressler's syndrome is usually seen 2–10 weeks after an MI. It is characterized by the triad of pericarditis, fever and pericaridal effusion. Features include central stabbing chest pain that is worse on inspiration and lying flat, fever, and lethargy. In the more serious cases, the patient may develop pericardial and pleural effusions. Examination is often unremarkable, although a pericardial rub is sometimes heard. Dressler's syndrome is thought to be an autoimmune condition secondary to the generation of new myocardial antigens after an MI. Patients often have a raised erythrocyte sedimentation rate (ESR) secondary to the inflammatory process. The condition usually settles with simple non-steroidal anti-inflammatory drugs (NSAIDs) and analgesia, although steroids are sometimes required.

Lucas Anton Dressler, German physician (1815–96).

3. G – Complete (third-degree) heart block

MI may damage the conduction system of the heart, with the result that atrial depolarization is unable to propagate to the atrioventricular node and down the bundle of His. Since the ventricles are unable to depolarize via the normal route, they enter an escape pacemaker rhythm with a rate of approximately 40 beats/min. On the ECG, there are both P-waves and QRS complexes, but no association between the two. Complete heart block following MI usually requires intravenous atropine and emergency pacing, followed by the insertion of a permanent pacemaker when the patient is haemodynamically stable. The exception is when complete heart block follows inferior MI, as the block is often transient.

4. F – Cardiac tamponade

In cardiac tamponade, there is rapid accumulation of fluid within the pericardial space, which compresses the heart, causing pump failure and cardiogenic shock. The patient is usually hypotensive, with distended neck veins and quiet heart sounds – features described by Beck's triad (not to be confused with Beck's cognitive triad: negative view of oneself, negative interpretation of past experiences and negative expectation of the future). Cardiac tamponade can be confirmed by echocardiography, but the rapidly fatal cardiogenic shock usually necessitates a clinical diagnosis and immediate treatment with pericardial aspiration by pericardiocentesis.

Claude Schaeffer Beck, American cardiac surgeon (1894–1971).

Aaron Temkin Beck, American psychiatrist (b1921).

5. J – Subacute left ventricular failure

Chronic left ventricular failure may be seen following MI due to irreversible damage of the myocardium, which compromises the heart's pumping mechanism. The symptoms of chronic left ventricular failure include shortness of breath, cough, reduced exercise tolerance, orthopnoea and paroxysmal nocturnal dyspnoea. Left ventricular failure is usually investigated using echocardiography. Management options include lifestyle changes, angiotensin-converting enzyme (ACE) inhibitors, β-blockers and diuretics.

Theme 4: Cutaneous lesions 2

1. D – Granuloma annulare

Granuloma annulare is a condition characterized by small reddish papules arranged in a ring. It usually occurs on the backs of the hands or feet, and is often associated with diabetes mellitus. Granuloma annulare is usually asymptomatic, and lesions fade after a year. Although its aetiology is unknown, it is thought to be due to a T-cell-mediated reaction.

Annulare, from Latin *anus* = ring.

2. H – Neurofibroma

Neurofibromas are benign neoplasms of the nerve sheaths of central or peripheral nerves that feel firm and rubbery. Neurofibromas may be single or multiple, as in neurofibromatosis (NF). NF is an autosomal dominant disorder characterized by multiple neurofibromas, coffee-coloured macules (café-au-lait patches) and axillary freckling, with a risk of developing CNS tumours (acoustic neuroma, optic glioma or meningioma), iris fibromas (Lisch nodules) and phaeochromocytomas. There are two types of NF: NF1 (von Recklinghausen's disease) is the 'peripheral' form, displaying the cutaneous manifestations; and NF2 is the 'central' form, with bilateral CNS tumours and very few cutaneous features.

Freidrich von Recklinghausen, German pathologist (1833–1910).

3. A– Cellulitis

The features of erythema, swelling, local pain and blistering of an area of skin in the pyrexial, unwell patient suggest a diagnosis of cellulitis. Cellulitis is an infection of the subcutaneous tissues that is most commonly caused by *Streptococcus pyogenes*. Treatment is by broad-spectrum intravenous antibiotics, such as flucloxacillin and benzylpenicillin.

4. I – Pyogenic granuloma

A pyogenic granuloma is an acquired haemangioma (note that it is neither pyogenic nor a granuloma!) that occurs most often on the head, trunk, hands and feet. It develops at a site of trauma (e.g. a thorn prick) as a bright-red nodule that bleeds easily and enlarges rapidly over 2–3 weeks. It affects the young and old extremes of age, but is most common in pregnant women. These lesions are benign and are managed by excision, although smaller lesions may resolve spontaneously.

5. F – Kaposi's sarcoma

Kaposi's sarcoma is a malignant tumour of vascular endothelium that gives rise to plaques and nodules in the skin and mucous membranes that have a bruise-like appearance. It is associated with underlying infection by human herpesvirus-8 (HHV-8 – also known as Kaposi's sarcoma-associated herpesvirus, KSHV) in people who are immunosuppressed (such as those with AIDS or patients on immunosuppressants following organ transplantation). Before the advent of AIDS, Kaposi's sarcoma was a rare sporadic tumour that occurred in Italian males and Ashkenazi Jews. Biopsy of the lesions is required to confirm diagnosis and symptomatic treatment is with radiotherapy.

Moriz Kohn Kaposi, Hungarian dermatologist (1837–1902).

Theme 5: Dizziness

Vertigo is defined as the subjective sensation of movement (usually rotary), often accompanied by pallor, sweating, nausea and vomiting. The objective sign of vertigo is nystagmus. In nystagmus, the eye drifts off target and performs recurrent corrections to return fixation to an object. The drifts are slower than the corrections, and the direction of the fast phase is defined as the direction of nystagmus. Although nystagmus can be physiological (e.g. after spinning – known as optokinetic nystagmus), pathological nystagmus is seen in disorders of the vestibular system (peripheral) or the cerebellum/brain stem (central). Peripheral lesions cause nystagmus away from the affected side of the lesion. The nystagmus of peripheral lesions is transient and always accompanied by vertigo. Central lesions cause nystagmus towards the side of the lesion that is persistent and not accompanied by vertigo.

Nystagmus, from Greek *nystagmus* = to nod.

1. E – Ménière's disease

In Ménière's disease, there is distension of the membranous labyrinth by accumulation of endolymph. It is most common between 40 and 60 years, and a quarter of cases are bilateral. Patients present with intermittent rotational vertigo that lasts a few hours, with tinnitus and distorted hearing. Attacks may be precipitated by a feeling of fullness in the ear. Patients develop progressive sensorineural deafness that is apparent on examination and can become severe. Attacks of Ménière's disease are treated with antiemetics. Salt and water restriction may reduce the frequency of relapses. In patients with unilateral symptoms who already have developed a severe hearing impairment, labyrinthectomy can be performed.

Prosper Ménière, French physician (1799–1862).

Tinnitus, from Latin *tinnire* = to ring.

2. A – Benign paroxysmal positional vertigo

Benign paroxysmal positional vertigo (BPPV) occurs secondary to degeneration of the utricular neuroepithelium in the semicircular canals. This may be spontaneous or occur after head injury. The degenerate material affects the free flow of endolymph in the labyrinth. Attacks of vertigo are precipitated by turning the head so that the affected ear is undermost (the vertigo appears after a latent period and is brief). Affected patients become reluctant to move their heads. Diagnosis of BPPV is by the Hallpike test: the patient is sat upright with the legs extended, the head is rotated 45°, then the patient is made to lie down quickly and the head held in extension. The patient's eyes are then observed. A positive test will result in nystagmus towards the affected side after a 5–10 s latent period.

Steady resolution usually occurs within weeks, but the Epley manoeuvre effectively treats most cases. In this manoeuvre, the patient sits upright with legs extended, and their head is rotated towards the affected side. With the head still turned, the patient is laid flat past the horizontal (as in the Hallpike test). This position is held for 30 s. The patient's head is then turned to the opposite side in the reclined position (and held for 30 s). The patient is now rolled onto their side (the side opposite to the affected ear) with the head still turned for 30 s. They are then sat upright, still with the head turned, to the opposite side of the lesion (for 30 s). Finally, the head is turned back to the midline with the neck flexed 45° (for 30 s).

Charles Skinner Hallpike, English otologist (1900–79).

3. B – Drug-induced ototoxicity

Certain drugs are ototoxic and can result in a variety of symptoms, including dizziness, tinnitus, sensorineural deafness and loss of balance. Drugs that are ototoxic include gentamicin, streptomycin, quinine and high doses of aspirin.

4. G – Ramsay Hunt syndrome

Ramsay Hunt syndrome is caused by herpes zoster infection of the geniculate ganglion, affecting the facial nerve and sometimes the vestibulocochlear nerve, which is in close proximity. Features include paralysis of the facial muscles on the affected side, with a herpetic eruption on the ear canal. Patients may also suffer with tinnitus, hearing loss and vertigo. Oral aciclovir improves the prognosis and reduces the risk of post-herpetic neuralgia.

James Ramsay Hunt, American neurologist (1872–1937).

5. D – Labyrinthitis

Labyrinthitis (also known as vestibular neuronitis) is the most common cause of vertigo, and may be viral in origin. Patients present with explosive severe vertigo, vomiting and ataxia (without tinnitus and deafness). Symptoms settle down over a few days. Management is with antiemetics, often prochlorperazine.

Theme 6: Diagnosis of joint pain 2

1. D – Gout

Gout occurs secondary to the deposition of uric acid crystals in the joint. It is most common in older, obese male drinkers with hypertension, ischaemic heart disease and diabetes. Other risk factors include cytotoxic drugs, diuretic use and Lesch–Nyhan syndrome (gout + learning difficulties + self-mutilating behaviour). Acute episodes of gout can be precipitated by trauma, illness, stress and thiazide diuretics. Acute gout usually presents with sudden pain, swelling and redness in the first metatarsophalangeal joint, although 25% of cases occur in the knee. Diagnosis is by joint aspiration, which shows negatively birefringent needle-shaped crystals. Acute gout is treated with NSAIDs (e.g. indometacin and diclofenac). Prophylaxis is with allopurinol, a xanthine oxidase inhibitor that slows the production of uric acid. This is offered to patients who have recurrent or chronic gout, who are using cytotoxic therapy, or who have Lesch–Nyhan syndrome. Allopurinol should not be prescribed within 1 month of an attack of gout, as it may precipitate a further attack. In patients allergic to allopurinol, probenecid is used as prophylaxis.

Other forms of gout are chronic tophaceous gout (the accumulation of urate in cartilage – often the ear and Achilles' tendon) and gout nephropathy (urate deposition in the kidneys resulting in acute renal failure and the formation of urate stones).

Gout, from Latin *gutta* = a drop. The ancient physician Galen thought that gout was caused by a small drop of the four humours in unbalanced proportions leaking into the joint space. The four humours – black bile, yellow bile, phlegm and blood – were thought to be the four basic substances of the human body, disturbances of which resulted in disease.

2. A – Ankylosing spondylitis

Ankylosing spondylitis (AS) is an inflammatory disorder of the back that is more common in males. Patients present with insidious-onset lower back pain and stiffness that is worse in the morning and gets better with exercise. There is poor spinal flexion, and in severe cases patients develop a rigid lower spine with a hunch (known as the 'question mark posture' or 'hang dog posture'). AS may also affect the large joints asymmetrically. AS is associated with a number of extra-articular features, which are remembered by the 'five As': **A**pical lung fibrosis, **A**nterior uveitis, **A**chilles' tendonitis/plantar fasciitis, **A**ortic regurgitation and **A**myloidosis.

This diagnosis of AS is made using Schober's test: two fingers are placed 10 cm apart on the lower back of the patient (5 cm above and below the L5 vertebra in the midline), and the patient is asked to flex. An increase between the fingers of <5 cm indicates spinal stiffness. X-ray of the hip shows blurred margins of the sacroiliac joints (sacroiliitis). Characteristic radiological features of the spine in AS include erosion of the corners of the vertebral bodies (Romanus lesions), the development of bony spurs (syndesmophytes) and calcification of the spinal ligaments (bamboo spine). Treatment options in AS are physiotherapy, exercise and slow-release NSAIDs, e.g. indometacin. Most patients manage to lead a normal life, although severe cases may impair ventilation.

AS is an example of a seronegative spondyloarthropathy, i.e. a disease associated with HLA-B27 that is characterized by a lack of rheumatoid factor (hence 'seronegative'). Other spondyloarthropathies are psoriatic arthritis, Reiter's disease and enteropathic arthritis.

Ankylosing spondylitis, from Greek *ankylos* = bent + *spondylos* = vertebra.

3. B – Enteropathic arthritis

Enteropathic arthritis is an asymmetrical oligoarthritis predominantly affecting the larger joints of the lower limb. It occurs with underlying inflammatory bowel disease. It is difficult to distinguish between ulcerative colitis (UC) and Crohn's disease from the history, although UC is more commonly associated with bloody stools. Other extraintestinal features of inflammatory bowel disease include clubbing, erythema nodosum (painful lesions on the lower legs), anterior uveitis (inflammation of the anterior eye causing acute pain, photophobia and blurring), ankylosing spondylitis, hepatobiliary disease (primary biliary cirrhosis), pyoderma gangrenosum (deep, necrotic ulcers with a dark red border usually occurring on the leg) and perianal disease (skin tags, fissures, fistulae). Management of enteropathic arthritis is by treating the underlying bowel disease.

4. I – Rheumatoid arthritis

This woman has rheumatoid arthritis, as characterized by symmetrical arthritis of the small joints of the hands that is worse in the morning. For more information on rheumatoid arthritis, see 'Features of rheumatoid arthritis' (Paper 8 Answers, Theme 7).

5. K – Still's disease

Juvenile idiopathic arthritis (JIA) was previously referred to as juvenile chronic arthritis or juvenile rheumatoid arthritis. JIA is defined as joint inflammation persisting for 6 weeks or more, with initial onset in a person under 16 years of age, in the absence of another specific cause. Diagnosis is clinical and relies on ruling out other causes of arthritis. JIA is classified according to the number of joints affected:

- monoarticular: single joint
- pauciarticular: ≤4 joints
- polyarticular: >4 joints.

Pauciarticular JIA usually occurs in younger children, affecting the knees, ankles and wrists most commonly. Polyarticular JIA is more common in girls of all ages, usually symmetrically involving the hands and wrists. Complications of JIA include chronic anterior uveitis, flexion contraction of the joints and amyloidosis. Management options include physiotherapy, simple analgesia (NSAIDs), intra-articular steroid injections and disease-modifying antirheumatic drugs (e.g. methotrexate and ciclosporin).

Still's disease is a systemic form of juvenile arthritis that is thought to be an autoimmune disorder. It usually begins at the age of 3–4 years and is more common in girls. Features of Still's disease include intermittent high pyrexia and a salmon-pink rash, with aches and pains of the joints and muscles. Other features are hepatosplenomegaly, lymphadenopathy and pericarditis. Inflammatory markers such as C-reactive protein are raised; however, antinuclear antibody and rheumatoid factor are usually negative. Management options include physiotherapy, resting splints, NSAIDs, disease-modifying drugs (e.g. methotrexate and ciclosporin) and steroids. The younger the age of onset of Still's disease, the worse the prognosis.

Sir George Freidrich Still, English physician (1861–1941).

Theme 7: Complications of drug therapy

1. G – Oculogyric crisis

Oculogyric crisis is a dystonic reaction that is often associated with drugs such as metoclopramide, neuroleptic agents and tricyclic antidepressants. It is most commonly seen in young females, who present with restlessness, agitation and confusion preceding the development of a fixed upward deviation of the eyes. The patient may also develop a fixed flexion deformity of the neck (spasmodic torticollis) in association with an opened mouth and protruding tongue. Treatment requires withdrawal of the offending drug. In severe or prolonged cases, an antimuscarinic agent (e.g. procyclidine) with or without a benzodiazepine is indicated.

2. H – Reye's syndrome

Reye's syndrome is associated with aspirin use in children, and causes fatty infiltration of the liver and severe encephalopathy. Children can initially present with a mild illness, but often progress to coma. Treatment is directed at managing complications such as raised intracranial pressure and hypoglycaemia. This condition is fatal in up to 40% of cases. For this reason, aspirin should never be given to children.

Douglas Reye, Australian pathologist (1912–78).

3. E – Nausea and vomiting

Morphine has a number of adverse effects that can limit its use and effectiveness. One of the most feared adverse affects of opiate use is nausea and vomiting, which can cause distress and, if severe, can lead to dehydration and electrolyte imbalance. It is therefore important to identify this complication early on and manage it appropriately. Early use of antiemetics may prevent the onset of nausea and vomiting and improve the patient's quality of life. Other complications of opiate therapy include pruritis, constipation and respiratory depression.

4. I – Vomiting after alcohol

Metronidazole is an antibiotic used to treat infections caused by anaerobic pathogens (e.g. *Clostridium difficile*). Patients should be warned not to consume alcohol while taking metronidazole, as it inhibits the enzyme aldehyde dehydrogenase, resulting in facial flushing, tachycardia and vomiting on consumption of alcohol.

5. B – Bronchospasm

Propranolol is a non-selective β-blocker that is commonly used to treat hypertension, anxiety, arrhythmia, heart failure and oesophageal varices. β-blockers inhibit the actions of catecholamines at the β_1-adrenergic receptors within the heart, producing a negative inotropic and chronotropic effect (i.e. they reduce the force and speed of contraction). They also block peripheral β_2-receptors in the vascular smooth muscle and bronchioles, causing peripheral vasodilatation and bronchoconstriction respectively. β-Blockers, especially non-selective agents such as propranolol, are contraindicated in people with asthma, as they may precipitate a life-threatening exacerbation of asthma. As an alternative, selective β_1-blockers (e.g. atenolol) have been developed that have minimal affects on the bronchiole β_2-receptors and are therefore less likely to cause bronchospasm. They may be safer in asthma compared with non-selective agents, but should still be avoided in patients with severe or brittle asthma.

Theme 8: Interpretation of liver function tests

Alkaline phosphatase is an enzyme found in the bile duct. Alkaline phosphatase levels that are raised three times above the normal limit are strongly indicative of biliary tract disease. A raised serum bilirubin is seen in hepatic and post-hepatic disease. Jaundice is defined as an elevation of serum bilirubin. Alanine transaminase (ALT) and aspartate transaminase (AST) – also known as alanine aminotransferase and aspartate aminotransferase – are enzymes of the liver, and levels above ten times the normal limit are strongly suggestive of hepatocellular disease.

Jaundice, from Latin *galbinus* = yellowish-green.

1. C – Gilbert's syndrome

Gilbert's syndrome is an autosomal dominant partial deficiency in glucuronosyltransferase, the enzyme that is required to conjugate bilirubin. People with this condition have a mildly raised, non-haemolytic, unconjugated hyperbilirubinaemia, especially when they are acutely unwell. The rest of the liver function tests are unaffected. This condition requires no treatment. Another congenital cause of hyperbilirubinaemia is Crigler–Najjar syndrome, an autosomal recessive total deficiency in glucuronosyltransferase resulting in unconjugated jaundice. This condition causes severe brain damage in the early years of life. Dubin–Johnson and Rotor's syndromes both result in impaired excretion of bile with a consequent conjugated hyperbilirubinaemia.

Nicholas Augustin Gilbert, French physician (1858–1927).

2. B – Biliary tract obstruction

This patient gives a history of biliary colic, which is caused by the contraction of the gallbladder against a blocked cystic duct or common bile duct and is usually secondary to gallstones. It commonly presents with a history of intermittent right upper quadrant pain that is exacerbated by fatty foods. Liver function tests in patients with uncomplicated biliary colic are often normal. If the common bile duct becomes occluded, conjugated bilirubin spills into the circulation and the damaged biliary canaliculi release alkaline phosphatase. Patients with biliary tract obstruction secondary to hepatocellular disease may also have raised AST, ALT and γ-GT (see below) levels.

3. H – Short-term alcohol abuse

γ-Glutamyltranspeptidase (γ-GT) is a liver enzyme that rises with hepatocellular damage. It is an extremely sensitive marker of liver disease, but has very poor specificity, i.e. it is often raised in well patients following alcohol intake. Its lack of specificity and inability to differentiate between diseases makes γ-GT a controversial test. γ-GT does have a role in differentiating the aetiology of a raised alkaline phosphatase level. Alkaline phosphatase is an enzyme that is found in a number of tissues throughout the body (biliary tract, bone and placenta). Therefore, if a patient is shown to have a raised alkaline phosphatase level in association with a raised γ-GT, it is likely that the liver is the source. Alternatively, if the γ-GT is within normal limits, the patient should be investigated for bone disease such as Paget's disease. In this case, the history of alcohol intake in association with a raised γ-GT and normal liver function tests indicates that the patient has consumed too much alcohol. The most appropriate action in this case would be to advise the patient to drink in moderation and to repeat the test in several weeks' time.

4. F – Hepatocellular inflammation

The history of jaundice and globally deranged liver function tests suggests hepatocellular disease. ALT is found mainly in the hepatocytes. When the hepatocytes are damaged by conditions such as alcoholic liver disease and viral hepatitis, ALT is released into the circulation. AST is similar to ALT, with the exception that it is also found in a number of other tissues, such as erythrocytes and the myocardium. AST can therefore also be raised in a number of other disease processes, such as haemolysis and myocardial infarction. The presence of significant hepatocellular disease can disrupt the liver parenchyma, causing obstruction of the biliary canaliculi and release of alkaline phosphatase into the circulation. An elevated alkaline phosphatase can therefore occur in biliary obstruction, hepatocellular disease and non-hepatic disease.

5. D – Haemolytic anaemia

In haemolytic anaemia, the excessive production of bilirubin caused by the destruction of erythrocytes surpasses the liver's ability to conjugate, resulting in large amounts of insoluble unconjugated bilirubin entering the circulation. Because unconjugated bilirubin is not water soluble, it does not enter the urine, and therefore causes acholuric jaundice (jaundice in association with normal coloured urine). Unconjugated bilirubin has a greater lipid solubility compared with conjugated bilirubin and, in hyperbilirubinaemic states, is more likely than conjugated bilirubin to cross the blood–brain barrier and cause encephalopathy. Lactate dehydrogenase (LDH) and AST are found in many tissues throughout the body, including the liver, myocardium and erythrocytes. Haemolysis thus results in the release of large amounts of LDH and AST into the serum. Other useful tests in the investigation of haemolysis include a full blood count, blood film analysis, Coombs' test and urinary urobilinogen levels, which are often raised.

Theme 9: Diagnosis of respiratory conditions 2

1. D – Chronic obstructive pulmonary disease

This man has an acute exacerbation of chronic obstructive pulmonary disease (COPD), as evidenced by a decreasing exercise tolerance, increased sputum production and increased sputum purulence. COPD is a chronic progressive disorder characterized by airflow obstruction. The obstruction may be partially (but not completely) reversible with bronchodilators. COPD encompasses bronchitis and emphysema. Chronic bronchitis is defined as cough with sputum for most days of a 3-month period on 2 consecutive years. Emphysema is a pathological diagnosis of permanent destructive enlargement of the alveoli. Smoking is the main risk factor, and 15% of smokers develop COPD. The pathology includes hypertrophy of the goblet cells and decreased cilia with loss of alveoli elastic recoil. The persistent hypoxaemia seen in COPD results in pulmonary vascular hypertension, which leads to cor pulmonale. Features of COPD include a productive cough (worse in the mornings), recurrent respiratory tract infections, exertional dyspnoea, expiratory wheeze and bibasal crepitations. Examination may also reveal tracheal tug, intercostal in-drawing, a barrel chest (increased anterior–posterior diameter), pursed lips, central cyanosis, carbon dioxide retention (flapping tremor, bounding pulse and warm peripheries) and right heart failure.

COPD is diagnosed by demonstrating a forced expiratory volume in 1 s (FEV_1) of <80% and an FEV_1/VC (vital capacity) ratio of <70% with little variation in peak flow. The lung capacity and residual volume are increased. Arterial blood gases typically show hypoxia and hypercapnia. A chest X-ray shows hypertranslucent lung fields, a flat diaphragm, bullae and prominent hila. Management options include stopping smoking, antibiotics for infections, regular anticholinergics (ipratropium) and a salbutamol inhaler as required. Smoking cessation can be helped by bupropion, which is prescribed 2 weeks before stopping. Long-term oxygen therapy (LTOT) of 1–4 L/min via nasal cannulae is given for patients with severe COPD who have given up smoking and who have a Po_2 <7.3 kPa and FEV_1 <1.5 L. Acute exacerbations of COPD are diagnosed when patients complain of worsening exercise tolerance, increasing sputum volume and increasing sputum purulence. Acute exacerbations of COPD are treated with 24–28% oxygen, nebulized salbutamol, oral prednisolone and prophylactic low-molecular-weight heparin. If CO_2 is rising or the patient is acidotic despite adequate oxygen therapy, consider ventilator support.

2. I – Open non-tension pneumothorax

A pneumothorax is air in the pleural space. It can occur with trauma or after rupture of a bulla. Spontaneous pneumothoraces are more common in young males who are tall and thin. Clinical features of spontaneous pneumothorax are sudden-onset unilateral chest pain and dyspnoea. Examination findings include reduced chest wall movements, hyper-resonance and reduced breath sounds on the affected side.

This man has a chest wound that is resulting in an open pneumothorax, as suggested by the respiratory distress, reduced breath sounds and hyper-resonance to percussion. The undisplaced trachea means that the pneumothorax is not under tension. Management of an open pneumothorax is initially by occluding the wound with a sterile dressing and taping down three sides only. The resulting 'flutter valve' allows air to leave the chest on expiration but prevents it being sucked into the chest on inspiration. Subsequent management is by chest drain insertion at a different site. Because air can flow freely between the lungs and the pleura in the open pneumothorax, infection is common. A closed pneumothorax occurs when the communication between the lungs and pleura is closed. The pleural air reabsorbs spontaneously within a few days and infection is uncommon. A chest X-ray in pneumothorax shows a deflated lung with a defined edge.

3. K – Pneumonia

Pneumonia is an acute respiratory illness with recent radiological pulmonary shadowing. A chest infection without chest X-ray changes is known as a lower respiratory tract infection. Community-acquired pneumonias are spread by droplet inhalation, and present with cough, fever and pleuritic chest pain. Cough is initially dry, but later becomes productive and may be blood stained. Examination reveals bronchial breath sounds in the affected area (due to consolidation) and coarse crepitations. Severity of pneumonia is assessed using the CURB-65 score – for details, see 'Scoring the severity of pneumonia' (Paper 10, Theme 8).

The most common pathogens involved in community-acquired pneumonia are *Streptococcus pneumoniae* (30%), *Mycoplasma pneumoniae*, *Staphylococcus aureus* and *Chlamydophila pneumoniae* (previously known as *Chlamydia pneumoniae*). The resulting infection may be lobar pneumonia (homogeneous consolidation of one or more lobes) or bronchopneumonia (patchy alveolar consolidation that commonly affects both lower lobes). Investigations include chest X-ray and sputum culture. Treatment is with relevant antibiotics. Empirical regimens include oral amoxicillin for uncomplicated cases and intravenous clarithromycin plus co-amoxiclav for severe disease. Seven to ten days of treatment is normally sufficient.

Pneumonia, from Greek *pneuma* = breath.

4. L – Pulmonary embolism

Pulmonary embolism (PE) is a blood clot in the lung vasculature. Most PEs (75%) derive from a deep vein thrombosis. Features include acute-onset pleuritic chest pain and shortness of breath, often with fever and tachycardia. The chest X-ray may show a wedge-shaped opacity due to consolidation associated with pulmonary infarction (Hampton's hump). The Westermark sign is a focus of oligaemia on X-ray distal to an occluded blood vessel. The ECG most commonly demonstrates a sinus tachycardia, although the S1Q3T3 pattern is characteristic (S-wave in lead I, Q-wave and inverted T-wave in lead III). An arterial blood gas reveals type I respiratory failure (normal pH, low Po_2). D-dimers are a breakdown product of clots: a low D-dimer can be used to exclude a PE, but a high level does not confirm it. The next investigation in PE depends on the chest X-ray: if the chest X-ray is clear, a ventilation–perfusion ($\dot{V}/\dot{Q}$) scan is performed to look for areas that are getting air but not blood. If the chest X-ray is not clear, or if a $\dot{V}/\dot{Q}$ scan is inconclusive, a spiral CT (CT pulmonary angiography) is the best investigation. Patients with a confirmed PE are started on heparin or low-molecular-weight heparin and then warfarinized for 6 months (aiming for an INR between 2 and 3). Patients who have suffered a massive PE need urgent thrombolysis.

5. N – Tension pneumothorax

This woman has the typical features of a tension pneumothorax: unilaterally decreased breath sounds, hyper-resonance to percussion, respiratory distress and tracheal deviation away from the affected side. A raised jugular venous pressure (JVP) may also be seen. If a tension pneumothorax is suspected then management should be immediate, without ordering a chest X-ray. A large-bore cannula is inserted in the second intercostal space in the midclavicular line. This is later followed by formal chest drain insertion into the fourth/fifth intercostal space, mid-axillary line.

Theme 10: Renal investigations

1. G – Midstream urine sample for microscopy, culture and sensitivity

This woman gives a typical history of cystitis. Common features of cystitis include dysuria, frequency, hesitancy, suprapubic discomfort, fever, and the production of dark and offensive urine. The first-line investigation of a suspected urinary tract infection (UTI) is urine dipstick analysis. A urine dipstick can be considered positive if it shows the presence of nitrites and leucocyte esterase. In addition, patients with a UTI may also have protein and blood in their urine. Urine dipstick analysis is not 100% accurate; for example, a significant proportion of elderly patients have nitrites and protein in their urine without infection. If the history and urine dipstick analysis suggest a UTI, it is usual to prescribe a relatively broad-spectrum antibiotic such as trimethoprim or cefradine. A midstream sample of urine should be sent for microscopy, culture and sensitivity prior to commencing antibiotics. Once the sensitivity of the organism is known, the antibiotic therapy can be adjusted. It is important that a *midstream* sample be sent, in order to reduce the risk of genital and distal urethral organisms and debris contaminating the sample.

2. E – Kidney–ureter–bladder X-ray

This patient is likely to be suffering from renal colic, which is usually caused by the presence of a calculus or calculi obstructing the ureter. Renal colic presents with severe loin pain that radiates to the groin and causes the patient to writhe around in agony. Patients may also suffer from vomiting, pallor, sweating, pyrexia and haematuria. The early investigation of renal colic involves urine dipstick analysis, full blood count, urea and electrolytes, and a kidney–ureter–bladder (KUB) X-ray. Approximately 90% of calculi are radio-opaque (i.e. visible on X-ray), and are often seen in the renal pelvis, at the pelviureteric junction or where the ureter enters the bladder. Some renal calculi (urate and xanthine stones) are radio-translucent and cannot be seen on X-ray. KUB is usually the quickest and easiest investigation to organize. Other investigations that may be indicated include the intravenous urogram, CT urogram and renal tract ultrasound. Initial treatment is supportive with analgesia and fluid resuscitation. Diclofenac, a strong non-steroidal anti-inflammatory drug, is particularly effective in the treatment of renal colic. If it is thought that the stone will not pass spontaneously, or there is evidence of hydronephrosis, a surgical opinion should be sought. Treatment options include extracorporeal shock wave lithotripsy, cystoscopy/ureteroscopy and percutaneous nephrolithotomy. Occasionally, open surgery is required for very large stones.

3. I – Renal biopsy

Deteriorating renal function in a patient with a transplanted kidney should always be taken seriously, as there is a possibility of organ rejection. Other causes include vessel thrombosis, infection and recurrence of existing disease, e.g. immunoglobulin A (IgA) nephropathy. A percutaneous renal biopsy will reveal the presence, aetiology and severity of any rejection process. Acute rejection is usually treated with pulsed steroid therapy (methylprednisolone). In severe episodes of rejection, antithymocyte globulin, which destroys T lymphocytes, can be given to slow the rejection process. Chronic rejection is often due to the fibrosis of the microcirculation within the graft and is usually irreversible. Chronic rejection usually means that the patient is re-listed for transplantation.

4. J – Renal tract ultrasound scan

A UTI in children usually presents with generalized symptoms such as fever, poor feeding, vomiting, lethargy and abdominal pain. Important causes of a UTI in children include vesicoureteric reflux, urinary tract obstruction, duplex ureters, constipation and sexual abuse. In this scenario, it likely that the child has vesicoureteric reflux, which causes urine to enter the ureters and renal pelvis during micturition. Vesicoureteric reflux usually presents in childhood with recurrent UTIs and failure to thrive, and can lead to renal scaring and renal failure. It is important to identify any anatomical or physiological abnormality that predisposes to the development of infection, and all children should have a renal tract ultrasound following a UTI. An urgent renal tract ultrasound scan should be performed if there is a history of recurrent UTI or if there are atypical features, e.g. non-coliform organisms, systemic illness and failure to respond to treatment. Following ultrasound, the next investigation is usually a *DMSA scan*, which highlights areas of renal scarring using a radioisotope-labelled compound (technetium-99m-labelled dimercaptosuccinic acid). If the ultrasound scan shows evidence of hydronephrosis, or if there is a family history of vesicoureteric reflux, a *micturating cystourethrogram* should be performed to confirm reflux.

5. K – Three early morning urine samples for microscopy, culture and Ziehl–Neelsen staining

Renal tuberculosis (TB) is a cause of sterile pyuria, i.e. the presence of leucocytes in association with a negative culture. It is usually seen in patients from the Asian subcontinent. The features of renal TB are non-specific and may mimic a simple UTI. In this case, the patient has some of the features of general TB, including lethargy, weight loss and night sweats. A positive Mantoux test would strongly indicate TB infection. To confirm the diagnosis of renal TB, three early morning samples of urine are taken for microscopy and Ziehl–Neelsen staining for acid-fast bacilli. Treatment is the same as for pulmonary TB.

The Ziehl–Neelsen stain identifies acid-fast mycobacteria, such as *Mycobacterium tuberculosis*.

Franz Ziehl, German bacteriologist (1857–1926).

Friedrich Neelsen, German pathologist (1854–94).

Theme 11: Study design

1. C – Case series

A case series is an in-depth descriptive report of observed clinical features and findings in a limited series of patients with a similar condition – in other words, a group of *case reports*. Case series are often published with respect to unusual conditions to help others recognize patterns in presentation, treatment or outcomes. A famous example is the case series reporting phocomelia (short limbs) in babies born to mothers who took thalidomide during pregnancy.

2. H – Systematic review

A systematic literature review aims to summarize all the available literature on a certain topic using a rigorous methodology. For example, if you wanted to look at the association between abdominal aortic aneurysms and diabetes, you would start by searching for all papers on article databases (e.g. PubMed) using relevant key words and gradually filter out non-relevant studies using a set of exclusion criteria (e.g. 'did not report prevalence data'). A *non-systematic review* would not use such a methodology.

3. D – Cohort study

A cohort study is a longitudinal analytical study where individuals with one or more common factors are observed and subsequent outcomes recorded. They are used to test associations between exposures and adverse health effects. Cohort studies can involve a control group. An example of a cohort study is a follow-up of women who use, and do not use, the oral contraceptive pill in order to compare the risk of venous thromboembolism.

Case–control studies start with individuals who already have the disease in question and a comparison control group. The observer then records retrospectively and compares the history of risk factors, exposure and other characteristics between the two groups. An example of a case–control study is a comparison of smoking histories between people with and people without lung cancer.

4. G – Randomized controlled trial

A randomized controlled trial (RCT) is a prospective, longitudinal study that uses randomly selected groups (including a control arm) designed to compare the role of 'intervention' against 'no intervention' or the current gold standard. Because they are randomized, controlled and prospective, thus reducing bias, RCTs are widely seen as the best way to perform interventional studies and provide the best evidence of causal relationships.

5. E – Meta-analysis

A meta-analysis combines the results of several studies that have looked at a similar hypothesis. By combining the results of multiple data-sets, the statistical power of the outcome is increased and the validity of the conclusion improved.

Theme 12: Management of neurological conditions

1. A – Amphetamines

This woman has narcolepsy, characterized by frequent sleep attacks, cataplexy (loss of muscle tone with strong emotion), hypnagogic and hypnopompic hallucinations (hallucinations on going to sleep and waking up respectively) and sleep paralysis (paralysis on waking). Management is with central nervous system stimulants, such as dexamfetamine (dexamphetamine).

2. I – Penicillin

This woman has tertiary syphilis (specifically neurosyphilis). The treatment of choice is penicillin.

3. E – Donepezil

This woman has Alzheimer's disease. The mainstay of drug treatment is with acetylcholinesterase inhibitors, which increase levels of the neurotransmitter acetylcholine and have been shown to slow disease progression in a proportion of patients. Examples of acetylcholinesterase inhibitors are donepezil, galantamine and rivastigmine.

4. K – Rifampicin and isoniazid

The history in this patient indicates meningitis. The long duration of symptoms and the presence of focal neurology suggest an underlying cause of tuberculosis. Treatment of tuberculosis meningitis is with antituberculous therapy, usually for 12 months (e.g. rifampicin, isoniazid, pyrazinamide and ethambutol for 6 months, followed by just rifampicin and isoniazid for a further 6 months).

5. D – Chlordiazepoxide

This man is suffering alcohol withdrawal – delirium tremens. This is treated with regular chlordiazepoxide.

Theme 13: Anaemia

1. H – Iron-deficiency anaemia secondary to gastrointestinal bleeding

Iron-deficiency anaemia (IDA) is defined as a haemoglobin concentration below 13.5 g/dL in males or 11.5 g/dL in females, in association with a low MCV and evidence of depleted iron stores (i.e. a low ferritin and a raised total iron-binding capacity). In the developed world, IDA is usually secondary to chronic blood loss from gastrointestinal, uterine and urinary tract sources. (Worldwide, hookworm infection and schistosomiasis are common causes.) In cases where the source of bleeding is obvious, further investigation is usually not necessary and treatment can begin. However, in many instances, bleeding goes unnoticed and is secondary to a more sinister cause such as gastrointestinal malignancy.

Therefore, patients with IDA without an obvious cause must be referred for investigation of the upper and lower gastrointestinal tracts in the first instance.

To treat IDA, the underlying cause must be corrected and iron stores replenished. The most appropriate method of replacing iron is with oral supplementation (e.g. ferrous sulphate 200 mg three times daily). Haemoglobin should rise by 1 g/dL every 7 days. Treatment is given until haemoglobin concentrations return to normal and for a further 3–6 months in order to replenish the depleted iron stores. If the haemoglobin fails to respond as expected, you must consider non-compliance/concordance with treatment, malabsorption and misdiagnosis. Intramuscular and intravenous preparations of iron do exist, but are usually reserved for cases of refractory anaemia secondary to malabsorption and chronic disease. Blood transfusion should be considered only in severe and symptomatic anaemia. Expect the haemoglobin concentration to increase by 1 g/dL per unit of red blood cells given.

2. K – Megaloblastic macrocytic anaemia secondary to vitamin B_{12} deficiency

Vitamin B_{12} is an essential water-soluble vitamin required for DNA synthesis and red blood cell production. It is absorbed in the terminal ileum only after binding intrinsic factor, which is secreted by gastric parietal cells. The liver is able to store approximately 1 mg of vitamin B_{12}, which is sufficient for 3–4 years; hence vitamin B_{12} deficiency takes years to manifest. The main causes of vitamin B_{12} deficiency are pernicious anaemia, poor dietary intake (vegans) and malabsorption secondary to disease of the terminal ileum. Pernicious anaemia describes the autoimmune loss of parietal cells and/or intrinsic factor, thus preventing the absorption of vitamin B_{12}. It is most common in women over 60 years. Around 90% of patients demonstrate antiparietal antibodies (but some normal women also have these) and 60% are found to have anti-intrinsic factor antibody (which is a more specific marker).

Patients with bowel pathology, such as Crohn's disease (this scenario), have normal levels of intrinsic factor but cannot absorb the vitamin B_{12}–intrinsic factor complex due to disease of the terminal ileum. Although most patents with pernicious anaemia complain of lethargy and general malaise, specific features of vitamin B_{12} deficiency include peripheral neuropathy, smooth tongue, angular stomatitis, depression, dementia and subacute degeneration of the spinal cord. The blood film is likely to show a macrocytic (increased MCV), megaloblastic anaemia with hypersegmented neutrophil nuclei (>6 lobes). In addition, serum vitamin B_{12} levels are low and ferritin levels are normal, reflecting normal iron stores. The two-part Schilling test distinguishes pernicious anaemia from intestinal causes of vitamin B_{12} deficiency – look it up if you feel keen! Treatment is with hydroxocobalamin (an intramuscular preparation of vitamin B_{12}), which is given as a 1 mg dose every other day until the blood film and symptoms improve, followed by 1 mg injections every 3 months.

The term 'megaloblast' describes an abnormally large nucleated erythrocyte precursor found in people deficient in vitamin B_{12} or folate.

3. D – Anaemic of chronic disease

Anaemia of chronic disease is associated with chronic inflammatory conditions (inflammatory bowel disease, rheumatoid arthritis), malignancy and chronic renal failure. Patients have a normocytic anaemia (although 25% of cases are microcytic) with normal or raised ferritin levels. Iron supplementation is not indicated, as body stores are normal, and treatment is of the underlying conditions. If anaemia is secondary to chronic renal failure (reduced erythropoietin secretion), exogenous erythropoietin administration may be used to stimulate red cell production.

4. B – β-Thalassaemia major

β-Thalassaemia major is an autosomal recessive disorder in which there is a complete lack of production of the haemoglobin β-globin chain. It occurs mainly in Mediterranean and Middle Eastern families and is due to a point mutation on chromosome 11. Because patients with β-thalassaemia major have mutations on both alleles and cannot synthesize any β-globin, they cannot produce functioning adult haemoglobin (HbA: $\alpha_2\beta_2$). This condition typically presents within the first year of life when the production of fetal haemoglobin (HbF: $\alpha_2\gamma_2$) begins to fall. Affected children become generally unwell and fail to thrive secondary to a severe microcytic anaemia. Ferritin levels are normal since there is no iron deficiency. A compensatory increase in the synthesis of HbF and haemoglobin A_2 (HbA_2: $\alpha_2\delta_2$) occurs, which can be detected on serum electrophoresis.

Clinical features include failure to thrive, lethargy, pallor and jaundice. On examination, there is often hepatosplenomegaly (secondary to extramedullary haematopoiesis), with bossing of the skull and long bone deformity (due to excessive intramedullary haematopoiesis). The treatment of β-thalassaemia major is with regular blood transfusions, aiming to maintain the haemoglobin concentration above 10 g/dL, or with allogeneic bone marrow transplantation. Regular iron chelation therapy (with desferrioxamine) is required to prevent iron overload and deposition in vital organs such as the heart, liver and endocrine glands. If untreated, death is inevitable in the first years of life.

β-Thalassaemia trait (β-thalassaemia minor) describes people heterozygous for the β-chain chromosomal mutation. Those affected have only a mild anaemia and are usually asymptomatic. *α-Thalassaemia* is common in south-east Asia. There are four α genes, and therefore four variants of α-thalassaemia. Affected people can be asymptomatic (one gene corruption), have mild hypochromic anaemia (two corruptions), have HbH disease (three corruptions) or can die in utero (all four genes corrupted). HbH is a β-chain tetramer that is functionally useless. Treatment options are as for β-thalassaemia.

Thalassaemia, from Greek *thalassa* = sea + *haima* = blood. It is so called as the disease is especially prevalent in 'countries by the sea' (i.e. the Mediterranean).

5. E – Autoimmune haemolytic anaemia

Autoimmune haemolytic anaemia occurs when autoantibodies are produced against antigens found on erythrocytes. The antigen–antibody complex triggers an immune response resulting in the premature destruction of antibody-coated erythrocytes in the spleen. Autoimmune haemolytic anaemia may be idiopathic or secondary to an underlying process such as infection, lymphoproliferative disease or malignancy. A number of drugs are also known to trigger an autoimmune haemolytic anaemia, including methyldopa, penicillin, cephalosporins and quinine. Patients have a severe normocytic or macrocytic anaemia with normal ferritin levels. Autoimmune haemolytic anaemia can be due to 'warm' antibodies (IgG, which binds best at 37°C) or 'cold' antibodies (IgM, which binds best at 4°C or 37°C). Warm autoimmune haemolysis accounts for 80% of cases and is most common in middle-aged women. Cold autoimmune haemolysis usually affects older patients with low-grade B-cell lymphoma, or following mycoplasma or Epstein–Barr virus infection. Patients with cold autoimmune haemolysis may suffer from acrocyanosis (cold and blue extremities).

The direct Coombs' test detects erythrocytes that are coated with autoantibodies. If positive, this test confirms an autoimmune cause for haemolysis as opposed to a non-immune-mediated haemolysis, e.g. glucose-6-phosphate dehydrogenase deficiency, hereditary spherocytosis and microangiopathic haemolytic anaemia. Treatment of autoimmune haemolytic anaemia involves managing the underlying condition, stopping any suspected causative drugs and immunosuppression with steroid therapy. Splenectomy may be considered in severe and refractory disease.

Yvonne Barr, British virologist (b1932).

Sir Michael Epstein, British pathologist (b1921).

Theme 14: Diagnosis of thyroid disease 1

1. H – Papillary carcinoma

The majority (70%) of thyroid tumours are papillary adenocarcinomas; 20% are follicular carcinomas. Both of these tumours occur most commonly in adolescents and young adults, who present with a discrete thyroid nodule. Papillary tumours may be multifocal and they spread to lymph nodes (as in this case). Follicular tumours occur as a single encapsulated lesion, and they spread via blood to the lungs and bone. Treatment is by total thyroidectomy (except for tumours <1 cm, which can be treated by a thyroid lobectomy). Papillary and follicular carcinomas may be thyroid-stimulating hormone (TSH) dependent (i.e. the presence of TSH stimulates their growth). For this reason, after thyroid surgery, patients take lifelong thyroxine, in order to suppress endogenous TSH secretion and reduce the risk of recurrence.

2. I – Reidel's thyroiditis

Reidel's thyroiditis is characterized by idiopathic fibrosis of the thyroid gland. Patients present with a slowly growing goitre that is firm and irregular, and for this reason it is difficult to distinguish from cancer without a biopsy. Initially, thyroid function tests are normal, but 30% of affected patients will develop hypothyroidism and hypoparathyroidism. Complications of the fibrosis include tracheal/oesophageal compression and recurrent laryngeal nerve palsy. There is no treatment for Reidel's thyroiditis, but palliative surgery can be performed if there are compressive symptoms (e.g. dysphagia or stridor).

3. E – Hashimoto's thyroiditis

Hashimoto's thyroiditis (or 'chronic thyroiditis') is an autoimmune condition of the thyroid, which most commonly affects women. Patients present with a diffusely enlarged, rubbery goitre. People with Hashimoto's thyroiditis typically become hypothyroid, although many are euthyroid in the early stages of the disease. Autoantibodies to thyroid peroxidase (an enzyme required to make thyroxine) may be found. Treatment of Hashimoto's thyoriditis is with thyroxine, which improves the goitre as well as the symptoms.

4. K – Toxic multinodular goitre

Multinodular goitres are most common in middle-aged women. They can present in many ways, including with an unsightly swelling or dysphagia. In some cases, one nodule in a multinodular goitre will become an autonomous thyroxine-secreting adenoma, resulting in features of hyperthyroidism. This scenario is known as a toxic multinodular goitre, or 'Plummer's disease'. Cardiac features, such as atrial fibrillation and palpitations, often predominate in toxic multinodular goitre. Treatment is with radio-iodine or subtotal thyroidectomy (antithyroid medications such as carbimazole have little effect).

Henry Stanley Plummer, American physician (1874–1937)

5. A – Anaplastic carcinoma

This woman has anaplastic carcinoma as indicated by her advanced age and acute presentation. Anaplastic carcinoma accounts for <5% of thyroid tumours but is the most aggressive. It presents in older patients with a hard, symmetrical, rapidly enlarging goitre. Spread is to lymph nodes and local structures, e.g. the trachea (resulting in stridor) and the recurrent laryngeal nerve (leading to hoarseness). There is no effective treatment for anaplastic thyroid tumours, although palliative radiotherapy or debulking surgery can be performed if there is tracheal compression. Most patients (>90%) with anaplastic carcinoma are dead within 1 year.

Theme 15: Secondary hypertension

1. F – Conn's syndrome

Conn's syndrome is caused by an aldosterone-secreting tumour within the adrenal cortex. Patients with hyperaldosteronism usually present with a prolonged non-specific illness associated with polyuria and polydipsia. Aldosterone causes retention of sodium at the distal tubule of the nephron at the expense of potassium ions, which are lost in the urine. The retained sodium causes water reabsorption, resulting in fluid retention, hypervolaemia and hypertension. The typical biochemical picture in hyperaldosteronism is hypernatraemia with hypokalaemia in the presence of normal renal function. Diagnosis can be confirmed by finding a raised plasma aldosterone and suppressed plasma renin levels (the renin:aldosterone ratio is typically less than 0.05). Treatment of Conn's syndrome requires surgical excision of the neoplasm and the use of an aldosterone antagonist such as spironolactone. The aldosteronoma of Conn's syndrome is typically found to be 'canary-yellow' in colour – this is in contrast to the grey shades of a phaeochromocytoma (see below).

Jerome Conn, American endocrinologist (1907–81).

2. J – Phaeochromocytoma

This woman presents with the typical features of a phaeochromocytoma. A phaeochromocytoma is a catecholamine-secreting neuroendocrine tumour of the adrenal medulla and is a rare cause of secondary hypertension. As a rough guide, 10% are malignant, 10% are bilateral, 10% are extra-adrenal and 10% are hereditary. The sporadic release of vast amounts of catecholamines, i.e. adrenaline, noradrenaline and dopamine, into the systemic circulation leads to paroxysmal episodes of tachycardia, hypertension, anxiety and weight loss. Diagnosis is usually based on a 24-hour urine collection demonstrating the presence of excess catecholamine degradation products (such as vanillylmandelic acid) and CT imaging. The management of phaeochromocytoma usually involves surgical excision. Surgery must be carried out under α- and β-blockade to protect against the potential release of large amounts of catecholamines into the circulation that can occur when the tumour is manipulated.

3. E – Coarctation of the aorta

Coarctation of the aorta is a relatively rare condition that is often associated with Turner's syndrome. The aorta is locally narrowed, causing proximal hypertension, reduced or absent femoral pulses, radiofemoral delay and an interscapular systolic murmur. The hypertension seen in coarctation is due to mechanical obstruction of blood flow, with resulting hypoperfusion of the kidneys causing activation of the renin–angiotensin–aldosterone cascade. In most cases, the lesion is distal to the origin of the left subclavian artery, so the blood pressure is equal in both arms. If the coarctation occurs between the origins of the right and left subclavian arteries, radioradial delay will be present on examination. Pharmacological treatment of hypertension is essential, but curative vascular surgery is often required, although hypertension may not resolve if the kidney has been irreversibly damaged.

Henry Turner, American endocrinologist (1892–1970).

4. B – Adult polycystic disease

Adult polycystic disease is an autosomal dominant condition with a prevalence of approximately 1/1000. In early adulthood, the patient develops multiple large cysts, predominantly in the kidneys but also in the liver, pancreas and spleen. The condition results in renal failure and hypertension. Adult polycystic disease is also associated with berry aneurysms in the circle of Willis, which may rupture causing a potentially fatal subarachnoid haemorrhage. On examination, the patient is hypertensive and usually has palpable cystic kidneys with or without hepatosplenomegaly. Diagnosis is usually confirmed by radiological investigation. The management of adult polycystic disease includes treating the hypertension and providing renal replacement therapy such as peritoneal dialysis, haemodialysis and eventually renal transplantation.

Thomas Willis, English physician (1621–73).

5. G – Cushing's disease

Adrenocorticotropic hormone (ACTH; also known as corticotropin) is secreted from the anterior pituitary gland in response to corticotropin-releasing hormone (CRH) from the hypothalamus. ACTH acts on the adrenal cortex to stimulate the release of glucocorticoids and androgens into the circulation. In Cushing's disease, a pituitary adenoma secretes large amounts of ACTH into the circulation, causing uninhibited glucocorticoid secretion. Patients with glucocorticoid and androgen excess suffer from *Cushing's syndrome*, which consists of a vast array of clinical features, including hypertension, central weight gain, a moon face, poor quality skin, bruising, poor wound healing, hirsutism, acne, abdominal striae, oligomenorrhoea, osteoporosis, hyperglycaemia, polyuria, polydipsia, myopathy, depression and psychosis.

Cushing's syndrome can also be caused by iatrogenic steroid prescriptions or the presence of an ectopic ACTH-secreting tumour such as a small cell lung carcinoma. Treatment of Cushing's syndrome requires correction of the underlying condition (e.g. removal of the pituitary adenoma in Cushing's disease) and management of any complications such as hypertension. In cases of iatrogenic disease caused by excess steroid therapy, the offending drug should be gradually reduced over a number of weeks and replaced by an alternative 'steroid-sparing' drug (e.g. the immunosuppressant azathioprine).

Harvey William Cushing, American neurosurgeon (1869–1939).

Practice Paper 4: Questions

Theme 1: Investigation of respiratory disease

Options

A. Bronchoscopy and biopsy
B. Chest X-ray
C. CT pulmonary angiography
D. D-dimers
E. Lung function tests
F. Kveim–Siltzbach test
G. Mantoux test
H. No investigation required
I. Pleural biopsy
J. Sputum culture
K. Sweat test
L. Ventilation–perfusion scan

For each of the following scenarios, select the most appropriate investigation. Each option may be used once, more than once or not at all.

1. A 12-year-old boy is brought to the GP by his mother. Over the last couple of years, he has suffered from repeated chest infections and his mother is worried that he is not putting on any weight. On examination, there are coarse crepitations throughout both lung lobes and his fingers are clubbed.

2. A 67-year-old man complains of a long history of shortness of breath on exertion and a productive cough. He has been coughing up sputum for the last 4 months, but has had symptoms on and off for a few years. He attributed his symptoms to smoking, but he stopped last year.

3. A 59-year-old man presents to the GP with worsening shortness of breath and a cough productive of bloody sputum. He has lost a stone in weight over the last month and has been having night sweats. A chest X-ray shows scarring at the apices.

4. A 67-year-old man presents with a 3-week history of a cough productive of blood-stained sputum. He has lost 2 stone (12 kg) in weight over the last 2 months. Auscultation of the lungs is unremarkable, and a chest X-ray shows a 2 cm density in the left lower lobe.

5. A 58-year-old man complains of left-sided chest discomfort that has been progressing over the last fortnight. He is otherwise well. On examination, the left lower lobe is dull to percussion, and a chest X-ray confirms a left-sided pleural effusion. A pleural tap is performed and reveals blood-stained fluid.

Theme 2: Nerve lesions of the lower limb

Options

A. Common peroneal nerve
B. Femoral nerve
C. Lateral femoral cutaneous nerve
D. Lateral plantar nerve
E. Medial plantar nerve
F. Obturator nerve
G. Sciatic nerve
H. Saphenous nerve
I. Sural nerve
J. Tibial nerve

For each of the following scenarios, select the most likely nerve lesion. Each option may be used once, more than once or not at all.

1. A 25-year-old man is taken to theatre after fracturing his hip in a motorbike accident. Postoperatively, it is noticed that he is unable to flex his left foot either up or down. There is no sensation below the left knee except over the medial aspect of the leg.

2. A 28-year-old woman is involved in a road traffic collision. Her right knee had hit the dashboard of the car. On arrival at the emergency department, she is unable to flex her toes on the right side. Examination reveals an absence of the ankle jerk and loss of sensation over the sole of the foot.

3. A 32-year-old man is stabbed in the groin during a fight. He attends the emergency department as he is unable to extend his knee afterwards. On examination, the knee jerk is absent and there is loss of sensation over the front of the thigh and the medial aspect of the leg.

4. A 46-year-old woman attends the GP complaining of intermittent pain in her right thigh. The pain is sharp and is relieved by sitting down. On examination, you note that she is obese. There is no deficit in tone or power in the lower limbs.

5. A 16-year-old boy was previously admitted to the orthopaedic ward with an ankle fracture, which was treated with a plaster cast. When the cast is removed, the boy is unable to dorsiflex his foot.

Theme 3: Mechanism of action of common drugs

Options

A. Cimetidine
B. Heparin
C. Hyoscine
D. Ibuprofen
E. Losartan
F. Morphine
G. Naloxone
H. Omeprazole
I. Paracetamol
J. Ramipril
K. Warfarin

For each of the following statements, select the most appropriate drug. Each option may be used once, more than once or not at all.

1. A drug that inhibits the γ-carboxylation of vitamin K-dependent clotting factors.

2. A drug that blocks cholinergic activity.

3. A drug that blocks the angiotensin II receptor.

4. A drug that inhibits the gastric parietal cell H^+/K^+ ATPase pump.

5. A non-steroidal anti-inflammatory drug.

Theme 4: Investigation in diabetes mellitus

Options

A. A single fasting venous blood glucose >7.0 mmol/L
B. A single random capillary blood glucose >7.0 mmol/L
C. A venous blood glucose between 7.8 and 11.1 mmol/L 2 hours after a 75 g oral glucose bolus
D. A venous blood glucose >11.1 mmol/L 2 hours after a 75 g oral glucose bolus
E. Fasting plasma cholesterol
F. Fructosamine
G. Glycosuria
H. HbA_{1c}
I. Ophthalmoscopy
J. Proteinuria
K. Two random blood glucose levels >11.1 mmol/L

For each of the following descriptions, select the best answer from the list above. Each option may be used once, more than once or not at all.

1. Which criterion should be used to diagnose diabetes in a 13-year-old boy with a 3-week history of lethargy, polyuria and polydipsia?

2. Which criterion is used to diagnose diabetes in an asymptomatic 57-year-old woman?

3. Which oral glucose tolerance test result indicates a diagnosis of glucose intolerance?

4. Which test is used to evaluate long-term glucose control in a patient with known diabetes?

5. Which test is required to evaluate a diabetic patient's cardiovascular risk?

Theme 5: Glasgow Coma Scale

Options

A. 0
B. 3
C. 4
D. 5
E. 6
F. 7
G. 8
H. 9
I. 11
J. 13
K. 14
L. 15

For each of the following scenarios, select the most appropriate Glasgow Coma Scale score. Each option may be used once, more than once or not at all.

1. You are called to see a 43-year-old woman following an open cholecystectomy. She is making noises but no understandable words. Her eyes open in response to speech and she withdraws appropriately from painful stimuli.

2. A 32-year-old intravenous drug user is brought to the emergency department following a suspected opiate overdose. He opens his eyes in response to pain and is making incomprehensible sounds. He withdraws from painful stimuli.

3. Following a road traffic collision, a patient is brought to the emergency department. On arrival, there is no respiration or cardiac output, so cardiopulmonary resuscitation is commenced.

4. A pedestrian is brought to the emergency department after being involved in a hit-and-run accident. He is not opening his eyes or making any sounds. He flexes abnormally in response to pain.

5. A 76-year-old man presents with shortness of breath and a productive cough. Although he is sitting up, with his eyes open and moving spontaneously, his speech is occasionally confused and muddled.

Theme 6: Investigation of liver disease

Options

A. α_1-Antitrypsin level
B. α-Fetoprotein
C. Antimitochondrial antibody
D. Antinuclear antibodies
E. Ceruloplasmin level
F. Cytomegalovirus PCR
G. Hepatitis A antigen
H. Hepatitis A IgG
I. Hepatitis A IgM
J. Hepatitis C RNA
K. Hepatitis C antibody
L. Total iron-binding capacity

For each of the following scenarios, select the most appropriate investigation. Each option may be used once, more than once or not at all.

1. A 12-year-old girl presents with jaundice. Her mother says that she has been behaving differently over the last few weeks. Investigation shows deranged liver function tests, and an ultrasound scan confirms cirrhotic changes within the liver.

2. A 34-year-old man presents with a 1-month history of vague upper abdominal pain. He is on insulin for diabetes, but is otherwise well. On examination, there appears to be a bronzed tan to the skin, although the patient denies having been on holiday.

3. A 42-year-old woman presents with a 4-week history of generalized itching. She has developed yellow lesions in the skin around her eyes. Blood tests reveal deranged liver function tests.

4. A 32-year-old man has recently returned from holiday in India, where he stayed with locals and dined with them. Two weeks later, he presents with jaundice and lethargy. Liver function tests reveal a massively raised ALT and a significantly raised bilirubin.

5. A 27-year-old nurse sustained a needlestick injury 4 months ago. She attends an occupational health appointment, where a blood test is done to exclude hepatitis C infection.

Theme 7: Complications of renal failure

Options

A. Advise exercise
B. Alfacalcidol
C. Intravenous bisphosphonate infusion
D. Intravenous calcium gluconate
E. Intravenous erythropoietin
F. Iron sulphate supplementation
G. Low-potassium diet
H. Oral ACE inhibitor and fluid restriction
I. Oral calcium channel blocker and fluid restriction
J. Oral erythropoietin
K. Phosphate supplements
L. Statin therapy
M. Stop phosphate binders
N. Urgent dialysis

For each of the following scenarios, select the most appropriate treatment. Each option may be used once, more than once or not at all.

1. A 56-year-old man with chronic renal failure has become gradually more lethargic over the last 2 months. On examination, he has pale palmar creases and pale conjunctivae. Auscultation reveals an ejection systolic murmur. His full blood count shows a haemoglobin concentration of 8.2 g/dL and a mean cell volume of 85 fL. The ferritin level is normal.

2. A 60-year-old woman with chronic renal failure mentions that she is becoming more generally lethargic. Blood tests show a calcium of 1.73 mmol/L, a phosphate of 2.7 mmol/L and an albumin of 45 g/L.

3. A 45-year-old man with chronic renal failure is found to have a blood pressure of 180/95 mmHg during an outpatient assessment. On reviewing the records, it is apparent that his blood pressure has been climbing for a number of weeks.

4. A 14-year-old boy with congenital nephrotic syndrome is found to have a total cholesterol of 9.3 mmol/L.

5. A 48-year-old man with end-stage renal failure presents to the emergency department after having a fit. Over the last few days, according to his wife, he has been suffering from fluctuating confusion and jerking movements in his arms and legs. Blood tests show a urea of 35.6 mmol/L, a creatinine of 600 μmol/L, a potassium of 5.4 mmol/L and a sodium of 147 mmol/L. An urgent head CT is requested, and demonstrates no abnormality.

Theme 8: Emergency management

Options

A. Head tilt and chin lift
B. High-dose steroids
C. Insert a cannula into the second intercostal space in the midclavicular line
D. Insert chest drain
E. Insert nasopharyngeal airway
F. Intramuscular benzylpenicillin and call ambulance
G. Intravenous benzylpenicillin
H. Intravenous lorazepam
I. Intravenous phenytoin
J. Intubate
K. Jaw thrust
L. Oral diazepam

For each of the following scenarios, select the next step in the management. Each option may be used once, more than once or not at all.

1. A 26-year-old woman presents to the emergency department with severe shortness of breath following a road traffic collision. On examination, she has reduced air entry over her left lung field and her trachea is deviated to the right.

2. A 12-year-old girl is seen in the community by her GP. She is lethargic, irritable and 'not feeling her usual self' according to her parents. On examination, she has a stiff neck and a non-blanching purpuric rash on her abdomen.

3. A 67-year-old woman presents to the emergency department complaining of lethargy, fever and a left-sided temporal headache. Examination reveals tenderness of the left temple, and there is no obvious pulsation of the temporal artery.

4. A 25-year-old man is brought to the emergency department while fitting. His airway has been secured using an oropharyngeal airway. He has oxygen saturations of 99% on 15 L of oxygen and a capillary refill time of 2 s. Intravenous access has been gained.

5. On your way home from work, you notice an unconscious cyclist lying in the street after apparently being involved in a road traffic collision. He was not wearing a helmet and appears to have a head injury. When you assess his airway, you hear grunting sounds.

Theme 9: Investigation of endocrine disease

Options

A. 17-Hydroxyprogesterone levels
B. 24-hour urinary vanillylmandelic acid
C. 24-hour urinary 5-hydroxyindole acetic acid
D. Aldosterone and renin levels
E. Dexamethasone suppression test
F. Parathyroid hormone and calcium levels
G. Serum calcitonin
H. Short Synacthen test
I. Vitamin D levels

For each of the following people, select the best distinguishing investigation. Each option may be used once, more than once or not at all.

1. A 42-year-old man is referred to the general medical clinic by his GP for uncontrollable hypertension. He is presently on ramipril and bendroflumethazide. On further questioning, he admits to having paroxysms of anxiety, sweating and palpitations that are brought on by stress and that he describes as 'panic attacks'.

2. A 44-year-old woman presents following a faint after standing up from a sitting position. She did not lose consciousness during this episode, but merely reported feeling 'dizzy and lightheaded'. She has no significant past medical history. On examination, you notice multiple areas of skin depigmentation but increased pigmentation in the palmar creases and on the elbows.

3. A 65-year-woman with known small cell lung cancer presents with hirsutism that she finds embarrassing. On examination, you note that she has a plethoric face, acne, abdominal striae and multiple bruises.

4. A 5-year-old girl is referred to the paediatric clinic by her GP with precocious puberty. On examination, she is found to have clitoromegaly and some pubic hair. She is above the 98th centile for height and weight.

5. A 50-year-old man attends the emergency department complaining of episodes of flushing and diarrhoea associated with difficulty in breathing. On further questioning, you find that these episodes are precipitated by stress and alcohol. On examination, his blood pressure is 130/86 mmHg and his heart rate is 82 beats/min.

Theme 10: Dementia 2

Options

A. Alzheimer's disease
B. Creutzfeldt–Jakob disease
C. Depressive pseudodementia
D. HIV dementia
E. Huntington's disease
F. Lewy body dementia
G. Neurosyphilis
H. Normal-pressure hydrocephalus
I. Parkinson's disease
J. Pick's disease
K. Vascular dementia
L. Wernicke's encephalopathy

For each of the following scenarios, select the most appropriate cause of dementia. Each option may be used once, more than once or not at all.

1. A 48-year-old man is brought to the GP by his wife. She says that he has been confused over the last 7 days and has been falling over a lot. Examination reveals a nystagmus but no other neurological signs.

2. A 71-year-old woman presents to the GP with a 12-month progressive decline in her memory function. She has no other symptoms. Her husband says that she now gets lost trying to find the bathroom at home. She has previously been fit and well, and physical examination is unremarkable. She scores 23/30 on a Mini-Mental State Examination.

3. A 34-year-old woman presents to the GP complaining of memory problems. At the surgery, she makes no attempt at eye contact with the doctor. When asked simple questions such as 'Where do you live?' and 'How old are you?', she answers that she does not know.

4. A 25-year-man presents to the GP with worsening memory and depression. He is also complaining of twitching movements in his upper and lower limbs. He is worried, as his mother told him that his father died of movement problems when he was young.

5. A 39-year-old man presents to the GP feeling generally lethargic. He has also noticed problems with his memory over the past few months. He has no documented past medical history. On examination, there are several white lesions in his mouth.

Theme 11: Heart sounds

Options

A. Austin Flint murmur
B. Continuous murmur radiating to the back
C. Ejection systolic murmur heard at the right second intercostal space only
D. Ejection systolic murmur heard best in the right second intercostal space that radiates into the right carotid artery
E. Graham Steell murmur
F. Muffled heart sounds
G. Mid-diastolic click loudest at the apex
H. Midsystolic murmur
I. Normal heart sounds
J. Opening snap best heard at the apex
K. Pansystolic murmur heard best at the apex with radiation into the axilla
L. Physiological splitting of the second heart sound
M. Reverse splitting of the second heart sound
N. Summation gallop rhythm

For each of the following scenarios, select the most appropriate heart sound. Each option may be used once, more than once or not at all.

1. A 67-year-old man presents with symptoms of acute left ventricular failure. On examination, you notice that his heart rate is 120 beats/min. On auscultation, there are more than two heart sounds present, but you cannot distinguish them from each other.

2. A 55-year-old man presents to the emergency department with a severe headache. He is known to have mitral valve regurgitation.

3. You are called to see an 87-year-old female inpatient who is complaining of chest pain. On examination, you notice a murmur. A brief look in her hospital notes confirms that she has known ischaemic heart disease, hypertension and aortic valve sclerosis.

4. A 65-year-old woman with known systemic lupus erythematosus presents with central chest pain that is very similar to the pain that she feels when suffering from pericarditis. Echocardiography demonstrates a pericardial effusion that is likely to be chronic. On auscultation, the heart sounds do not sound as they should.

5. A 45-year-old man presents with abdominal pain. He is known to have Marfan's syndrome with advanced aortic valve regurgitation.

Theme 12: Management of skin disease

Options

A. 5-Fluorouracil
B. Analgesia
C. Cryotherapy
D. Fluid resuscitation
E. Intravenous antibiotics
F. Oral antibiotics
G. Surgical debridement and intravenous antibiotics
H. Surgical excision
I. Reassurance

For each of the following presentations, select the most appropriate management plan. Each option may be used once, more than once or not at all.

1. A 52-year-old woman presents to the emergency department with redness and swelling of her right cheek. On examination, the area of erythema is well demarcated and is warm to the touch. Her temperature is 38.1°C and she feels unwell.

2. A 37-year-old man presents to his GP with a lesion on his back. On examination, the lesion is 1 cm in size, painless and mobile. It is attached to the overlying skin, but not to the underlying subcutaneous tissue, and it has a central punctum. There is no palpable cervical lymphadenopathy. The man is worried about the cosmetic appearance.

3. A 73-year-old woman presents with a raised temperature and feeling unwell. She has a large area of erythema and swelling on her left leg that is becoming necrotic. This started when she hit her leg on a stool a few days ago, but since then the erythema and necrosis have spread rapidly.

4. A 7-year-old boy is brought by his father to the emergency department with multiple, yellow, crusty, blistering lesions on his face and arms. The lesions are itchy and occasionally bleed. The boy's older brother is suffering similar complaints.

5. A 5-year-old girl is brought to the GP by her mother because she has longstanding freckling in her mouth. On examination, the child has multiple bluish-black macular lesions around the lips and nose. She is otherwise well.

Theme 13: Connective tissue disease

Options

A. Antiphospholipid syndrome
B. Dermatomyositis
C. Diffuse cutaneous systemic sclerosis
D. Limited cutaneous systemic sclerosis
E. Overlap syndromes
F. Polymyositis
G. Sjögren's syndrome
H. Systemic lupus erythematosus

For each of the following scenarios, select the most likely underlying connective tissue disease. Each option may be used once, more than once or not at all.

1. A 45-year old woman presents with a 2-month history of hip and shoulder weakness. She is finding it especially difficult to climb stairs. The weakness is demonstrable on examination and she is tender over the proximal joints. No skin lesions are visible.

2. A 32-year-old woman presents with sudden-onset shortness of breath with a cough productive of blood. She has had two pulmonary emboli in the past. On examination, the chest is clear and no skin lesions are seen.

3. A 49-year-old woman has noticed that the skin on her face and hands is becoming tight and uncomfortable. She denies any other symptoms. On examination, there are multiple telangiectasia on her face. The skin on both her hands and her face is tight and shiny, but the skin of the proximal arms is unaffected.

4. An 18-year-old woman presents with a long history of dry, itchy eyes. She denies having any problems with her vision. There is no abnormality on examination.

5. A 27-year-old woman has developed a red, scaly rash on her checks and nose that is worse in the sunlight. She also complains of pain in the small joints of her hands. On examination, there are no additional cutaneous lesions, and no deformity is seen in the hands.

Theme 14: Diagnosis of haematological disease

Options

A. Chronic myeloid leukaemia
B. Dehydration
C. Essential thrombocythaemia
D. Hodgkin's lymphoma
E. Monoclonal gammopathy of uncertain significance
F. Multiple myeloma
G. Myelofibrosis
H. Non-Hodgkin's lymphoma
I. Osteoporosis
J. Polycythaemia rubra vera
K. Secondary polycythaemia
L. Waldenström's macroglobulinaemia

For each of the following scenarios, select the most appropriate underlying diagnosis. Each option may be used once, more than once or not at all.

1. A 74-year-old man is being investigated following a crush fracture of his T8 vertebra. He is found to have a monoclonal band on serum electrophoresis and free immunoglobulin light chains in his urine.

2. A 25-year-old man presents to his GP complaining of a mass in his neck. The mass is generally painless, although it occasionally aches after alcohol. He admits to losing a significant amount of weight over the last month and also complains of excessive sweating and general itching. A biopsy of the mass reveals the presence of Reed–Sternberg cells.

3. A 74-year-old woman presents to her GP complaining of headaches and itching that is much worse after a warm bath. On examination, she has a normal cardiovascular and respiratory system. While palpating the abdomen, the doctor feels a vague fullness in the left upper quadrant. A full blood count shows a haemoglobin concentration of 22.1 g/dL.

4. A 65-year-old man on long-term oxygen therapy for chronic obstructive pulmonary disease is found to have a haemoglobin concentration of 18.4 g/dL.

5. An 83-year-old man is referred for bone marrow aspiration after presenting with hepatomegaly, splenomegaly and pancytopenia. No marrow could be aspirated during the first attempt. A trephine biopsy is successfully performed, and histology reveals hypercellular marrow containing many abnormal megakaryocytes.

Theme 15: Conditions of the vessel wall

Options

A. Annual ultrasound monitoring
B. Elective surgical repair
C. Intravenous antibiotics
D. Maintain systolic blood pressure above 150 mmHg with fluid resuscitation while awaiting emergency surgical repair
E. Maintain systolic blood pressure at approximately 100 mmHg with fluid resuscitation while awaiting emergency surgical repair
F. No intervention necessary
G. Oral antihypertensive medication and close blood pressure monitoring
H. Reduce systolic blood pressure to 100 mmHg using an intravenous antihypertensive agent and refer for emergency surgical repair
I. Urgent abdominal ultrasound scan
J. Urgent CT scan
K. Urgent magnetic resonance angiography
L. Urgent ultrasound scan and compression

For each of the following scenarios, select the most appropriate course of action. Each option may be used once, more than once or not at all.

1. A fit and well 67-year-old man attends his GP for an annual check-up. On examination, the doctor notices an expansile pulsatile mass in the patient's abdomen. An outpatient ultrasound scan is requested, and shows a 6.5 cm abdominal aortic aneurysm.

2. A 77-year-old man from a nursing home complains of back pain. He is known to have prostate cancer as well as ischaemic heart disease, chronic heart failure, type 2 diabetes and chronic obstructive pulmonary disease. A staging CT, which demonstrates spinal metastases, also finds a 7 cm abdominal aortic aneurysm.

3. A 60-year-old man presents to the emergency department following a collapse that was preceded by a sudden-onset abdominal pain that radiated to his back. His wife informs you that he is on the waiting list to 'have an operation on his main artery', but can tell you no more. He appears pale and his blood pressure is 70/35 mmHg. On examination, his abdomen is tender and rigid.

4. A 67-year-old woman presents to the emergency department complaining of a tearing central chest pain that is radiating to her back. Her ECG shows sinus tachycardia and her physical examination is normal. Her blood pressure is 170/90 mmHg and her heart rate is 90 beats/min. A portable chest X-ray demonstrates a widened mediastinum. An urgent CT is requested, and shows that both the ascending and the descending aorta have a false lumen.

5. You are called to see a 55-year-old man on the ward who has developed a painful pulsatile mass in his groin while awaiting discharge following an elective angiogram.

Practice Paper 4: Answers

Theme 1: Investigation of respiratory disease

1. K – Sweat test

This child has cystic fibrosis. The gold standard investigation for cystic fibrosis is the sweat test. The abnormal function of sweat glands results in an excess concentration of sodium chloride (NaCl) in sweat. Sweat is stimulated by pilocarpine iontophoresis, collected on filter paper and analysed.

Normal sweat NaCl concentration = 10–14 mmol/L

Sweat NaCl concentration in CF = 80–125 mmol/L.

At least two sweat tests should be performed, as diagnostic errors and false positives are common.

2. E – Lung function tests

This man has chronic obstructive pulmonary disease (COPD), a chronic progressive disorder characterized by airflow obstruction caused by smoking. Features of COPD include a productive cough (worse in the morning), recurrent respiratory tract infections, exertional dyspnoea, expiratory wheeze and bibasal crepitations. COPD is diagnosed by using lung function tests to demonstrate a forced expiratory volume in 1 s (FEV_1) <80% and an FEV_1/VC (vital capacity) ratio <70% with little variation in peak flow.

3. J – Sputum culture

This patient has tuberculosis (TB). The diagnosis of TB can be made by sputum staining (using Ziehl–Neelsen stain) and culture (on Lowenstein–Jensen media). Sputum cultures of TB can take up to 6 weeks to grow.

4. A – Bronchoscopy and biopsy

This patient presents with typical features of a lung tumour. This should be followed up with a bronchoscopy with washings and a biopsy to confirm histological diagnosis. A CT scan should be performed to assess staging of disease.

5. I – Pleural biopsy

Mesothelioma is a malignant tumour of the pleura. The effusion of mesothelioma tends to be blood stained, but the definitive diagnosis is made by pleural biopsy.

Theme 2: Nerve lesions of the lower limb

1. G – Sciatic nerve

The sciatic nerve can be damaged with fracture dislocations of the hip or by misplaced gluteal injections. Sciatic nerve palsy results in paralysis of the hamstrings and all the muscles of the leg and foot. Sensation is lost below the knee, except for the medial leg (supplied by the saphenous nerve, a branch of the femoral nerve) and the upper calf (supplied by the posterior femoral cutaneous nerve).

2. J – Tibial nerve

The tibial nerve is particularly vulnerable to damage during posterior dislocations of the knee. It can also be compressed in the posterior tarsal tunnel behind the medial malleolus. A branch of the sciatic nerve, the tibial nerve supplies the flexor compartment of the leg (calf muscles). It also gives rise to the medial and lateral plantar nerves, which supply the intrinsic muscles of the foot as well as plantar sensation. Tibial nerve palsy results in loss of toe flexion, ankle inversion and the ankle jerk. Sensation over the plantar surface of the foot is lost. Affected patients walk with a shuffling gait, as the take-off phase of walking is impaired. There is loss of the lateral longitudinal arch of the foot, and atrophy of the intrinsic foot muscles eventually results in a claw foot.

3. B – Femoral nerve

The femoral nerve enters the thigh via the femoral triangle, where it lies lateral to the femoral artery. It can easily be damaged by penetrating wounds, hip dislocations or thigh haematomas. The femoral nerve supplies motor branches to the quadriceps and sensory branches to the anterior thigh and medial calf (via the saphenous nerve). Femoral nerve palsies result in a loss of knee extension and loss of sensation over the anterior thigh and medial leg.

4. C – Lateral femoral cutaneous nerve

The lateral femoral cutaneous nerve can become trapped at the inguinal ligament, especially in obese people or pregnant women. Nerve entrapment causes pain or a burning sensation in the lateral thigh (known as meralgia paraesthetica) with no motor abnormality. Pain is often caused by long periods of standing.

Meralgia, from Greek *meros* = thigh + *algos* = pain.

5. A – Common peroneal nerve

The common peroneal nerve (or common fibular nerve) is a branch of the sciatic nerve that supplies the dorsiflexors and evertor muscles of the foot and sensation to the lateral lower leg and upper foot. The common peroneal nerve lies in close proximity to the fibula, and may become trapped by below-knee plaster casts or damaged with fibular fractures. Features of common peroneal nerve lesions include lack of dorsiflexion (with a resulting foot drop) and loss of sensation in the anterolateral lower leg and dorsum of the foot (except for the lateral aspect of the foot, which is supplied by the sural nerve). The inability to dorsiflex the foot will result in a 'high-stepping' gait to ensure that the foot is not scraped along the ground.

The *saphenous nerve* can be damaged during surgery on the long saphenous vein, particularly when the vein is stripped below the knee, resulting in loss of sensation to the medial aspect of the calf. The *sural nerve* is a cutaneous sensory branch of the tibial nerve, and can be damaged during surgery on the short saphenous vein. Lesions of the sural nerve result in a loss of sensation to the lateral side of the foot and little toe. The *obturator nerve* can be damaged in obstetric procedures and pelvic disease. Features of obturator nerve palsy include loss of hip adduction and loss of sensation to the upper inner thigh. *Superior gluteal nerve* lesions result in loss of hip abduction and a pelvic dip on walking (Trendelenburg gait). *Inferior gluteal nerve* lesions lead to loss of hip extension and to buttock wasting.

Theme 3: Mechanism of action of common drugs

1. K – Warfarin

Warfarin is used as an anticoagulant in deep vein thrombosis and pulmonary embolism. In addition, it is used to prevent thrombosis and embolism in patients with atrial fibrillation, valvular heart disease and mechanical heart valves. Warfarin inhibits the γ-carboxylation of vitamin K-dependent clotting factors (factors II, VII, IX and X). The inhibition of γ-carboxylation produces factors that are unable to promote coagulation, resulting in an overall hypocoagulable state. Warfarin usually takes around 3 days to exert its effect; therefore, patients who require immediate anticoagulation should be started on heparin at the same time as warfarin. The heparin can then be discontinued once the warfarin has produced the desired anticoagulation as measured by the international normalized ratio (INR).

2. C – Hyoscine

Hyoscine is an antimuscarinic (anticholinergic) drug used in the treatment of irritable bowel syndrome, abdominal cramping and motion sickness. It also has a role in reducing respiratory and gastric secretions in palliative and preoperative care. Unfortunately, since the actions of hyoscine are not selective, it has a large side-effect profile, which includes dry mouth, blurred vision, photophobia (secondary to pupil dilatation), urinary retention, constipation and tachycardia.

3. E – Losartan

Losartan is an angiotensin II receptor antagonist. In health, the activation of angiotensin II receptors by angiotensin II results in peripheral vasoconstriction, stimulation of aldosterone release, and reabsorption of sodium and water from the renal tubules. Inhibition of these actions by angiotensin II receptor antagonists helps reduce blood pressure in hypertensive patients. They are usually used as second-line agents in patients who are intolerant to the side-effects of angiotensin-converting enzyme (ACE) inhibitors, e.g. ramipril.

4. H – Omeprazole

Omeprazole is a proton pump inhibitor (PPI). By inhibiting parietal proton (H^+/K^+ ATPase) pumps, PPIs reduce gastric acid secretion. They are used to treat dyspepsia, gastro-oesophageal reflux disease and *Helicobacter pylori* infection. They can also be used to reduce the risk of developing gastritis and peptic ulcers in patients taking non-steroidal anti-inflammatory drugs (see below) or steroids, and following surgery. They have largely superseded H_2-receptor antagonists, e.g. cimetidine, in the treatment and prophylaxis of gastro-oesophageal disease.

5. D – Ibuprofen

Ibuprofen is a non-steroidal anti-inflammatory drug (NSAID). Other drugs belonging to this class include aspirin, diclofenac, ketorolac and naproxen. They have multiple actions, but are mainly used for their analgesic, antipyretic and anti-inflammatory properties. NSAIDs work by inhibiting the enzyme cyclooxygenase, which is responsible for the synthesis of proinflammatory prostaglandins. Prostaglandins are also important in regulating mucosal protection by gastric acid secretion and renal blood flow. Because of this role of prostaglandins, if their synthesis is inhibited by NSAIDs, the loss of regulation promotes gastric acid mucosal damage (increasing the risk of gastritis and peptic ulcer disease) and reduced renal blood flow (increasing the risk of renal failure). Therefore, patients prone to gastritis, peptic ulcer disease and renal impairment should not be prescribed NSAIDs, and individuals who require long-term treatment should be prescribed gastroprotective agents such as omeprazole. NSAIDs are also contraindicated in asthmatic patients, along with β-blockers, as they can trigger bronchospasm in sensitive individuals.

Theme 4: Investigation in diabetes mellitus

1. A – A single fasting venous blood glucose >7.0 mmol/L

Diabetes mellitus in young individuals usually presents with a history of general lethargy, polyuria, polydipsia and weight loss. Alternatively, the first presentation may be with diabetic ketoacidosis. In symptomatic patients, a fasting venous blood glucose >7.0 mmol/L or a random blood glucose >11.1 mmol/L is considered to be diagnostic of diabetes mellitus. A capillary blood glucose level obtained from a finger test or evidence of glucose in the urine should not be used for diagnosis, but can be used in the assessment of short-term glucose control.

Diabetes mellitus, from Greek *diabainein* = to siphon + Latin *mellis* = sweet.

In other words, to pass sweet urine.

2. K – Two random blood glucose levels >11.1 mmol/L

Type 2 diabetes is caused by peripheral insulin resistance and is usually asymptomatic until complications arise late on in the disease process. The diagnostic criteria for type 2 diabetes are the same as for type 1 diabetes. In symptomatic patients, a fasting venous blood glucose >7.0 mmol/L or a random blood glucose >11.1 mmol/L is required for diagnosis. In asymptomatic patients, the same criteria are used, but must be demonstrated on two separate occasions. In cases where a diagnosis cannot be confirmed or excluded, an oral glucose tolerance test can be performed. The patient is given a 75 g oral glucose bolus following a 12-hour fast. A venous blood glucose >11.1 mmol/L 2 hours after the glucose bolus indicates diabetes.

3. C – A venous blood glucose between 7.8 and 11.1 mmol/L 2 hours after a 75 g oral glucose bolus

Impaired glucose tolerance is a diagnosis that implies impaired glucose regulation that does not reach the diagnostic criteria for diabetes mellitus. It is diagnosed on the basis of a fasting venous blood glucose < 7.0 mmol/L in association with a 2-hour venous blood glucose level between 7.8 and 11.1 mmol/L following a 75 g glucose bolus as part of the oral glucose tolerance test. Patients with impaired glucose tolerance run the risk of developing diabetes, and also have a significant risk of morbidity and mortality secondary to cardiovascular disease. Therefore, patients with this diagnosis should be followed up on a yearly basis to assess their glucose levels and cardiovascular risk.

4. H – HbA_{1c}

Adult haemoglobin (HbA_1) becomes irreversibly glycated to form HbA_{1c} when exposed to prolonged periods of hyperglycaemia. Since haemoglobin has a half-life of 8 weeks, HbA_{1c} can be used to assess long-term glucose control in a diabetic patient. High levels of HbA_{1c} indicate poor long-term glucose control and should prompt a review of the patient's lifestyle and management. The HbA_{1c} level should be <7.5% in diabetic patients, unless there is significant cardiovascular risk, in which case the target should be <6.5%. In patients who are prone to significant episodes of hypoglycaemia, a higher level of HbA_{1c} can be acceptable. Fructosamine, produced by the glycation of plasma proteins in the presence of high plasma glucose levels, may used to assess glucose control over a period of 2–3 weeks. It is not as reliable as HbA_{1c}, and has a more limited clinical role. Special circumstances in which fructosamine is preferred to HbA_{1c} include the assessment of glucose control in gestational diabetes and in patients with haemoglobinopathies such as thalassaemia, when HbA_{1c} levels are likely to be unreliable.

5. E – Fasting plasma cholesterol

The lipid profile is essential for evaluating and modifying cardiovascular risk in diabetic patients. A high total plasma cholesterol and a high ratio of total cholesterol to high-density lipoprotein (HDL)-cholesterol places a patient at risk of macrovascular disease such as myocardial infarction, stroke and peripheral vascular disease. The lipid profile should be evaluated in conjunction with the patient's blood pressure, family history and lifestyle, and the presence of microalbuminuria/proteinuria. All diabetic patients should be educated as to the need for a healthy diet, regular exercise and smoking cessation. Specific pharmacological treatments include statin therapy for hyperlipidaemia, antihypertensives for persistent hypertension and ACE inhibitors for microalbuminuria/proteinuria. Antiplatelet therapy with low-dose aspirin should be considered in all diabetic patients with cardiovascular disease and those at significant risk of developing cardiovascular disease.

Theme 5: Glasgow Coma Scale

The Glasgow Coma Scale (GCS) is a subjective way of assessing and recording a patient's consciousness. The scale compromises three components: eyes, verbal and motor response. The scores for each are as follows:

Best eye response (E):

4 Eyes open spontaneously
3 Eyes open to speech
2 Eyes open to pain
1 No eye opening.

Best verbal response (V):

5 Coherent speech
4 Confused/disorientated speech
3 Inappropriate words without conversational exchange
2 Incomprehensible sounds
1 No verbal response.

Best motor response (M):

6 Obeys commands
5 Localizes to pain
4 Withdraws from pain
3 Abnormal flexion in response to pain (decorticate response)
2 Abnormal extension in response to pain (decerebrate response)
1 No motor response.

The maximum score is 15 (E4, V5, M6) and the minimum is 3 (E1, V1, M1).

The scale was first published in 1974 by Teasdale and Jennett, two professors of neurosurgery at the University of Glasgow.

1. H – 9

This woman is opening her eyes in response to speech (E3), is making noises but no words (V2) and withdraws from painful stimuli (M4): GCS = 3 + 2 + 4 = 9.

2. G – 8

This man opens his eyes with pain (E2), is making noises but no words (V2) and withdraws from painful stimuli (M4): GCS = 2 + 2 + 4 = 8.

3. B – 3

This patient has no pulse or respiratory effort. Therefore, he will have no eye opening (E1), verbal output (V1) or motor response (M1): GCS = 1 + 1 + 1 = 3. Remember that the lowest GCS is 3, not 0!

4. D – 5

This man is not opening his eyes (E1) or making any sound (V1); he flexes abnormally in response to pain (M3): GCS = 1 + 1 + 3 = 5.

5. K – 14

This man's eyes are open spontaneously (E4), but he has confused speech (V4); he is also moving spontaneously (M6): GCS = 4 + 4 + 6 = 14.

Theme 6: Investigation of liver disease

1. E – Ceruloplasmin level

Wilson's disease is an autosomal recessive disease of copper metabolism. In health, copper is transported in the serum bound to ceruloplasmin (ferroxidase) and is excreted in the bile. In Wilson's disease, there is a defect in copper metabolism such that it is not excreted in the bile and instead accumulates in the tissues. This process suppresses the synthesis of ceruloplasmin, which allows unbound (free) copper to enter the circulation. The high levels of free serum copper accumulate in vital organs such as the liver (resulting in cirrhosis), eye (causing Keiser–Fleischer rings), kidney and basal ganglia of the brain (leading to personality changes). If left untreated, the patient is at risk of developing cirrhosis, renal tubular disease, neurological disease and neuropsychiatric complications. Patients with Wilson's disease have elevated serum free copper, urinary copper and hepatic copper (via biopsy). Paradoxically, total serum copper is usually low.

Samuel Alexander Wilson, British neurologist (1878–1937).

2. L – Total iron-binding capacity

Hereditary haemochromatosis is a common autosomal recessive disease in which there is excessive intestinal absorption of iron. The excess iron is deposited in tissues such as the liver (resulting in cirrhosis), myocardium (leading to heart failure), endocrine organs (causing diabetes), skin (giving a tanned appearance) and joints. Patients often present in middle age, with males presenting earlier than females owing to the protective effect of menstruation. Investigations will usually show a raised ferritin, a reduced total iron-binding capacity (due to saturation) and a transferrin saturation >60%. Liver biopsy will often reveal parenchymal iron overload with or without cirrhosis.

3. C – Antimitochondrial antibody

Primary biliary cirrhosis is thought to be an autoimmune disease in which chronic granulomatous inflammation of the interlobular bile ducts causes cirrhosis, portal hypertension and liver failure. It tends to affect middle-aged women, who usually present with pruritis and deranged liver function tests. Xanthelasmas are a recognized feature (as in this case). Up to 98% of patients with primary biliary cirrhosis are positive for the highly specific antimitochondrial antibody M2 subtype. Other investigations used to diagnose primary biliary cirrhosis include hepatic ultrasound imaging, endoscopic retrograde cholangiopancreatography (ERCP) and liver biopsy. The treatment of primary biliary cirrhosis is largely symptomatic. Cholestyramine is used to treat pruritis, and ursodeoxycholic acid may improve ascites and jaundice but is unlikely to prolong life. Without liver transplantation, most patients will die approximately 2 years after the development of jaundice.

4. I – Hepatitis A IgM

Hepatitis A is caused by an RNA virus that is transmitted by the faecal–oral route. It often presents with a non-specific lethargic illness that is followed by the development of jaundice. The earliest serological marker of acute infection is hepatitis A immunoglobulin M (IgM) antibody. Hepatitis A IgG antibodies develop later in the course of the disease, and remain for many years. Hepatitis IgG antibodies usually convey immunity to the disease.

5. K – Hepatitis C antibody

Hepatitis C is caused by an RNA virus that is transmitted through sexual activities and blood products, including the sharing of needles among intravenous drug users. The acute infection is often silent, with many individuals being completely asymptomatic. Hepatitis C antibodies can be used to diagnose previous infection, but take up to 3 months to develop. Approximately 85% of patients with acute hepatitis C infection go on to become chronic carriers, which carries a significant risk of developing cirrhosis, liver failure and hepatocellular carcinoma.

Theme 7: Complications of renal failure

1. E – Intravenous erythropoietin

This patient has a normocytic anaemia secondary to chronic renal failure. This form of anaemia is likely to have a multifactorial aetiology, but is mainly due to the reduced secretion of erythropoietin from the damaged kidneys. This anaemia cannot be corrected by iron supplementation alone, as iron stores are usually normal. Recombinant erythropoietin can be given as intravenous and subcutaneous infusions to patients with normocytic anaemia secondary to chronic renal failure to stimulate erythrogenesis. When erythropoietin is prescribed, ferritin levels should be closely monitored. If ferritin levels are low then oral or intravascular iron may be given.

2. B – Alfacalcidol

This patient is hypocalcaemic. Hypocalcaemia in chronic renal failure is due to reduced synthesis of vitamin D. In health, cholecalciferol is formed within the skin in response to sunlight. Cholecalciferol is hydroxylated in the liver to form 25-hydroxycholecalciferol, which is then hydroxylated again in the kidney by 1α-hydroxylase to form 1,25-dihydroxycholecalciferol. This is the active form of vitamin D, which increases the absorption of calcium from the gastrointestinal tract, increases the reabsorption of calcium and phosphate from the kidneys, and reduces parathyroid hormone secretion. The hypocalcaemia of renal failure is treated by supplementing the active form of vitamin D with calcitriol (1,25-dihydroxycholecalciferol) and alfacalcidol (1-hydroxycholecalciferol).

3. I – Oral calcium channel blocker and fluid restriction

Hypertension is an important and common complication of chronic renal failure. Hypertension is largely due to fluid retention, although increased renin secretion may play a role, especially when renal vascular disease is present. Fluid restriction may be enough to reduce the patient's blood pressure. Oral antihypertensive agents such as calcium channel blockers or β-blockers may also be prescribed. Caution should be taken in prescribing ACE inhibitors, as they can worsen renal failure and promote hyperkalaemia. In patients receiving dialysis, the regimen can be altered to remove fluid as well as waste products in a process known as ultrafiltration.

4. L – Statin therapy

Patients with nephrotic syndrome lose large amounts of protein in the urine. The low serum oncotic pressure that results from the loss of albumin stimulates the liver to increase lipoprotein synthesis, causing hyperlipidaemia and accelerated atherosclerosis. Hypercholesterolaemia in nephrotic syndrome should be treated with a statin such as simvastatin or atorvastatin.

5. N – Urgent dialysis

This patient is suffering from uraemic encephalopathy. The high levels of serum urea cross the blood–brain barrier, causing fluctuating confusion, cognitive impairment, myoclonic jerks and seizures. The actual mechanism by which urea induces encephalopathy is likely to be much more complex than simply interfering with neurotransmitter release, although there is thought to be an element of this. The ultimate treatment of uraemic encephalopathy is with dialysis (haemodialysis or peritoneal dialysis), which removes urea and other waste products from the plasma. In an emergency when haemodialysis cannot be performed, it is possible to remove urea from the plasma using haemofiltration, which is available in most intensive care units.

Theme 8: Emergency management

1. C – Insert a cannula into the second intercostal space in the midclavicular line

This patient has a tension pneumothorax requiring urgent decompression. In tension pneumothorax, air enters the pleural space with each breath but cannot escape. Eventually, the pressure is sufficient to displace the mediastinum and compress the great vessels, resulting in circulatory collapse, cardiogenic shock and eventual death. Clinical findings in tension pneumothorax include tachypnoea, tachycardia, a trachea displaced away from the affected side, reduced chest wall movement on the affected side, hyper-resonance to percussion on the affected side and reduced breath sounds on the affected side. If a tension pneumothorax is suspected, it must be treated immediately without further investigation. To decompress the pneumothorax, a large-bore cannula should be inserted into the second intercostal space in the midclavicular line. When the cannula is in situ and the needle is removed, there should be a hiss of air to indicate decompression. Once the patient is stabilized, a formal chest drain with a water seal should be inserted.

2. F – Intramuscular benzylpenicillin and call ambulance

This child has the clinical features of meningitis with septicaemia (neck stiffness in association with general illness and a non-blanching purpuric rash). It is essential that this patient be given antibiotics as soon as possible and admitted to a paediatric high-dependency unit. If the patient is seen in the community, they should be given an intramuscular dose of benzylpenicillin while transport to hospital is being arranged. Once in hospital, the patient will require intravenous antibiotics (e.g. cefotaxime) for at least 7 days, in addition to supportive measures.

3. B – High-dose steroids

It is likely that this patient has giant cell arteritis (GCA). GCA is a form of vasculitis that affects the medium and large arteries of the head and neck. It commonly affects the temporal artery and presents with general illness, scalp tenderness, jaw claudication and temporal headache. Later features include optic nerve neuropathy and sudden blindness. All patients in whom giant cell arteritis is suspected should have their erythrocyte sedimentation rate (ESR) measured and receive high-dose oral steroids, e.g. 60 mg prednisolone daily. A temporal artery biopsy should be arranged, but may not be diagnostic, since the lesions within the artery may 'skip', leaving some areas with normal histology. It is important to get an early ophthalmological opinion if the eyes are involved (as in this case).

4. H – Intravenous lorazepam

In any situation, it is essential to ensure that the patient's airway, breathing and circulation are intact before progressing to the management of any underlying condition. The first-line antiepileptic medication used in seizure is intravenous lorazepam. It is important to have full resuscitation equipment available when administering intravenous benzodiazepines, since there is a risk of respiratory arrest. If intravenous access is not possible, alternative options include rectal diazepam or buccal midazolam. If the benzodiazepines fail to stop the seizure, an intravenous infusion of phenytoin should be started. If this fails, an anaesthetist should be called to initiate general anaesthesia.

5. K – Jaw thrust

This patient has potentially sustained a cervical spine injury that, if manipulated, could result in significant neurological disability or death. The patient also has a partial upper airway obstruction, indicated by the snoring respiratory noises. In line with the ABC approach, it is essential to secure the airway first. The most appropriate manoeuvre to open the airway of a patient with potential cervical spine injury is the jaw thrust. The jaw thrust requires the rescuer to grip the angle of the mandible with the index and middle fingers and lift using counter-traction, achieved by placing the thumbs on the cheek bones. This manoeuvre will open the upper airway while maintaining the stability of the cervical spine. The other commonly used airway manoeuvre is the head tilt/chin lift. This manoeuvre involves significant manipulation of the cervical spine, and is therefore contraindicated in patients with potential cervical spine injury. However, if a jaw thrust has failed to open the airway of a patient with potential cervical spine injury, the lone rescuer can use the head tilt/chin lift. In this situation, the angle of head tilt should be gradually increased until the airway is opened.

Theme 9: Investigation of endocrine disease

1. B – 24-hour urinary vanillylmandelic acid

This man presents with uncontrollable hypertension and attacks of anxiety, sweating and palpitations. Along with facial flushing and headaches, these are classic presenting features of phaeochromocytomas.

Phaeochromocytomas are tumours of the adrenal medulla (the central part of the adrenal gland). They arise from chromaffin cells and secrete large amounts of catecholamines. Breakdown products of catecholamines include vanillylmandelic acid (VMA), which is excreted in the kidney. Therefore, the suspicion of phaeochromocytoma can be strengthened by finding an increased concentration of urinary VMA over a 24-hour period. An abdominal CT will help localize the tumour.

Phaeochromocytomas are associated with a '10% rule': 10% are malignant, 10% are extra-adrenal, 10% are familial and 10% are bilateral. Familial phaeochromocytomas can be associated with three main conditions: neurofibromatosis, multiple endocrine neoplasia and von Hippel–Lindau syndrome (which is characterized by phaeochromocytomas, retinal haemangioblastomas, clear-cell renal carcinomas and pancreatic neuroendocrine tumours). The treatment of phaeochromocytomas is by surgical excision, but, prior to this, α-blockers need to be given for 6 weeks to inhibit the effects of a sudden surge of catecholamines that may occur intraoperatively. A normal life expectancy is expected if treatment is successful.

2. H – Short Synacthen test

This woman presents with postural hypotension. She has vitiligo and some areas of increased skin pigmentation, making her likely to have Addison's disease. The best investigation to perform is the short Synacthen test.

Addison's disease is primary autoimmune-mediated adrenocortical failure. The action of the adrenal cortex can be described in simplified terms as the secretion of three things: glucocorticoids, mineralocorticoids and adrenal androgens. These usually feed back to the anterior pituitary to reduce ACTH (adrenocorticotropic hormone, also known as corticotropin) secretion. Therefore, failure of the adrenal cortex has many consequences: reduced glucocorticoids (leading to hypoglycaemia and weight loss), reduced mineralocorticoids (leading to hyperkalaemia, hyponatraemia and hypotension), reduced adrenal androgens (leading to decreased body hair and libido) and ACTH excess (leading to increased pigmentation in sun-exposed areas, pressure areas, palmar creases, buccal mucosa and recent scars). The diagnosis of Addison's disease is by the short Synacthen test. In this investigation, plasma cortisol levels are measured before and half an hour after administration of a single intramuscular dose of ACTH. Normally, the ACTH will result in a rise in cortisol. If there is no rise in cortisol on the second reading, adrenal insufficiency is indicated. Management of Addison's disease is with the replacement of glucocorticoids and mineralocorticoids (with hydrocortisone and fludrocortisone).

Thomas Addison, English physician (1795–1860).

3. E – Dexamethasone suppression test

This woman presents with hirsutism, striae, acne, plethora and bruising, all of which are features of Cushing's syndrome. Other features include psychosis, cataracts, poor skin healing, hyperglycaemia and proximal myopathy. Because the patient has a small cell lung tumour, the cause of her Cushing's syndrome could be ectopic ACTH secretion from the malignancy. The diagnosis of Cushing's syndrome is by finding a raised 24-hour free urinary cortisol or with the dexamethasone suppression test (not a random cortisol, which is useless as cortisol has a natural diurnal variation). In the dexamethasone suppression test, there is a high serum cortisol level that is not suppressed by dexamethasone.

Harvey Cushing, American neurosurgeon and endocrinologist (1869–1939).

4. A - 17-Hydroxyprogesterone levels

The presentation of clitoromegaly, precocious puberty and accelerated growth in this young girl is indicative of congenital adrenal hyperplasia (CAH). This is an autosomal recessive deficiency of the enzyme 21-hydroxylase. This enzyme is required to synthesize mineralocorticoids and glucocorticoids (but not adrenal androgens) from the hormone precursor 17-hydroxyprogesterone. Because there is a lack of mineralocorticoids and glucocorticoids, there is no negative feedback on the anterior pituitary, resulting in increased ACTH secretion. The high ACTH then causes an increased secretion of adrenal androgens, since this does not require the deficient hormone. The androgens result in the physical features of CAH, namely ambiguous genitalia (in girls), precocious puberty (in girls), accelerated growth in childhood and virilization. The diagnosis of CAH is suggested by finding a raised concentration of the precursor 17-hydroxyprogesterone. Treatment is with hydrocortisone and fludrocortisone to replace the deficient steroids.

5. C - 24-hour urinary 5-hydroxyindole acetic acid

The features of paroxysmal flushing, diarrhoea, bronchospasm and abdominal pain precipitated by stress, alcohol and caffeine strongly suggest carcinoid syndrome.

Carcinoid tumours are tumours of enterochromaffin cells of the gastrointestinal tract (most commonly of the appendix, ileum or rectum) that secrete serotonin (5-hydroxytryptamine, 5-HT). The secreted 5-HT is carried from the bowel, via the portal vein, to the liver, where it is harmlessly broken down. However, when carcinoid tumours metastasize to the liver, they can secrete 5-HT directly into the bloodstream, bypassing liver metabolism and resulting in the symptoms described above. The presence of carcinoid metastases in the liver that result in symptoms is known as *carcinoid syndrome*. The diagnosis of carcinoid syndrome is by measuring 24-hour urinary 5-hydroxyindole acetic acid (5-HIAA), a breakdown product of 5-HT. Management is by resection or, in widespread disease, symptomatic treatment with octreotide (a somatostatin analogue that inhibits 5-HT release). Carcinoid tumours are slow growing so, even if disseminated disease is present, patients can live for many years.

Theme 10: Dementia 2

1. L – Wernicke's encephalopathy

Wernicke's encephalopathy is a reversible condition caused by a severe deficiency of thiamine (vitamin B_1). It is often associated with alcohol abuse, the processes involved being a lack of adequate oral intake, hyperemesis and malabsorption caused by gastrointestinal lesions. The triad of features in Wernicke's syndrome is confusion, ataxia and nystagmus. Ophthalmoplegia is also an important feature. If untreated, Wernicke's encephalopathy can lead to the irreversible *Korsakoff's syndrome*, characterized by confusion, anterograde and retrograde amnesia, and confabulation.

Karl Wernicke, German psychiatrist (1848–1905).

Sergei Korsakoff, Russian neuropsychiatrist (1854–1900).

2. A – Alzheimer's disease

Alzheimer's disease is the most common type of dementia. There is global brain atrophy, with deposition of β-amyloid protein in the brain. Features include gradual progressive cognitive decline, apathy/lability of mood, personality deterioration, paranoia and parkinsonian features. The diagnosis is made by excluding other causes of dementia. The mainstay of treatment is with acetylcholinesterase inhibitors (donepezil, galantamine and rivastigmine) which increase concentrations of the neurotransmitter acetylcholine, although these drugs may only be effective in a select proportion of cases. Early onset Alzheimer's disease (<65 years) can occur in people with Down's syndrome and in those who inherit the amyloid precursor or presenilin proteins.

Alois Alzheimer, German psychiatrist (1864–1915).

The *Mini-Mental State Examination* (published by Marshal Folstein, an American psychiatrist, in 1975) is a useful cognitive test marked out of 30 points. A score of 23–26 demonstrates mild cognitive impairment, 16–22 moderate and <15 severe. A quicker method of assessing cognitive function is the Hodkinson Abbreviated Mental Test Score (AMTS), which requires individuals to provide answers to the following 10 items:

(a) Age?
(b) Time to the nearest hour?
(c) Remember and recall an address (e.g. '42 West Street').
(d) Year?
(e) Name of the hospital?
(f) Recognize two people (e.g. doctor, nurse).
(g) Date of birth?
(h) Dates of the First World War?
(i) Name of the present monarch?
(j) Count backwards from 20 to 1.

An AMTS of 6 or less is often used to indicate cognitive impairment.

3. C – Depressive pseudodementia

Pseudodementia is recognized in people with severe depression. Their apparent cognitive dysfunction is heavily affected by their lack of motivation. The mood disturbance precedes the cognitive impairment, and patients may not try during formal assessments, often providing 'don't know' responses to questions asked. They are more likely to complain of memory loss, whereas someone with true dementia is more likely to confabulate and try to hide it. Depressive pseudodementia is a diagnosis of exclusion in someone with depression, and management aims to treat the underlying mood disorder.

4. E – Huntington's disease

Huntington's disease is an autosomal dominant disorder with excess CAG trinucleotide repeats on chromosome 4. This results in the destruction of certain extrapyramidal areas in the brain. Onset is usually in mid-adulthood. Features include choreiform movements, with an increased rate of depression, schizophrenia and suicide. Seizures may be a late feature. Insight tends to be maintained for much of the early course. Diagnosis is clinical, but can be confirmed by DNA analysis. Management is symptomatic.

George Huntington, American physician (1850–1916).

Choreiform, from Greek *chorea* = dance.

5. D – HIV-related dementia

HIV-related dementia (also known as AIDS dementia complex) occurs years after initial infection. It presents with reduced cognitive function, low energy and libido, general apathy, and eventually muscle spasticity with hyperreflexia, incontinence and ataxia. It is caused by the virus itself rather than an opportunistic infection. Diagnosis is based on clinical probability.

Theme 11: Heart sounds

1. N – Summation gallop rhythm

A gallop rhythm is heard when the first (S_1) and second (S_2) heart sounds are followed by a pathological third (S_3) and/or fourth (S_4) heart sound. It is most commonly associated with left ventricular failure. When this rhythm is associated with tachycardia, the heart sounds cannot be individually distinguished and therefore 'summate' into a single sound. The third heart sound occurs in early diastole, and is caused by the rush of blood entering the ventricle as it relaxes. The presence of a third heart sound can be a normal finding in those below 40 years of age, but when pathological is associated with cardiac failure, mitral regurgitation and dilated cardiomyopathy. On auscultation, the presence of a third heart sound is thought to resemble the phonetic pronunciation of the word 'Kentucky'.

The fourth heart sound occurs just before the first heart sound in the cardiac cycle. It is caused by the atria contracting against abnormally stiff ventricles, and is always pathological. A fourth heart sound can be heard in left ventricular hypertrophy, e.g. caused by aortic stenosis, systemic hypertension, amyloidosis and hypertrophic obstructive cardiomyopathy. On auscultation, the presence of a fourth heart sound is thought to resemble the phonetic pronunciation of the word 'Tennessee'. Both third and fourth heart sounds are best auscultated with the bell, with the patient leaning to the left.

2. K – Pansystolic murmur heard best at the apex with radiation into the axilla

Mitral regurgitation is usually associated with valvular heart disease such as rheumatic fever; however, it may also be secondary to functional dilatation of the left ventricle as seen in conditions such as dilated cardiomyopathy and Marfan's syndrome. Acute mitral regurgitation can occur in the setting of myocardial infarction, when there is necrosis and rupture of the chordae tendineae that usually anchor the valve leaflets in place. Other features of mitral regurgitation include the presence of atrial fibrillation, a systolic thrill, a displaced thrusting apex beat and a quiet first heart sound. Chest X-ray and ECG both show signs of left atrial and ventricular hypertrophy. Valve replacement should be considered in the case of worsening and refractory symptoms prior to the development of irreversible left ventricular damage.

3. C – Ejection systolic murmur heard at the right second intercostal space only

Aortic sclerosis is caused by age-related degeneration of the aortic valve. The condition is asymptomatic and is usually picked up incidentally. On auscultation, there is an ejection systolic murmur heard only in the aortic area, with no associated radiation or ejection click. Aortic stenosis, on the other hand, is usually symptomatic, causing a classic triad of exertional dyspnoea, exertional angina and exertional syncope. Sudden death may also be precipitated. The symptoms of aortic stenosis are due to left ventricular outflow obstruction and myocardial ischaemia secondary to left ventricular hypertrophy. It is a pathological condition caused by rheumatic fever, senile calcification of the valve or a congenital bicuspid aortic valve. On auscultation, there is an ejection systolic murmur that is best heard with the diaphragm in the aortic area (second right intercostal space) and that radiates into the carotid arteries. This may or may not be associated with an ejection click. Other signs of aortic stenosis include a non-displaced left ventricular heave and a slow-rising carotid pulse.

An ECG may show signs of left ventricular hypertrophy and strain (ST depression and inverted T-waves in leads II, III, aVL, V5 and V6). In the presence of worsening symptoms, patients may be considered for valve replacement. In those with multiple comorbidities, a percutaneous valvuloplasty may be more appropriate.

4. F – Muffled heart sounds

This patient has a pericardial effusion secondary to systemic lupus erythematosus. The fluid that has accumulated in the pericardium distorts the heart sounds, making them appear muffled on auscultation. Other signs of pericardial effusion include a globular heart on chest X-ray and complexes of reduced amplitude on ECG. Definitive diagnosis is usually with echocardiography. The chronic nature of this effusion has allowed the patient time to compensate and remain haemodynamically stable. In patients presenting with an acute pericardial effusion (e.g. haemopericardium secondary to trauma), relatively small amounts of fluid may restrict the heart, resulting in cardiogenic shock and death unless the effusion is drained rapidly via pericardiocentesis.

5. A – Austin Flint murmur

Causes of aortic regurgitation include aortic dilatation (in Marfan's syndrome), infective endocarditis and rheumatic fever. The Austin Flint murmur is heard in patients with significant aortic regurgitation. It is a mid-diastolic low-pitched rumbling murmur best heard at the apex. The murmur is caused when a regurgitated jet of blood passes through the damaged aortic valve and strikes the anterior leaflet of the mitral valve. The more common murmur of aortic regurgitation is a high-pitched early diastolic murmur best heard along the left sternal border with the patient leaning forward at the end of expiration (which is not an option in the present case).

Other signs of aortic regurgitation include a collapsing pulse, capillary pulsation in the nail beds (Quincke's sign), 'pistol shot' femoral bruits (Traube's sign) and visible carotid pulsation (Corrigan's sign). A Graham Steell murmur describes an early diastolic crescendo murmur that may be heard if pulmonary valve regurgitation complicates an underlying mitral stenosis.

Austin Flint, American physician (1812–86)

Theme 12: Management of skin disease

1. E – Intravenous antibiotics

Erysipelas is a superficial streptococcal infection that is confined to a fascial compartment and is often found on the face or legs. It presents as a painful red swelling with a characteristically well-defined edge. Erysipelas is treated initially with 2 days of intravenous antibiotics followed by a 1- to 2-week oral course. If it is not treated early, then infection can spread deeper and wider to become cellulitis or necrotizing fasciitis.

Erysipelas, from Greek *erusi* = red + *pelas* skin.

2. H – Surgical excision

This man has a sebaceous cyst (also known as an 'epidermal cyst'). Sebaceous cysts arise from hair follicles in any part of the body (especially the scalp, face, ears, back and upper arms) and contain keratin. They are painless and mobile and often have a central punctum. Although they are not attached to the subcutaneous tissues below, sebaceous cysts are fixed to the overlying skin. They are benign and can be ignored, but, if the patient is worried about cosmesis, excision is performed.

3. G – Surgical debridement and intravenous antibiotics

Necrotizing fasciitis (also known as the 'flesh-eating bug') is a deep infection of the skin most often caused by a group A streptococcus (e.g. *S. pyogenes*). Infection often starts in an area of trauma or surgery. Affected areas become erythematous and swollen, and tissue soon becomes necrotic. Patients feel systemically unwell and have a high fever. The infection spreads rapidly, and the mortality rate is as high as 30%. Management is therefore aggressive, with intravenous broad-spectrum antibiotics and extensive surgical debridement of infected tissues to prevent further spread. Without surgery, necrotizing fasciitis is fatal.

4. F – Oral antibiotics

Impetigo is a superficial skin infection caused by staphylococci or streptococci. It generally occurs in children, and presents with thin-walled blisters that itch and bleed and have a superficial golden-yellow crust. These lesions eventually heal without scarring. Impetigo is contagious and requires treatment. If there are only a few lesions, treatment is with bactericidal ointment, such as fusidic acid. If there are many lesions, topical therapy would be inappropriate, so oral flucloxacillin is given instead.

Impetigo, from Latin *impetere* = to assail, referring to its aggressively contagious nature.

5. I – Reassurance

This boy has Peutz–Jeghers syndrome, a condition characterized by multiple bluish-black freckles around the lips, nose, oral mucosa and fingers, as well as multiple gastrointestinal hamartomatous polyps. These polyps are benign and have only a very low malignant potential. The polyps may predispose to gastrointestinal bleeding or intussusceptions, but, in the asymptomatic patient, reassurance is sufficient.

Johannes Augustinus Peutz, Dutch physician (1886–1957).

Harold Joseph Jeghers, American physician (1904–90).

Theme 13: Connective tissue disease

1. F – Polymyositis

Polymyositis is a rare inflammatory disorder of skeletal muscle. Patients present with proximal muscle weakness (hips and shoulder), which may manifest as difficulty in climbing stairs or in standing up from a sitting position. This may be accompanied by swelling, tenderness and wasting of the affected muscle. Blood tests reveal a raised creatine kinase (CK), but the definitive investigation is muscle biopsy, which demonstrates inflammation and necrosis. Polymyositis is associated with underlying malignancy. Anti-Jo-1 antibodies may be present. Treatment is with steroids and immunosuppressants.

Some cases of polymyositis are accompanied by characteristic skin changes – this combination is known as *dermatomyositis*. The skin features include a heliotrope (purple) discoloration of the eyelids, scaly red–purple raised papules over the knuckles and elbows (Gottron's papules), and periungual telangiectasia. If the skin features occur in the absence of muscle weakness, it is known as *amyopathic dermatomyositis*.

Heinrich Adolf Gottron, German dermatologist (1890–1974).

Heliotrope, from Greek *helios* = sun + *tropein* = to turn; so called as the leaves of this purple flower turn towards the sun.

2. A – Antiphospholipid syndrome

Antiphospholipid syndrome is characterized by recurrent arterial and venous thromboses (pulmonary embolism, deep vein thrombosis, stroke and peripheral thrombosis), recurrent miscarriage and thrombocytopenia. The diagnosis is confirmed by the presence of specific autoantibodies (anticardiolipin and lupus anticoagulase). Note that the presence of the anticardiolipin antibody will lead to a false-positive VDRL (Venereal Disease Reference Laboratory – syphilis) test. The management of antiphospholipid syndrome involves avoidance of thrombotic risk factors, including smoking and the contraceptive pill, and treating hypertension, hyperlipidaemia and diabetes. Patients who have no history of thrombosis should take low-dose aspirin. After the first thrombotic episode, lifelong warfarin is taken, aiming for an INR of 2.5. If a patient is planning on getting pregnant, warfarin should be stopped (as it is teratogenic) and subcutaneous heparin used instead.

3. D – Limited cutaneous systemic sclerosis

Systemic sclerosis is a connective tissue disorder characterized by thickening and fibrosis of the skin (scleroderma) with involvement of internal organs. There are two forms: a limited cutaneous type (60%) and a diffuse cutaneous type (40%). Limited cutaneous scleroderma is limited to the distal limbs (i.e. distal to the elbows and knees). Other features include a beaked nose and small, furrowed mouth (microstoma). Limited cutaneous scleroderma also encompasses the CREST syndrome, which is characterized by calcinosis, Raynaud's phenomenon, oesophageal dysmotility, sclerodactyly and telangiectasia. Calcinosis is the formation of calcium deposits in the soft tissues, often seen on the pulps of the fingers. Raynaud's phenomenon is an idiopathic condition with episodic digital vasospasm precipitated by a cold environment, as a result of which the affected fingers or toes become white and may be painful. Oesophageal dysmotility is manifested as dysphagia and reflux. Sclerodactyly describes the presence of tight, shiny skin over the fingers, producing a fixed flexion deformity. In limited cutaneous scleroderma, the anticentromere antibody is characteristically positive. Pulmonary hypertension is a common internal manifestation.

Diffuse cutaneous scleroderma can involve the whole skin of the body. Patients are characteristically positive for the anti-SCL-70 antibody (also known as antitopoisomerase II). In this form of the disease, patients are particularly at risk of a 'renal crisis' – a life-threatening malignant hypertension with rapid renal impairment. In contrast, pulmonary hypertension is less common. Diffuse cutaneous systemic sclerosis has a worse prognosis than limited cutaneous disease. The treatment of systemic sclerosis is with steroids and immunosuppressants. Penicillamine slows skin disease (steroids do not help the skin). Lung fibrosis is the main cause of death, followed by renal disease.

Scleroderma can occur without internal organ disease (localized scleroderma). If this occurs in plaques, it is known as morphea; if it occurs in lines it is termed *en coup de sabre*. 'Scleroderma *sine* scleroderma' is the term used when patients have typical vascular or internal organ features of systemic sclerosis but without the cutaneous sclerosis.

Morphea, from Greek *morpha* = shape.

En coup de sabre, from French = cut of the sword.

Scleroderma, from Latin *skleros* = hard + *dermis* = skin.

Maurice Raynaud, French physician (1834–81).

4. G – Sjögren's syndrome

The main features of Sjogren's syndrome are dry eyes (keratoconjunctivitis sicca) and dry mouth (xerostoma). Other features are corneal ulcers, oral candida, vaginal dryness, dyspareunia and respiratory hoarseness. Diagnosis is with Schirmer's test: a 35 mm-long piece of filter paper is placed under the lower eyelid for 5 minutes – if less than 10 mm becomes moist, it indicates Sjögren's syndrome. Anti-Ro and Anti-La antibodies may be present. Treatment is with artificial tears and artificial saliva.

Henrik Sjögren, Swedish ophthalmologist (1899–1986).

5. H – Systemic lupus erythematosus

Systemic lupus erythematosus (SLE) is most common in middle-aged women, and is characterized by arthralgia (joint pain) and rashes. Flare-ups of disease may be triggered by sunlight, the contraceptive pill, infection and stress. Common features are non-erosive arthritis (Jaccoud's arthritis), a discoid rash on the body, a rash over the cheeks and nose (butterfly rash), fever, depression and myalgia. Features can occur in many systems, and a diagnosis of SLE requires four or more of the following ('A RASH POINTs MD'):

Arthralgia
Renal disease: nephrotic syndrome
Antinuclear antibody
Serositis: pleurisy, pleural effusion, pericarditis
Haematological disorders: pancytopenia
Photosensitivity
Oral ulcers
Immunology (autoantibodies): anti-dsDNA, anti-Smith
Neurological problems: depression, psychosis
Malar rash
Discoid rash.

SLE is also associated with a non-infective endocarditis (Libman–Sacks endocarditis). Treatment of SLE is with analgesia, steroids and immunosuppressants. Lupus can be induced by certain drugs, e.g. isoniazid and penicillamine. Drug-induced lupus is associated with antihistone antibodies. Discoid lupus is a benign variant in which there is skin involvement only.

Sigismond Jaccoud, Swiss physician (1830–1913).

Overlap syndromes describe cases in which patients have more than one connective tissue disease simultaneously, e.g. SLE + scleroderma. Overlap syndromes are associated with anti-U1-RNP antibody.

Theme 14: Diagnosis of haematological disease

1. F – Multiple myeloma

In multiple myeloma, there is a malignant proliferation of plasma cells that secrete monoclonal antibodies and light immunoglobulin chains. Multiple myeloma is a multisystem disease that may present with lethargy, bone pain, pathological fracture, renal failure, amyloidosis and pancytopenia due to marrow infiltration. Diagnosis requires two of the following three criteria: marrow plasmacytosis, serum/urinary immunoglobulin light chains (Bence Jones protein) and skeletal lesions (osteolytic lesions, pepperpot skull and pathological fractures). People who have evidence of serum or urine monoclonal antibodies but do not fill the criteria for multiple myeloma are said to have *monoclonal gammopathy of uncertain significance*, which has a 2% annual risk of transforming into multiple myeloma. Treatment of multiple myeloma aims to improve symptoms and suppress disease activity. Bone pain may be controlled with analgesia, bisphosphonates and orthopaedic intervention. Renal failure, caused by the deposition of light chains within the kidney, is usually managed by promoting fluid intake, although renal replacement therapy may be required. Infection, anaemia and bleeding caused by pancytopenia secondary to marrow infiltration can be managed with broad-spectrum antimicrobials, erythropoietin therapy and blood product replacement, respectively. In patients less than 55 years of age, allogeneic stem cell transplantation offers a hope of cure, but has a treatment-related mortality rate of 30% and is associated with significant morbidity from treatment-related side-effects. Chemotherapy (melphalan and prednisolone) is often used to suppress disease activity, but is generally viewed as palliative. Survival is usually less than 4 years, with death occurring secondary to renal failure or infection.

Henry Bence Jones, English physician (1813–73).

2. D – Hodgkin's lymphoma

Hodgkin's lymphoma has a bimodal age distribution, with peak incidences occurring in the third and sixth decades. Is it usually of B-cell origin and is associated with a history of glandular fever. It classically presents with asymmetrical painless lymphadenopathy, usually in the form of a single rubbery lymph node in the cervical, axillary or inguinal region, which may become painful after alcohol ingestion. Disease spread to the mediastinal nodes may cause dyspnoea and superior vena caval obstruction. Approximately 20% of patients suffer systemic symptoms such as weight loss, sweating, fever, pruritis and general lethargy. These are known as 'B' symptoms and are associated with a worse prognosis. Diagnosis is usually based on lymph node biopsy showing pathognomonic Reed--Sternberg cells (large malignant B cells). CT is used to assess spread, and staging is by the Ann Arbor system (I = one node region involved; II = two or more ipsilateral regions; III = bilateral node involvement; IV = extranodal disease). Early stage disease is usually managed with radiotherapy alone. In advanced and bulky disease, a combination of radiotherapy and chemotherapy is often employed. The prognosis of Hodgkin's lymphoma is usually good, with a 70% chance of cure even in late-stage disease. Increasing age indicates a poorer prognosis.

Non-Hodgkin's lymphoma (NHL) is most common in people in their 70s and is associated with Epstein–Barr virus (EBV), HIV and *Helicobacter pylori* infection. It is usually of B-cell origin. NHL also presents with painless lymphadenopathy (with or without systemic symptoms) and is staged using the Ann Arbor classification. Diagnosis is with lymph node biopsy, and management is with chemotherapy (e.g. CHOP: cyclophosphamide, doxorubicin, vincristine, prednisolone). The median survival is 10 years.

Specific types of NHL include *Burkitt's lymphoma* (which frequently involves the jaw and is most often seen in African children with EBV infection) and *mycosis fungoides* (a cutaneous T-cell lymphoma).

Thomas Hodgkin, British physician (1798–1866).

Denis Parsons Burkitt, Irish surgeon (1911–93).

Ann Arbor, a city in the US state of Michigan, where a committee on Hodgkin's disease staging classification met and revised the staging of lymphoma.

3. J – Polycythaemia rubra vera

Polycythaemia rubra vera is a myeloproliferative disorder characterized by raised haemoglobin, red cell count and packed cell volume (haematocrit). The condition is caused by mutation of a single pluripotent stem cell that results in excessive production of erythrocytes and, to a lesser degree, platelets and neutrophils. As a result, the blood becomes extremely viscous, causing an increased risk of arterial and venous thrombosis and paradoxical bleeding. Patients often complain of headache, lethargy and pruritis, which is classically worse after bathing in warm water. Treatment of polycythaemia rubra vera involves venesection (bloodletting) and chemotherapy with hydroxyurea. If treated appropriately, patients tend to survive for many years and often die from unrelated causes. Approximately 30% of patients will develop myelofibrosis (below) and 5% will develop acute myeloid leukaemia (AML) as part of the disease's natural history.

Polycythaemia, from Greek *poly* = many + *kytos* = cell.

Rubra vera, from Latin *rubra* = red + *vera* = true.

4. K – Secondary polycythaemia

Secondary polycythaemia is usually caused by increased secretion of erythropoietin as part of the physiological response to hypoxia in conditions such as chronic obstructive pulmonary disease and cyanotic heart disease. Less frequently, erythropoietin is secreted ectopically from tumour cells (e.g. renal cell carcinomas). Occasionally, the condition is iatrogenic – caused by the overuse of artificial erythropoietin in the treatment of conditions such as anaemia of chronic renal failure. Treatment of secondary polycythaemia involves managing the underlying disease and symptomatic venesection.

5. G – Myelofibrosis

Myelofibrosis is a myeloproliferative disease characterized by the replacement of erythropoietic bone marrow with inert fibrotic material. The disease originates from a single abnormal pluripotent stem cell that populates the marrow with abnormal megakaryocytes, which in turn secrete factors known to stimulate fibrosis. Intramedullary fibrosis causes marrow failure and subsequent pancytopenia. In response to anaemia, extramedullary erythropoiesis in the liver and spleen produces the common finding of massive hepatosplenomegaly. Diagnosis is usually based on the combination of a pancytopenic blood film with characteristic tear-drop poikilocytes, a dry bone marrow aspirate and a trephine biopsy showing dense fibrosis of the bone marrow. Myelofibrosis is treated symptomatically with blood transfusion, chemotherapy and splenectomy in severe cases. The average survival time is less than 5 years, although some patients survive for many years. Death usually occurs due to the development of AML, infection or liver failure.

Waldenström's macroglobulinaemia is a lymphoproliferative disease similar to lymphoma and characterized by the production of immunoglobulin M (IgM) paraproteins. Clinical features are secondary to hyperviscosity (nosebleeds, blurred vision, retinal haemorrhage and confusion).

Poikilocyte, from Greek *poikilos* = irregular.

Jan Gosta Waldenström, Swedish physician (1906–96).

Theme 15: Conditions of the vessel wall

1. B – Elective surgical repair

A true aneurysm is defined as an abnormal dilatation of an artery involving all three layers of the arterial wall. Adverse events associated with aneurysm formation include rupture, occlusion, distal ischaemia and thromboembolic disease. Abdominal aortic aneurysms tend to affect those over 50 years of age and are often asymptomatic prior to rupture, although patients sometimes complain of back and abdominal pain. Diagnosis is often incidental, and is usually confirmed by an abdominal ultrasound or CT scan.

Trials have shown that abdominal aortic aneurysms less than 5.5 cm in diameter have a low rate of rupture (1% per year) and can be monitored with regular abdominal ultrasound or CT scans. Aneurysms larger than 6 cm in diameter are at significant risk of rupture (25% per year), as are those shown to be expanding at a rate of more than 1 cm/year. In such cases, the patient should be considered for elective surgical repair. Individuals with multiple comorbidities who would be placed at high risk during open surgery may be considered for endovascular repair, in which a stent is placed in the abdominal aneurysm via the femoral or iliac artery. Endovascular repair is associated with fewer postoperative complications and a reduced 30-day mortality rate compared with open repair, but has more long-term complications, requires more intensive follow-up and is more likely to require further intervention.

2. F – No intervention necessary

When assessing abdominal aortic aneurysms and the need for intervention, the risks of rupture must be weighed against the risks of intervention and the impact that it may have on the patient's quality of life. In this case, the patient has multiple comorbidities, including metastatic malignancy, ischaemic heart disease, COPD and diabetes that place him at significant risk of mortality from the anaesthetic alone. The most appropriate and ethical course of action would be to avoid all intervention and maintain the patient's lifestyle since it is likely that the metastatic malignancy would end his life prior to the rupture of his aortic aneurysm.

3. E – Maintain systolic blood pressure at approximately 100 mmHg with fluid resuscitation while awaiting emergency surgical repair

Ruptured aortic aneurysms usually present with collapse that may or may not have been preceded by severe abdominal pain (which typically radiates to the back). A number of patients present with a loin pain that is not dissimilar to that of renal colic. Since renal colic is rare in elderly people, individuals who present in this way should be viewed with suspicion and a ruptured or leaking aneurysm excluded. Patients who have ruptured an aortic aneurysm are hypotensive, tachycardic, tachypnoeic and appear peripherally shut down and anxious. Since the mortality rate is effectively 100% if untreated, a ruptured aortic aneurysm requires urgent open surgical repair if the patient is suitable (the arguments in Case 2 are still applicable). The mainstay of treatment, while surgery is being organized, is fluid resuscitation to provide adequate blood pressure to perfuse the vital organs. The systolic blood pressure should be maintained at approximately 90–100 mmHg, as higher pressures are likely to disrupt clot formation around the site of the rupture and exacerbate bleeding. Survival rates vary between centres and surgeons, but as a rule are approximately 50–60% following rupture (compared with survival rates of 90–98% following elective repair).

4. H – Reduce systolic blood pressure to 100 mmHg using an intravenous antihypertensive agent and refer for emergency surgical repair

In aortic dissection, there is a split in the layers of the aorta, resulting in a 'false' and a 'true' lumen – the false lumen being larger. Risk factors include hypertension (80%), male gender, atherosclerosis, collagen disorders and trauma. Dissecting aortic aneurysms usually present with sudden-onset tearing chest pain that refers to the interscapular region of the back. Other features include hypertension, tachycardia, a widened mediastinum on chest X-ray and the CT finding of a double lumen within the aorta.

This case is an example of a type A aortic dissection, since it involves the ascending aorta. Type A dissections always require emergency surgical repair. Type B dissections, which begin distal to the origin of the left subclavian artery, can often be managed conservatively. In order to prevent the dissection from extending, the systolic blood pressure must be maintained at approximately 100 mmHg using intravenous antihypertensive agents such as labetalol while awaiting surgical repair.

5. L – Urgent ultrasound scan and compression

This man has developed a false aneurysm, which, by definition, involves only one or two layers of the vessel wall. A false femoral artery aneurysm is a recognized complication of angiography, as this artery is often used to gain access to the vasculature. People who use illict drugs may cause a false femoral aneurysm by inadvertently piercing the artery instead of the vein. Initial management is by compression. Ultrasound confirms the diagnosis. Some cases of false aneurysm will require surgical correction because of the risk of rupture, thrombosis and infection.

Practice Paper 5: Questions

Theme 1: Management of type 2 diabetes

Options

A. Acarbose
B. Dietary and lifestyle advice
C. Gliclazide
D. Glucagon
E. Insulin
F. Islet cell transplantation
G. Metformin
H. Rosiglitazone

For each of the following patients with diabetes, select the most appropriate management option. Each option may be used once, more than once or not at all.

1. A 65-year-old man is newly diagnosed with type 2 diabetes. He has no apparent macrovascular complications and an HbA_{1c} level of 8.5%.

2. A 65-year-old overweight man is failing to adequately control his blood glucose levels despite having the importance of lifestyle changes explained to him on several occasions over a 6-month period. His last HbA_{1c} level was 8.5%.

3. A 65-year-old woman with a body mass index of 23 is failing to adequately control her blood glucose levels despite having the importance of lifestyle changes explained to her on several occasions over a 6-month period. Her last HbA_{1c} level was 8.5%.

4. A 65-year-old overweight woman has extremely poor glycaemic control and evidence of macrovascular disease despite taking metformin, gliclazide and rosiglitazone.

5. A 65-year-old overweight man is failing to control his blood glucose despite taking the maximum daily dose of metformin.

Theme 2: Speech problems

Options

A. Broca's aphasia
B. Bulbar palsy
C. Cerebellar speech
D. Dysphonia
E. Lesion of the arcuate fasciculus
F. Psudobulbar palsy
G. Wernicke's aphasia

For each of the following scenarios, select the most appropriate cause of the speech disturbance. Each option may be used once, more than once or not at all.

1. A 29-year-old man is brought to the emergency department after being involved in a fight. He is clearly under the influence of alcohol and is aggressive towards staff. It is difficult to understand what he is saying, as the words are coming out slurred and muddled. He understands what the doctor is saying to him, and provides appropriate answers.

2. A 65-year-old man has recently suffered an acute right-sided hemiparesis. His wife now says that he talks gibberish. There is no evidence of a change in quality or speed of his speech. When you ask him what his name is, he replies 'Pleased to breakfast you'. Apart from the hemiparesis, examination is unremarkable.

3. A 67-year-old man presents to the GP with difficulty speaking and swallowing. This has been getting worse since a stroke 4 months ago. He has no problems with comprehension and is able to answer questions appropriately. On examination, the tongue appears small and contracted. The jaw jerk is brisk.

4. A 25-year-old man has an urgent operation to resect a papillary thyroid tumour. After the operation, he complains of a hoarse voice. He otherwise feels well and has no problems understanding and answering questions.

5. A 73-year-old woman, who recently suffered a stroke, is now having problems speaking. Her husband says that her speech is laboured and that she finds it difficult to get the right words out. When you ask her how she is, she replies 'Me....Margaret.....doctors.....well....'. When you ask her to point to the clock, she promptly does so.

Theme 3: Gastrointestinal radiology

Options

A. Achalasia
B. Crohn's disease
C. Hiatus hernia
D. Ischaemic colitis
E. Oesophageal spasm
F. Oesophagitis
G. Pancreatitis
H. Primary sclerosing cholangitis
I. Toxic megacolon
J. Ulcerative colitis
K. Visceral perforation

For each of the following descriptions, select the most likely diagnosis. Each option may be used once, more than once or not at all.

1. A 56-year-old man presents with severe upper abdominal pain. A chest X-ray shows free air under the right hemidiaphragm.

2. A 47-year-old woman presents with a short history of difficulty swallowing and intermittent regurgitation. On a barium swallow study, she is shown to have a proximally dilated oesophagus that tapers distally.

3. A 65-year-old woman is admitted with worsening shortness of breath and sputum production. A chest X-ray shows an air–fluid level behind her heart, but no evidence of consolidation.

4. A 51-year-old man presents with acute abdominal pain and blood-stained diarrhoea. An abdominal X-ray reveals a 12 cm dilatation of his transverse colon with colonic wall thickening.

5. During endoscopic retrograde cholangiopancreatography, a 45-year-old man with ulcerative colitis and jaundice is found to have multiple strictures throughout his common bile duct and biliary tree.

Theme 4: Tumour markers

Options

A. α-Fetoprotein
B. Alkaline phosphatase
C. *BRCA-1*
D. CA 125
E. CA 15-3
F. CA 19-9
G. Calcitonin
H. Human carcinoembryonic antigen
I. Human chorionic gonadotropin
J. Neuron-specific enolase
K. Prostatic acid phosphatase
L. Prostate-specific antigen

For each of the following scenarios, select the most useful tumour marker. Each option may be used once, more than once or not at all.

1. A 56-year-old man has a 1-month history of weight loss, anorexia and worsening jaundice. A blood test shows a bilirubin of 300 μmol/L, an AST of 55 IU/L and an alkaline phosphatase of 760 IU/L.

2. A 67-year-old woman complaining of weight loss, abdominal pain and an increasing abdominal girth is found to have a large mass in her left lower abdomen and ascites on transvaginal ultrasound imaging.

3. A 58-year-old man who is a former intravenous drug user and has hepatitis C presents with a general deterioration in health. He has lost a significant amount of weight and has become increasingly jaundiced. He is also experiencing right upper quadrant abdominal pain. An urgent abdominal ultrasound scan shows a poorly circumscribed hypoechoic mass in the left lobe of his liver.

4. A 78-year-old man who presented to his GP with urinary frequency, hesitancy and nocturia is shown to have a craggy unilateral mass originating from the left lobe of his prostate gland on digital rectal examination.

5. A 54-year-old woman has a fixed, craggy mass in the right upper quadrant of her right breast. She is also tender in the right upper quadrant of her abdomen.

Theme 5: Conduction defects

Options

A. First-degree heart block
B. Second-degree: Mobitz type I heart block
C. Second-degree: Mobitz type II heart block
D. Third-degree (complete) heart block
E. Bifasicular block
F. Digitalis toxicity
G. Left bundle-branch block
H. Long-QT syndrome
I. Right bundle-branch block
J. Sick sinus syndrome
K. Sinus bradycardia

For each of the following scenarios, select the most likely conduction defect. Each option may be used once, more than once or not at all.

1. A 65-year-old woman is admitted for an elective cholecystectomy. She has no significant past medical history. The clerking house officer notices a PR interval of 0.24 s on her routine admission ECG.

2. A routine ECG is taken from a 72-year-old man for insurance purposes. The tracing shows that not all P-waves are followed by QRS complexes. The PR interval is constant throughout.

3. An ECG taken from an 82-year-old woman who had fractured the neck of her left femur shows an increasing PR interval from beat to beat. This is eventually followed by a P-wave without an associated QRS complex. The PR interval returns to normal in the next complex, and this cycle repeats.

4. A 55-year-old man presents with an episode of central crushing chest pain lasting 30 minutes. An ECG demonstrates widened QRS complexes, S-waves in lead V1, and an 'M' pattern in the QRS complex in leads V5 and V6 with associated T-wave inversion.

5. A tall 23-year-old medical student presents to his GP. Earlier that day, he had an ECG taken by a colleague while practising clinical skills for his final clinical examination. The tracing showed wide QRS complexes, an RSR1 pattern in V1 and V2, and large S-waves in V6. His colleague informed him that he had a conduction defect.

Theme 6: Skin manifestations of systemic disease 2

Options

A. Acrodermatitis enteropathica
B. Candidiasis
C. Circinate balanitis
D. Dermatitis herpetiformis
E. Erythema nodosum
F. Ichthyosis
G. Kaposi's sarcoma
H. Keratoderma blenorrhagicum
I. Leukoplakia
J. Linea nigra
K. Lupus pernio
L. Pyoderma gangrenosum
M. Scurvy
N. Spider naevi

For each of the following scenarios, select the most appropriate diagnosis. Each option may be used once, more than once or not at all.

1. A 14-year-old girl develops an intensely itchy blistering rash on her forearms. She is on a special diet for coeliac disease, but is otherwise well.

2. A 12-month-old baby develops a red, scaly, pustular eruption around his mouth and anus. He has also been passing frequent loose motions. His parents say that these symptoms began as he was weaned onto solids. He was previously well.

3. A 37-year-old man develops white lesions on his tongue. The lesions are present on both sides of his tongue, but do not rub off. He is otherwise well.

4. A 29-year-old woman develops a pigmented line on her abdomen that runs down from her navel. She is 34 weeks' pregnant, but has no medical problems.

5. A 39-year-old man develops a scaly, hyperkeratotic lesion on the soles of his feet. He also complains of pain in his left knee and pain on passing urine. He has no previous medical history.

Theme 7: Congenital and genetic diseases of the kidney

Options

A. Alport's syndrome
B. Autosomal recessive polycystic kidney disease
C. Autosomal dominant polycystic kidney disease
D. Bilateral renal agenesis causing Potter's syndrome
E. Congenital nephrotic syndrome
F. Cranial diabetes insipidus
G. Cystinosis
H. Diabetes mellitus
I. Down's syndrome
J. Duplex ureters
K. Nephrogenic diabetes insipidus
L. Posterior urethral valve obstruction
M. Unilateral renal agenesis

For each of the following scenarios, select the most likely underlying condition. Each option may be used once, more than once or not at all.

1. A 2-week-old boy is failing to thrive and is producing vast quantities of urine. Investigation shows that he is dehydrated and has a low urinary sodium concentration. He is referred for a water deprivation test, during which desmopressin fails to concentrate his urine.

2. A 2-year-old girl is referred to the community paediatrician by her GP for failure to thrive. Examination reveals a number of poorly defined masses in her distended abdomen. Blood tests show a potassium of 3.7 mmol/L, a sodium of 138 mmol/L, a urea of 9 mmol/L and a creatinine of 130 μmol/L. An abdominal ultrasound scan is requested, and shows enlarged, irregular kidneys on both sides.

3. A 23-year-old woman from Africa gives birth to a baby who has a flat face, low-set ears and many joint abnormalities, including club feet. On further questioning, the woman admits that the doctors in Africa were worried because she did not have enough amniotic fluid. The baby dies 2 hours after birth.

4. A 5-year-old boy is being investigated for an abdominal mass. An ultrasound scan shows a single hypertrophied kidney on the left.

5. A 2-day-old boy on the neonatal unit is referred for a renal tract ultrasound scan. He has not passed any urine since birth and has a palpable bladder on examination. The scan shows a full bladder, dilated ureters and bilateral hydronephrosis.

Theme 8: Hormones in endocrine disease

Options

A. Adrenocorticotropic hormone
B. Antidiuretic hormone
C. Follicle-stimulating hormone
D. Growth hormone
E. Insulin
F. Melanocyte-stimulating hormone
G. Oestrogen
H. Prolactin
I. Thyroid-stimulating hormone
J. Thyroxine

For each of the following cases, select the hormone that is most likely to be raised. Each option may be used once, more than once or not at all.

1. A 35-year-old woman has primary hypothyroidism.
2. A 54-year-old man with a known pituitary tumour develops lactating nipples.
3. A 25-year-old woman has Graves' disease.
4. A 57-year-old man has acromegaly.
5. A 25-year-old woman has premature ovarian failure.

Theme 9: Signs of cardiovascular disease

Options

A. First-degree heart block
B. Third-degree heart block
C. Acute aortic regurgitation
D. Aortic stenosis
E. Atrial fibrillation
F. Atrial flutter
G. Chronic aortic regurgitation
H. Heterozygous familial hypercholesterolaemia
I. Homozygous familial hypercholesterolaemia
J. Mitral regurgitation
K. Mobitz type II heart block
L. Myocardial infarction
M. Rheumatic fever
N. Secondary hypercholesterolaemia block
O. Subacute bacterial endocarditis

For each of the following scenarios, select the most appropriate underlying diagnosis. Each option may be used once, more than once or not at all.

1. On examination of a 75-year-old man who presented with shortness of breath, mild chest pain and palpitations, you note that he has an irregularly irregular pulse.

2. You are asked to see a 37-year-old man who presented to the emergency department with chest pain. He is extremely anxious, as both his father and grandfather died suddenly in their 30s. On examination, you notice a pale ring around his cornea and yellow plaques just below his eye. When you mention these findings to the patient, he says that he has similar lesions on his elbows and within his Achilles' tendon.

3. On examination of a 50-year-old man who presented with fever, weight loss and lethargy, you notice small linear red lesions beneath his fingernails.

4. While examining a 62-year-old man who presented in a state of collapse, you note that his heart rate is only 40 beats/min. Additionally, there appears to be an abnormally large wave within the jugular venous pressure waveform.

5. While examining a 65-year-old man who is currently being treated for a suspected aortic dissection and acute pulmonary oedema, you hear an early diastolic murmur. In addition, you notice an exaggerated pulsation of his carotid arteries and an abnormal, short, sharp, loud systolic sound on auscultation of the femoral arteries.

Theme 10: Haematological malignancy

Options

A. Acute lymphoblastic leukaemia
B. Acute myeloid leukaemia
C. Burkitt's lymphoma
D. Chronic lymphocytic leukaemia
E. Chronic myeloid leukaemia
F. Disseminated intravascular coagulation
G. Hodgkin's lymphoma
H. Myelofibrosis
I. Myeloma
J. Neutrocytosis
K. Neutropenic sepsis
L. Non-Hodgkin's lymphoma
M. Tumour lysis syndrome

For each of the following scenarios, select the most appropriate underlying cause. Each option may be used once, more than once or not at all.

1. A 9-year-old boy is brought to the GP by his mother, who feels that he is very lethargic and bruises easily. The doctor requested a full blood count, which showed a haemoglobin concentration of 9.3 g/dL, a white cell count of 80 × 10^9/L and a platelet count of 30 × 10^9/L.

2. A 2-year-old girl with Down's syndrome becomes generally unwell and develops multiple bruises during a 3-day illness. Blood tests show a haemoglobin concentration of 6.8 g/dL, a white cell count of 60 × 10^9/L and a platelet count of 10 × 10^9/L. Auer rods can be seen in blast cells on microscopy.

3. A 74-year-old man complains of a 6-month history of lethargy, itching and severe abdominal discomfort. On examination, the doctor notices several areas of bruising on the skin and what he thinks to be an enlarged spleen on palpation of the abdomen. A full blood count shows a white cell count of 100 × 10^9/L. He is later shown to possess the Philadelphia chromosome.

4. A 12-year-old girl receiving chemotherapy for acute lymphoblastic leukaemia becomes generally unwell on the ward. She complains of pins and needles around her lips and spasms in her hands and feet. Her urine output has also significantly decreased. Blood tests show that she is hyperkalaemic, hyperphosphataemic, hyperuricaemic and hypocalcaemic.

5. A 5-year-old-girl becomes febrile, hypotensive and tachycardic 1 week after receiving induction chemotherapy for an acute leukaemia. The full blood count shows a haemoglobin concentration of 8.9 g/dL, a white cell count of 0.5 × 10^9/l, a platelet count of 60 × 10^9/L and a neutrophil count of 0.1 × 10^9/L.

Theme 11: Headache 2

Options

A. Cluster headache
B. Coitus-induced headache
C. Giant cell arteritis
D. Ice-cream headache
E. Meningitis
F. Migraine
G. Sagittal sinus thrombosis
H. Sinusitis
I. Space-occupying lesion
J. Tension headache
K. Trigeminal neuralgia

For each of the following scenarios, select the most appropriate cause of headache. Each option may be used once, more than once or not at all.

1. A 52-year-old woman presents to the GP with a 2-month history of worsening headaches. The headaches are worse in the morning, and are exacerbated by coughing and laughing. More recently, she has been complaining of blurred vision and nausea.

2. A 64-year-old woman presents to the emergency department with malaise and a left-sided headache that has been getting worse over the last 24 hours. She also complains of some pain in her shoulders. On examination, she is tender over the left side of her head. Fundoscopy is unremarkable.

3. A 34-year-old man presents with a 6-month history of dull, generalized headache. He says that it feels as if someone is pressing on his head. He denies nausea, visual disturbance or focal neurological signs.

4. A 17-year-old girl presents with a 1-week history of headache and pain in her face that is worse on coughing. She is worried about failing her advanced level modules, as she has already had 2 weeks off school with a cold. On examination, she is tender over the left cheek. Fundoscopy is unremarkable.

5. A 32-year-old woman presents to the emergency department with a sudden-onset frontal headache and vomiting. Fundoscopy shows bilateral papilloedema, but examination is otherwise unremarkable. She has no significant medical history and takes the oral contraceptive pill. While in the department, she has a seizure.

Theme 12: Arterial blood gases

Options

A. Fully compensated metabolic acidosis
B. Fully compensated metabolic alkalosis
C. Fully compensated respiratory acidosis
D. Fully compensated respiratory alkalosis
E. Metabolic acidosis
F. Metabolic alkalosis
G. Respiratory acidosis
H. Respiratory alkalosis
I. Type I respiratory failure
J. Type II respiratory failure

Reference ranges: Po_2 >11.0 kPa, Pco_2 4.6–6.0 kPa, bicarbonate 22–28 mmol/L, pH 7.35–7.45.

For each of the following scenarios, select the most appropriate blood gas disturbance. Each option may be used once, more than once or not at all.

1. A 72-year-old man is returned to the ward following a transurethral resection of the prostate. You are called to see him because he is confused. Blood gases show pH 7.39, Po_2 7.0 kPa, Pco_2 5.1 kPa and bicarbonate 24 mmol/L.

2. A 17-year-old girl who has a history of polyuria and polydipsia presents with reduced consciousness and apparent shortness of breath. Her blood gases show pH 7.28, Po_2 15.7 kPa, Pco_2 2.5 kPa and bicarbonate 14 mmol/L.

3. A 26-year-old woman is admitted following a multiple overdose. She appears to be breathing heavily, so a blood gas is taken. The results show pH 7.36, Po_2 12.0 kPa, Pco_2 3.8 kPa and bicarbonate 18 mmol/L.

4. A 31-year-old man presents with severe epigastric pain and vomiting. His arterial blood gases are pH 7.49, Po_2 12.7 kPa, Pco_2 5.0 kPa and bicarbonate 34 mmol/L.

5. A 64-year-old woman is admitted with chest pain and a purulent cough. Her arterial blood gases are pH 7.31, Po_2 12.0 kPa, Pco_2 7.4 kPa and bicarbonate 26 mmol/L.

Theme 13: Management of rheumatological disease

Options

A. Allopurinol
B. Aspirin
C. Heparin
D. Indometacin
E. Interferon
F. Joint replacement
G. Methotrexate
H. Physiotherapy
I. Steroids
J. Sulfasalazine
K. Warfarin

For each of the following scenarios, select the most appropriate management option. Each option may be used once, more than once or not at all.

1. A 64-year-old man presents with sudden-onset severe pain in his left toe, which occurred at rest. He is otherwise well. On examination, the small joint of the great toe is swollen, red and tender.

2. A 52-year-old woman presents to the emergency department with malaise and a left-sided headache that has been getting worse over the last 24 hours. She also complains of some pain in her shoulders. On examination, she is tender over her left scalp.

3. A 47-year-old woman presents to the rheumatologist with a long history of pain in the small joints of her hands. The pain is worst in the mornings. She is taking regular analgesia, but this is not enough. On examination, there is a 3 cm hard nodule on the back of her left arm, near the elbow.

4. A 35-year-old man presents with a 6-month history of lower back pain and stiffness that is worse in the morning. He takes paracetamol for the pain, but with little effect. He has a past history of recurrent peptic ulcers.

5. A 28-year-old woman has had four miscarriages in the past. She is now pregnant again and is desperate to have the baby. She has a past history of two deep vein thromboses.

Theme 14: Jaundice

Options

A. Autoimmune hepatitis
B. Bacterial hepatitis
C. Common bile duct stone
D. Gilbert's syndrome
E. Haemolysis
F. Hepatic metastases
G. Opiate overdose
H. Pancreatic carcinoma
I. Paracetamol intoxication
J. Viral hepatitis

For each of the following scenarios, select the most likely underlying cause of jaundice. Each option may be used once, more than once or not at all.

1. A 58-year-old man presents to his GP with a 4-week history of worsening jaundice that is associated with dark urine and pale stools. He denies any pain, but has lost a stone in weight over the last month. There is no history of foreign travel, intravenous drug use or sexual activity with prostitutes.

2. A 40-year-old woman presents to the emergency department with severe right upper quadrant pain, vomiting and jaundice. She has had similar pains in the past that were triggered by fatty food.

3. A 67-year-old man presents to his GP with jaundice. On further questioning, he admits to a 5-month history of diarrhoea, bleeding per rectum and weight loss. On examination, the liver is palpable 4 cm below the costal margin and has an uneven border.

4. A 28-year-old woman presents to the emergency department with a 2-month history of lethargy, abdominal pain and jaundice. On further questioning, she admits to using intravenous drugs.

5. A 16-year-old girl presents to the emergency department complaining of severe lethargy, jaundice and bruising. On further questioning, she admits having taken 30 co-codamol tablets 72 hours ago. After 'sleeping off' the overdose, she initially felt well and did not seek medical attention.

Theme 15: Spinal cord lesions

Options

A. Anterior cord syndrome
B. Brown-Séquard syndrome
C. Cauda equina syndrome
D. Central cord syndrome
E. Posterior cord syndrome
F. Syringomyelia

For each of the following scenarios, select the most appropriate spinal cord lesion. Each option may be used once, more than once or not at all.

1. A 28-year-old man is stabbed in the back. He is now unable to move his left lower limb. On examination, you note that he cannot feel pain on the right leg, although motor function in this limb is preserved.

2. A 32-year-old woman presents with a long history of worsening neck and shoulder pain associated with sensory loss in both upper limbs. On examination, the patient is insensate to pain and temperature in the distal upper limbs, although joint position sense is intact. There is no other motor or sensory loss.

3. A 72-year-old woman attends the emergency department after falling down the stairs. She banged her forehead during the fall. On examination, she has bilateral upper limb weakness.

4. A 52-year-old woman describes sudden-onset back pain that occurred when she was trying to move her sofa earlier in the day. She now complains of an inability to pass urine and of pain going from her back to both legs. On examination, there is a loss of sensation around the perineum.

5. A 22-year-old builder falls from scaffolding and hits his head. He says that he felt his head tug backwards during the fall. On examination, there is no motor or sensory loss in the arms or legs, but he has difficulty coordinating his walking.

Practice Paper 5: Answers

Theme 1: Management of type 2 diabetes

1. B – Dietary and lifestyle advice

Many patients with newly diagnosed type 2 diabetes can be managed initially with diet and lifestyle changes, although many will later require treatment. A healthy diet with daily exercise should be advised to all patients. Furthermore, diabetic patients should be educated as to the importance of smoking cessation, blood pressure control, glycaemic control and foot care. All patients with type 2 diabetes should receive annual review, including assessment of long-term glycaemic control using HbA_{1c} glycated haemoglobin A_1) measurement, lipid profile, blood pressure, fundoscopy, urinalysis, and examination for signs of peripheral neuropathy and foot disease. If the HbA_{1c} is appropriate and there are no other concerns, the patient can be reviewed annually. If the HbA_{1c} is too high or there are other areas of concern, such as hypoglycaemia, hyperlipidaemia or hypertension, the patient should be reviewed at more regular intervals.

2. G – Metformin

The patient in this question is not responding to lifestyle changes and dietary advice and has poor long-term glycaemic control, as shown by the high HbA_{1c} level. To reduce the likelihood of this patient developing macro- and microvascular disease, he requires oral hypoglycaemic treatment to improve glycaemic control. Metformin, a biguanide, is the oral hypoglycaemic agent of choice in overweight patients (body mass index, BMI >25 kg/m^2), as it does not increase body weight. Metformin increases peripheral insulin sensitivity and inhibits gluconeogenesis, thus improving glycaemic control. It does not increase insulin secretion or cause hypoglycaemia, and therefore has no hypoglycaemic effect in non-diabetic people. Metformin can rarely cause a life-threatening lactic acidosis, and should therefore be avoided in patients with renal or hepatic impairment, or in those with an excessive alcohol intake.

3. C – Gliclazide

As in the previous question, the patient in this question is not adequately managed using dietary and lifestyle changes alone. The main difference between the two patients is their weight. The patient in this question has a BMI of 23 kg/m^2 – an appropriate weight. Gliclazide belongs to the sulphonylurea group of oral hypoglycaemics. Sulphonylureas are insulin secretagogues, i.e. they promote endogenous insulin secretion from pancreatic β-cells, and are the oral hypoglycaemics of choice in patients who are not overweight. The main side-effects of sulphonylureas are weight gain and hypoglycaemia. The risk of hypoglycaemia can be reduced by using short- and medium-term acting agents such as tolbutamide and gliclazide. Longer-acting sulphonylureas (glibenclamide and chlorpropamide) are more prone to causing hypoglycaemia.

4. E – Insulin

Insulin is indicated in patients with type 2 diabetes who have poor glycaemic control despite maximal education, lifestyle changes and oral hypoglycaemic therapy. Insulin is usually given in conjunction with maximum oral hypoglycaemic therapy. In type 2 diabetes, insulin is usually administered in a twice-daily regimen using premixed (biphasic) insulin preparations. In some patients, a once-daily dose of long-acting insulin at night time is preferable. The side-effects of insulin therapy include weight gain, hypoglycaemia and lipoatrophy/lipohypertrophy at injection sites.

5. C – Gliclazide

In patients who are not responding to maximum single-agent oral hypoglycaemic therapy, a second agent is added. If the patient was taking metformin, then a sulphonylurea such as gliclazide should be added. Conversely, if the patient was taking a sulphonylurea, then metformin should be added (if it is not contraindicated – see above). If, for some reason, the second-line agent is contraindicated, then the patient should be started on a thiazolidinedione such as *rosiglitazone* in addition to the original agent. Similarly, if the combination of metformin and a sulphonylurea is proving inadequate then a thiazolidinedione should be added as a third agent. The thiazolidinedione class of oral hypoglycaemic agents, also known as glitazones, increase peripheral insulin sensitivity. They are best used in combination with other oral hypoglycaemic medications as second- or third-line agents. Thiazolidinediones are potentially hepatotoxic, so patients should have their liver function tested on a regular basis during the first year of treatment. *Acarbose* is an example of an α-glucosidase inhibitor. These drugs delay absorption of carbohydrates in the gut by inhibiting disaccharidases.

Theme 2: Speech problems

1. C – Cerebellar speech

This man has dysarthria – poor articulation due to problems of the mouth and tongue. Alcohol intoxication results in cerebellar dysfunction, one of the features of which is slurred speech that has a 'sing-song' quality. Other features of cerebellar dysfunction include ataxia, nystagmus and poor coordination. Other causes of dysarthria are myopathies, spasticity (mumbling, breathy speech) and parkinsonism (rapid, stammering, quiet speech).

2. G – Wernicke's aphasia

Language processing is done predominantly in the left hemisphere. Wernicke's area (in the left temporal lobe near the primary auditory cortex) is responsible for recognizing and analysing spoken language. Broca's area (in the left frontal lobe near the primary motor cortex) is responsible for producing coherent speech. Wernicke's and Broca's areas are connected by the arcuate fasciculus.

In fluent aphasia, the normal number of words is produced, but the wrong words are spoken. In non-fluent aphasia, verbal output is reduced. Damage to Wernicke's area (*Wernicke's aphasia*) results in a fluent aphasia with poor comprehension and poor repetition. This is because the patient cannot analyse what has been said, but is still able to say something thanks to an intact Broca's area. Conversely, in *Broca's aphasia*, there is a non-fluent aphasia with good comprehension and poor repetition. In other words, the patient can wholly understand what is said, but, because they have problems with the motor side of speech, they are unable to repeat what you have said or indeed to say much at all. A *lesion in the arcuate fasciculus* (which joins the two areas) results in a fluent aphasia with good comprehension but poor repetition – i.e. an intact Wernicke's area means that the patient can understand what is said, an intact Broca's area means that they can speak, but the lack of a connection between the two means that they would not be able to repeat a phrase that is told to them.

Karl Wernicke, German neuropathologist and psychiatrist (1848–1905).

Pierre Paul Broca, French physician (1824–80).

3. F – Pseudobulbar palsy

The lower cranial nerves (IX to XII) supply the muscles involved in speech and swallowing. Damage to these nerves results in dysphagia and dysarthria. The lesions can either involve the lower motor neurons (leading to bulbar palsy) or the upper motor neurons (leading to pseudobulbar palsy). *Pseudobulbar palsy* results in a small, contracted tongue and a brisk jaw jerk. Causes include motor neuron disease, multiple sclerosis, brain-stem tumour and brain-stem stroke. *Bulbar palsy* results in a wasted, fasciculating tongue and a palate that moves very little. Causes include motor neuron disease, syringobulbia, Guillain–Barré syndrome and myasthenia gravis.

4. D – Dysphonia

In dysphonia, the vocal cords do not generate sound appropriately, and this can result in hoarse or whispering speech. In this case, the patient had thyroid surgery that damaged the recurrent laryngeal nerve (a branch of the vagus nerve that supplies the pharynx). Unilateral damage of this nerve presents with hoarseness. Bilateral damage would result in breathing difficulties and aphonia (the inability to speak). Laryngeal and bronchial tumours can invade the recurrent laryngeal nerve to produce similar symptoms.

5. A – Broca's aphasia

See Case 2 above.

Theme 3: Gastrointestinal radiology

1. K – Visceral perforation

The presence of free air under the diaphragm (pneumoperitoneum) on chest X-ray indicates a perforated abdominal viscus that has allowed air to enter the peritoneal cavity, e.g. a perforated peptic ulcer. In order to maximize the chance of seeing free air under the diaphragm, the chest X-ray should be taken with the patient in an erect position. A similar finding may be seen when the transverse colon is interpositioned between the superior border of the liver and diaphragm. This is known as Chilaiditi's syndrome, or hepatodiaphragmatic interposition of the colon, and is usually an incidental finding in an asymptomatic patient.

2. A – Achalasia

Achalasia is a progressive failure of relaxation of the lower oesophagus, with dilatation, tortuosity and hypertrophy of the oesophagus above. It occurs secondary to idiopathic degeneration of the nerve ganglia of the oesophagus, known as Auerbach's plexus. Achalasia is commonest in the third to fifth decades and is more prevalent in women. Patients experience worsening dysphagia, and regurgitation from the dilated oesophagus can result in aspiration pneumonia. Chest X-ray appearances include the lack of a gastric bubble (because the dilated oesophagus does not empty, so swallowed air cannot pass to the stomach). The dilated oesophageal sac with food in it gives rise to the air–fluid level and the 'double right heart border' appearance.

A barium swallow in achalasia shows a dilated oesophagus with a tapering lower segment resembling a bird's beak. Diagnosis of achalasia is by manometry, which shows an increased lower oesophageal pressure at rest, failure of the oesophagus to relax after swallowing and absence of useful peristalsis in the lower oesophagus. Management is by balloon dilatation of the oesophagus or by Heller's cardiomyotomy, in which the muscle of the oesophagus is cut longitudinally down to the mucosa. Achalasia predisposes to squamous cell carcinoma of the oesophagus.

Ernest Heller, German surgeon (performed the first cardiomyotomy in 1913).

3. C – Hiatus hernia

A hiatus hernia occurs when the stomach herniates through the diaphragm into the thorax. Some patients remain completely asymptomatic, whereas others suffer from intolerable gastro-oesophageal reflux disease and dyspepsia. Complications include weight loss, oesophagitis, oesophageal ulceration, oesophageal stricture and aspiration pneumonia. Diagnosis is usually made during endoscopy or with barium-swallow studies, although many cases are identified incidentally on chest X-ray as a shadow behind the heart with or without an air–fluid level (caused by the presence of gastric contents). Treatment is usually conservative, and involves lifestyle adaptations such as weight loss, smoking cessation and a healthy balanced diet. Proton pump inhibitors may be used to improve symptoms. Surgical repair of medically resistant reflux is with Nissen's fundoplication, where the fundus of the stomach is wrapped around the lower oesophagus.

Rudolph Nissen, German surgeon (1896–1981).

4. I – Toxic megacolon

Toxic megacolon refers to life-threatening dilatation of the colon secondary to infective or inflammatory colitis. Patients are usually known to have colitis, and present acutely with abdominal pain, abdominal distension, diarrhoea, blood-stained stools, fever and tachycardia. Abdominal X-ray shows colonic dilatation of >6 cm with or without colonic wall thickening, multiple air–fluid levels and disruption of the haustral pattern. Investigation will usually reveal significantly raised inflammatory markers and electrolyte imbalance. Patients with proven toxic megacolon should be managed in a high-dependency environment and receive fluid resuscitation, corticosteroids, antibiotics and daily abdominal X-rays to assess disease progression. If the dilatation is becoming worse or the patient is clinically deteriorating, a colectomy should be considered.

5. H – Primary sclerosing cholangitis

Primary sclerosing cholangitis is a condition in which chronic inflammation of the biliary tract results in the development of multiple strictures within the intra- and extrahepatic ducts. This condition is associated with inflammatory bowel disease, which is implicated in up to 75% of cases. It is usually seen in young men, and presents with lethargy and pruritis. As the disease progresses, the patient is at risk of developing the symptoms and complications of chronic liver disease, such as jaundice, cholangitis, hepatomegaly, coagulopathy, portal hypertension, oesophageal varices, ascites, encephalopathy and liver failure. There is also a 10% risk of developing cholangiocarcinoma. Diagnosis is based on the presence of deranged liver function tests, hypergammaglobulinaemia and biliary tract imaging – endoscopic retrograde cholangiopancreatography (ERCP) or magnetic resonance cholangiopancreatography (MRCP). Treatment is with steroids, ursodeoxycholic acid, cholestyramine and the supplementation of fat-soluble vitamins (A, D, E and K). If there is evidence of liver failure, oesophageal varices or ascites, the patient should be considered for liver transplantation. Without a transplant, death usually occurs within 12 years.

Theme 4: Tumour markers

1. F – CA 19-9

It is likely that this patient has a pancreatic tumour, for which CA 19-9 is a tumour marker. Painless jaundice, caused by the tumour obstructing the common bile duct, is a common presentation of pancreatic cancer. Other features include lethargy, weight loss, epigastric pain and liver capsule pain secondary to liver metastases. The diagnosis of pancreatic cancer usually involves abdominal ultrasonography, ERCP and CT. Tumour markers can be used as an adjunct to diagnosis and to measure the patient's response to treatment. They should not be used as a stand-alone diagnostic tool. The prognosis of pancreatic tumours is extremely poor, with most patients surviving less than 6 months and only 2% alive at 5 years. Treatment of pancreatic cancer is mostly palliative. On rare occasions, the tumour may be treated surgically by pancreaticoduodenectomy, more commonly referred to as Whipple's operation. It should be noted that CA 19-9 may also be raised in biliary tract malignancy.

Allen Oldfather Whipple, American surgeon (1881–1963).

2. D – CA 125

The most likely diagnosis in this case is ovarian carcinoma, for which CA 125 is a tumour marker. The clinical features of ovarian malignancy include weight loss, abdominal pain, increasing abdominal girth and ascites. Unfortunately, the symptoms of ovarian malignancy usually occur late, with the result that the disease is often advanced and metastatic at presentation. Diagnosis usually involves transvaginal ultrasonography, CT, ovarian biopsy and measurement of CA 125. Both chemotherapy and surgery are used in the management of ovarian cancer, and have both curative and palliative roles. Radiotherapy is now limited to the palliation of symptoms. Because ovarian malignancy usually presents late, the prognosis is poor. However, if the disease is diagnosed early and treated appropriately, 5-year survival rates for early stage disease can be as high as 95%.

3. A – α-Fetoprotein

It is likely that this patient has hepatocellular carcinoma secondary to chronic hepatitis C infection. α-Fetoprotein is the most important and widely used tumour marker for hepatocellular carcinoma, but may also be raised in a number of other conditions, including viral hepatitis, alcoholic hepatitis and germ cell tumours. Hepatocellular carcinoma is associated with a number of vague symptoms, such as lethargy, weight loss and right upper quadrant abdominal pain, with jaundice being a late sign. Sudden deterioration of liver function and clinical status in a patient with chronic hepatitis or cirrhosis can indicate the presence hepatocellular carcinoma. Investigation usually reveals deranged liver function tests and abnormal clotting. Ultrasonography shows a poorly defined hypoechoic mass. CT is likely to show a low-density lesion that does not enhance with contrast. MRI is currently the best method for radiological diagnosis. A liver biopsy is usually required to confirm the diagnosis, and may be performed under CT or ultrasound guidance. Surgical resection, chemotherapy and transplantation all have roles in the management of hepatocellular carcinoma, but, despite this, the prognosis remains poor, with many patients dying within 6 months of diagnosis.

4. L – Prostate-specific antigen

This is likely to be a prostatic carcinoma. The patient gives a clear history of prostatism and has a poorly defined mass on digital examination of the prostate. Prostate-specific antigen (PSA) has largely replaced prostatic acid phosphatase as the most widely used tumour marker of prostatic carcinoma. Despite being very sensitive, PSA has a relatively low specificity, meaning that it is often raised in patients without prostate cancer. Therefore, it should be used in conjunction with history, examination, imaging and biopsy results, and should never be used alone to diagnose prostate cancer.

5. E – CA 15-3

This woman has a breast mass that has a number of malignant characteristics. Features of breast malignancy include a poorly defined mass, tethering to the skin or underlying muscle, with associated skin changes such as dimpling, peau d'orange and Paget's disease (a scaly eczematous rash of the nipple). Breast cancer is usually diagnosed on the basis of history, examination, mammography and biopsy. The staging of breast cancer can be achieved with CT, chest X-ray and liver ultrasonography. CA 15-3 is a tumour marker for breast cancer that is used to assess the patient's response to treatment and to identify relapse of disease. High levels of CA 15-3 suggest metastatic disease. Because of its poor sensitivity, CA 15-3 cannot be used for screening or diagnosis. *BRCA-1* and *-2* are genes associated with a higher risk of breast and ovarian cancer, and are not tumour markers.

Other examples of tumour markers include:

- human chorionic gonadotropin, β subunit (βhCG): choriocarcinoma, testicular tumours
- calcitonin: medullary thyroid cancer
- carcinoembryonic antigen (CEA): colorectal tumours
- monoclonal immunoglobulin G (IgG) (paraprotein): multiple myeloma
- neuron-specific enolase (NSE): small cell lung cancer
- placental alkaline phosphatase: ovarian carcinoma, testicular tumours
- S-100: malignant melanoma
- thyroglobulin: thyroid tumours.

Theme 5: Conduction defects

1. A – First-degree heart block

In first-degree heart block, there is a delay in atrioventricular conduction. It is defined by a PR interval of greater than 0.2 s (five small squares on the standard ECG tracing). The PR interval, measured from the beginning of the P-wave (atrial depolarization) to the beginning of the QRS complex (ventricular depolarization) is normally 0.12–0.20 s. First-degree heart block is usually caused by fibrosis of the conduction pathways secondary to ischaemic heart disease, but it is also seen as a normal variant and in digitalis toxicity. It is asymptomatic, and requires no specific treatment apart from observation.

2. C – Second-degree: Mobitz type II heart block

In Mobitz type II second-degree heart block, atrial depolarization is not always followed by ventricular depolarization, i.e. not all P-waves are followed by a QRS complex. There is no specific pattern to the 'dropped' QRS complexes, and the PR interval remains constant, in contrast to Mobitz type 1 (Wenckebach) blockade (see below). This condition is usually secondary to significant ischaemic heart disease and may be a prelude to complete heart block. It warrants investigation by a cardiologist.

3. B – Second-degree: Mobitz type I heart block

In Mobitz type I second-degree heart block, also known as Wenckebach block, there is progressive lengthening of the PR interval culminating in an unconducted P-wave, i.e. it is not followed by a QRS complex. Following this 'dropped' beat, the PR interval returns to its shortest duration and the cycle repeats. The Wenckebach phenomenon occurs secondary to impaired conduction along the proximal bundle of His. It is usually a benign variant, occurring especially in athletes.

In third-degree heart block, there is no atrioventricular conduction, so the atria and ventricles beat independently. An ECG tracing will demonstrate regular P-waves and regular QRS complexes, but these will occur at differing rates. Ventricular activity depends upon escape rhythms, which tend to be slow (25–50 beats/min) and do not vary with exercise. Cannon *a*-waves may be seen on the jugular venous pressure (JVP) due to atrial contraction against a closed tricuspid valve (when atrial and ventricular contractions occur simultaneously). Causes of third-degree heart block include inferior myocardial infarction and sarcoidosis, and this condition requires permanent cardiac pacing.

Karel Frederik Wenckebach, Dutch anatomist (1864–1940).

4. G – Left bundle-branch block

Electrical activity from the atrioventricular node travels down the bundle of His. This soon divides into left and right branches. Injury of either bundle branch results in characteristic ECG changes secondary to altered pathways for ventricular depolarization.

The ECG findings in this scenario are classic for left bundle-branch block (LBBB). LBBB is always pathological, and is seen in ischaemic heart disease, myocardial infarction, hypertension and cardiomyopathy. In this scenario, it is likely to be a new finding secondary to acute myocardial infarction, in which case it is an indication for thrombolysis. Since the conduction down the left bundle branch is delayed, the QRS complex is prolonged (>0.12 s) and the myocardium depolarizes from right to left, producing dominant R-waves in V6. The subsequent delayed depolarization of the left ventricle produces deep S-waves in V1 and a further R-wave in V6, which completes the 'M' pattern in V6. It should be noted that LBBB makes interpretation of the remaining ECG impossible.

Wilhelm His Jr, Swiss cardiologist (1863–1934).

5. I – Right bundle-branch block

The ECG of right bundle-branch block (RBBB) shows a prolonged QRS complex (>0.12 s), an RSR pattern in V1 and prominent S-waves in V6. RBBB can be a normal variant in tall, thin adults (as in this case). More sinister causes of RBBB include pulmonary embolus, cor pulmonale and atrial septal defect. Both RBBB and LBBB have an RSR_1 pattern on one side (seen as an 'M'), with a 'W' pattern on the other. Remember 'MarroW' (RBBB has an 'M' in V1 and a 'W' in V6) and 'WilliaM' (LBBB has a 'W' in V1 and an 'M' in V6).

Theme 6: Skin manifestations of systemic disease 2

1. D – Dermatitis herpetiformis

Dermatitis herpetiformis is a blistering, intensely itchy rash that develops on the extensor surfaces. It is associated with coeliac disease and is treated with dapsone. There are many cutaneous features of gastrointestinal disease, including the following:

- malabsorption: ichthyosis (dry, scaly skin), eczema, oedema
- liver disease: jaundice, spider naevi, palmar erythema, leukonychia
- renal failure: itching, half white and half red nails
- Crohn's disease: perianal abscess, fistulae, skin tags, aphthous ulcers
- ulcerative colitis: erythema nodosum, pyoderma gangrenosum
- sarcoidosis: erythema nodosum, lupus pernio (purple indurated lesions).

2. A – Acrodermatitis enteropathica

Acrodermatitis enteropathica is a rare inherited defect of zinc malabsorption. Features develop during weaning, and include a perianal and oral red, scaly, pustular rash, failure to thrive, diarrhoea, and poor wound healing.

Other nutritional deficiencies can result in cutaneous features. Protein malnutrition causes growth retardation, muscle wasting, altered pigmentation, ulcers, dry/red hair (in Africans). Vitamin C deficiency (*scurvy*) causes bleeding gums, perifollicular purpura and a woody oedema. Niacin deficiency causes a photosensitive pigmentation. Iron deficiency can result in alopecia, koilonychias (spoon-shaped nails) and angular stomatitis.

3. I – Leukoplakia

Oral hairy leukoplakia is a white rash that develops along the sides of the tongue and that cannot be rubbed off (unlike candidiasis). It is caused by Epstein–Barr virus infection and may be a sign of underlying HIV infection. Other skin conditions seen with HIV include oral candidiasis (which can extend into the oesophagus), severe herpes simplex episodes, seborrhoeic dermatitis, Kaposi's sarcoma and molluscum contagiosum.

4. J – Linea nigra

This woman has developed linea nigra, a dark line of pigmentation running down from the umbilicus, which is a normal skin feature of pregnancy. Other skin lesions that can develop in pregnancy are spider naevi and abdominal striae. In pregnancy, psoriasis tends to improve, whereas eczema may get worse.

5. H – Keratoderma blenorrhagicum

This man has Reiter's syndrome, characterized by arthritis, urethritis and iritis. There are two skin features that can develop alongside this disease: keratoderma blenorrhagicum and circinate balanitis. *Keratoderma blenorrhagicum* describes the presence of pustular, crusty, yellow–brown papular lesions on the soles of the feet that are clinically and histologically indistinguishable from pustular psoriasis. It is seen in 15% of men with Reiter's syndrome. *Circinate balanitis* describes an annular, erythematous reaction on the glans penis, and occurs in 30% of men with Reiter's syndrome.

Theme 7: Congenital and genetic diseases of the kidney

1. K – Nephrogenic diabetes insipidus

Antidiuretic hormone (ADH, also known as arginine vasopressin) is synthesized in the hypothalamus and secreted from the posterior pituitary gland in response to rising serum osmolarity. ADH increases the permeability of the renal collecting ducts by opening protein gateways, called aquaporins, through which water is reabsorbed into the circulation. Diabetes insipidus (DI) describes a number of conditions where there is either a lack of ADH secretion or a peripheral resistance to its actions, resulting in the production of vast volumes of diluted urine, polydipsia and dehydration. DI is broadly divided into cranial and nephrogenic DI. In cranial DI, there is a lack of ADH secretion from the pituitary gland, usually caused by acquired disease such as pituitary neoplasm or following head injury. In nephrogenic DI, mutations in the ADH receptor or aquaporin II protein prevent the collecting tubules from responding to ADH despite normal or raised levels of ADH. The most common mutation is in the *AVPV2* gene and is X-linked recessive, meaning that nephrogenic DI is typically a disease of males. Nephrogenic DI may also be seen secondary to other diseases that affect the kidney, such as sickle cell anaemia and polycystic kidney disease.

The investigation of choice in DI is the water deprivation test. In this test, the patient has their urine and plasma osmolarity measured at hourly intervals while being deprived of fluid. The patient's weight is also measured, and the test is stopped if the patient loses over 3% of their body weight. In normal individuals, fluid restriction causes the plasma osmolarity to rise, which in turn stimulates ADH secretion and water reabsorption. In DI, the patient continues to produce large volumes of dilute urine despite being dehydrated. Patients who do not concentrate their urine during the test are given a dose of desmopressin, which is a synthetic ADH analogue. If the diabetes insipidus is due to a lack of ADH secretion, i.e. cranial DI, the desmopressin causes the kidney to reabsorb water and concentrate the urine. If the patient has nephrogenic DI, their kidneys cannot respond to the desmopressin, and therefore the patient continues to produce large volumes of dilute urine. Thus, cranial DI can be treated with desmopressin, whereas nephrogenic DI cannot. In nephrogenic DI, the urine output can be slowed by using thiazide diuretics and non-steroidal anti-inflammatory drugs, although the most important treatment is good fluid management.

2. B – Autosomal recessive polycystic kidney disease

Autosomal recessive polycystic kidney disease (ARPKD) is a genetic condition caused by mutations in the *PKD1* or *PKD2* genes that result in the formation of multiple fluid-filled cysts within the collecting ducts of the kidney and the liver. Severe ARPKD can present during labour with respiratory difficulties and acute renal failure. More insidious presentations are common, and typically combine failure to thrive, hypertension and worsening renal function. Patients who present earlier tend to have more renal disease in proportion to hepatic disease, whereas the opposite is true of those who present later on in life. The majority of patients with ARPKD eventually require renal replacement therapy. This condition should not be confused with *autosomal dominant polycystic kidney disease*, which presents later in life and is associated with berry aneurysms and subarachnoid haemorrhage.

3. D – Bilateral renal agenesis causing Potter's syndrome

Bilateral renal agenesis is a condition that is not compatible with life and usually results in stillbirth or death in the early neonatal period. Women carrying a fetus with bilateral renal agenesis have low amounts of amniotic fluid (oligohydramnios). This is because the fetal kidneys and urogenital tract are essential for the production of amniotic fluid, which protects the fetus from trauma in utero. Bilateral renal agenesis is one of the causes of Potter's syndrome. Potter's syndrome occurs when severe oligohydramnios results in facial deformities, epicanthic folds, low-set ears, pulmonary hypoplasia and joint deformities. Other causes of Potter's syndrome include ARPKD and congenital obstructive uropathy.

Edith Louise Potter, American pathologist (1901–93).

4. M – Unilateral renal agenesis

Unilateral renal agenesis is a relatively common condition in which one kidney does not develop. The remaining kidney hypertrophies and compensates for the missing kidney. Patients are often completely asymptomatic and are diagnosed incidentally during the investigation of other disease or *post mortem*. Sometimes the condition is discovered during the investigation of hypertension or an abdominal mass.

5. L – Posterior urethral valve obstruction

In posterior urethral valve obstruction, remnants of embryological membranes remain in the urethra, causing urinary tract obstruction. The obstruction causes dilatation of the bladder, bilateral vesicoureteric reflux and bilateral hydronephrosis. Patients may be diagnosed antenatally by ultrasonography. Severe disease that is not noticed antenatally is usually discovered during the first days of life with anergia, a palpable bladder and deteriorating renal function. Occasionally, children with posterior urethral valves may not be diagnosed until infancy, when they present with recurrent urinary tract infection, diurnal enuresis or renal failure. Diagnosis is usually based upon the findings of a micturating cystourethrogram, which allows visualization of the valves and demonstrates any bladder and ureteric abnormalities. Treatment is with surgical correction. Severe disease may lead to end-stage renal failure, the need for renal replacement therapy and eventual renal transplantation.

Theme 8: Hormones in endocrine disease

1. I – Thyroid-stimulating hormone

Primary hypothyroidism is caused by pathology of the thyroid gland itself, e.g. primary atrophic hypothyroidism, Hashimoto's thyroiditis, post-thyroidectomy and post-radioactive iodine treatment. In primary hypothyroidism, the low levels of circulating thyroid hormones are insufficient to inhibit the secretion of thyroid-stimulating hormone (TSH) from the anterior pituitary gland. This lack of negative feedback results in high serum levels of TSH in association with low thyroxine (T_4) and triiodothyronine (T_3) levels. *Secondary hypothyroidism* is due to a lack of stimulating factors, i.e. thyrotropin-releasing hormone and/or TSH, which is caused by disease of the hypothalamus and pituitary gland, respectively. In secondary hypothyroidism, there is a normal or low TSH in association with low T_4 and T_3 levels.

2. H – Prolactin

This patient is complaining of galactorrhoea (inappropriate lactation). When not associated with pregnancy, this condition is usually caused by hyperprolactinaemia. Hyperprolactinaemia is often associated with pituitary tumours, in which case it is either due to the presence of a prolactin-secreting adenoma (a prolactinoma) or secondary to the mass effect of the tumour. The latter causes hyperprolactinaemia by compressing the pituitary stalk, thereby preventing dopamine, an inhibitor of prolactin release, from reaching the pituitary gland. Other features of hyperprolactinaemia include menstrual disturbance in women, impotence in men, infertility and osteoporosis. The treatment of hyperprolactinaemia secondary to pituitary disease involves dopamine agonists (bromocriptine) followed by surgery to remove the tumour if indicated.

3. J – Thyroxine

Graves' disease is an autoimmune disease in which autoantibodies activate the TSH receptor to trigger the synthesis and release of thyroxine into the circulation. The high levels of circulating thyroxine feed back to the anterior pituitary gland to suppress the secretion of TSH. Thus, in Graves' disease, thyroxine levels are elevated and TSH levels are suppressed.

4. D – Growth hormone

Acromegaly is caused by excessive secretion of growth hormone (GH) in adulthood. Most cases are caused by the presence of a GH-secreting pituitary adenoma. Rarely, acromegaly can be caused by the ectopic secretion of GH-releasing hormone or GH secretion from non-pituitary tumours. GH can be measured in the serum, but, owing to its unreliable nature, this is rarely used as a stand-alone diagnostic tool.

5. C – Follicle-stimulating hormone

Premature ovarian failure is when the menopause occurs before 40 years of age due to ovarian pathology and is often idiopathic. The clinical features of premature ovarian failure include amenorrhoea, vaginal dryness, loss of pubic hair, osteoporosis and loss of libido. Since the ovary cannot synthesize oestrogen or progesterone, the lack of negative feedback on the anterior pituitary gland results in the increased secretion of luteinizing hormone (LH) and follicle-stimulating hormone (FSH). Treatment of premature ovarian failure involves the replacement of oestrogen and progesterone until the time when menopause would have occurred naturally.

Summary of the pituitary hormones

- Anterior pituitary gland: adrenocorticotropic hormone (corticotropin)
  growth hormone
  thyroid-stimulating hormone
  follicle-stimulating hormone
  luteinizing hormone
  prolactin
- Posterior pituitary gland: antidiuretic hormone (arginine vasopressin)
  oxytocin.

Theme 9: Signs of cardiovascular disease

1. E – Atrial fibrillation

Atrial fibrillation is a common supraventricular arrhythmia that is seen in up to 10% of patients over 65 years of age. It is usually secondary to ischaemic heart disease, but may occur in a number of other conditions, such as mitral stenosis, pericarditis, thyrotoxicosis, acute alcohol intoxication and pulmonary embolism. In atrial fibrillation, the sinoatrial node depolarizes in a rapid and disorganized manner, causing the atria to contract at a rate of 300–600 beats/min. Only sporadic impulses from the sinoatrial node depolarize the atrioventricular node and ventricular myocardium, causing the ventricles to contract in an irregular rhythm. The pulse in atrial fibrillation is said to be *irregularly irregular* in nature, since the irregularity follows no specific pattern.

Other features of atrial fibrillation include palpitations, dyspnoea, syncope, and the sequelae of systemic emboli such as stroke and acute limb ischaemia. The ECG usually shows a fibrillating baseline, irregularly spaced QRS complexes and an absence of P-waves. Treatment usually includes the use of an anticoagulant (warfarin) or an antiplatelet drug (aspirin) to reduce the likelihood of thrombosis and emboli. In addition, the patient should receive a rate-controlling medication such as digoxin/β-blockers, or rhythm-controlling agents such as amiodarone. A holistic approach should be used when deciding which treatment is most appropriate, since the complications of treatment may be more disabling than their intended benefits.

2. H – Heterozygous familial hypercholesterolaemia

Familial hypercholesterolaemia (FH) is an autosomal dominant disease caused by a mutation in the low-density lipoprotein (LDL) receptor located on chromosome 19. The defective receptor prevents LDL-cholesterol from being taken up and metabolized by the liver. As a result, there is a high level of circulating LDL, which leads to premature atherosclerosis. The patient is therefore at significant risk of premature vascular disease, including myocardial and cerebral infarction.

Heterozygous FH affects approximately 1 in 500 of the UK population. Patients have one functioning LDL allele in addition to the mutated allele, and are therefore able to produce some functioning LDL receptors. Presentation is usually in middle age with significantly raised plasma cholesterol that is unresponsive to dietary and lifestyle changes. Patients may or may not exhibit the external stigmata of hypercholesterolaemia, such as corneal arcus, tendon xanthomas and skin xanthelasma.

Homozygous FH is much rarer than heterozygous FH, and is associated with the complete absence of functioning LDL receptors in the liver. The patient has a significantly raised plasma cholesterol, external stigmata of hypercholesterolaemia and early ischaemic heart disease. Adolescent death usually occurs secondary to atherothrombotic events.

All patients with FH should receive lifestyle and dietary advice and undergo regular endocrine review. High-dose statin therapy is usually given in heterozygous FH, but is of limited use in homozygous FH. This is because statins require functioning LDL receptors for much of their action. A number of other lipid-lowering drugs are available, and are often used as adjuncts to statin therapy. They include fibrates, nicotinic acid and cholestyramine, which promote the excretion of cholesterol in bile and prevent its reabsorption. Plasmapheresis (removal, treatment and return of blood plasma from the circulation, in this case in order to improve the lipid profile) and liver transplantation may be considered in severe homozygotic disease to prolong life.

Plasmapheresis, from Greek *plasma* = something moulded + *aphaeresis* = taking away.

Xanthelasma, from Greek *xanthos* = yellow.

3. O – Subacute bacterial endocarditis

Subacute bacterial endocarditis usually presents with a generalized febrile illness associated with a new cardiac murmur. The patient usually has pre-existing valvular disease, and may have experienced recent bacteraemia secondary to an invasive procedure, instrumentation or intravenous drug use. There are a number of signs of endocarditis that are seldom seen but are often referred to in final examinations. Hand signs include clubbing, linear splinter haemorrhages in the nail bed (this scenario), flat painless macules on the palm (Janeway's lesions) and painful nodes in the finger pulp (Osler's nodes). Fundoscopy may demonstrate small boat-shaped lesions, which are caused by retinal immune complex deposition (Roth's spots). More common features of subacute bacterial endocarditis include a vasculitic rash and microscopic haematuria. Diagnosis is confirmed by blood cultures and echocardiographic evidence of vegetations on the valve leaflets.

The Duke criteria can be used to help diagnose endocarditis. This requires the presence of the two major criteria *or* one major criterion and three minor criteria *or* the presence of all five minor criteria.

Duke criteria for infective endocarditis

Major criteria

1. Positive blood culture defined as:
    - typical organisms in two culture bottles *or*
    - persistently positive blood cultures
2. Echocardiographic evidence defined as:
    - positive echocardiogram *or*
    - new valve regurgitation.

Minor criteria

1. Presence of risk factors, e.g. rheumatic fever
2. Fever >38°C
3. Evidence of vasculitic disease
4. Positive blood culture (not meeting major criteria)
5. Positive echocardiogram (not meeting major criteria).

Duke criteria, named after Duke University, North Carolina, USA.

Edward Janeway, American cardiologist (1872–1917).

Sir William Osler, Canadian physician (1849–1919).

Moritz Roth, Swiss pathologist (1839–1914).

4. B – Third-degree heart block

In third-degree heart block, also known as complete heart block, there is no conduction between the atria and ventricles, due to a block within or below the atrioventricular node. The atria continue to contract at their normal rate of 70–90 beats/min, whereas the ventricles depolarize at a rate of 40 beats/min or less under the control of a ventricular escape pacemaker rhythm. There is thus complete atrioventricular disassociation, meaning that there is no relationship between atrial and ventricular contraction. This is shown on ECG as a complete lack of relationship between the P-waves and the abnormally wide QRS complexes. The lack of atrial–ventricular coordination means that the atria often contract against closed atrioventricular valves. When the right atrium contracts against a closed tricuspid valve, blood is forced back along the superior vena cava and jugular veins, producing so-called 'cannon *a*-waves' in the JVP waveform.

Complete heart block is usually secondary to ischaemic heart disease, but is also seen following inferior and anterior myocardial infarction. Systemic illness, including connective tissue disease and digitalis toxicity, may also precipitate complete heart block. Many sufferers are asymptomatic, whereas others experience recurrent episodes of syncope (known as Stokes–Adams attacks), shortness of breath and hypotension. Definitive treatment is with a dual-chamber artificial pacemaker, although temporary pacing and atropine may be used in emergency situations when the patient is haemodynamically compromised.

5. C – Acute aortic regurgitation

This is a case of acute aortic regurgitation secondary to a type A (i.e. involving the ascending aorta) dissecting aortic aneurysm. Since this is an acute event, the left ventricle has had no time to compensate for the increased demands placed upon it, resulting in left ventricular failure and cardiogenic shock. On auscultation of aortic regurgitation, there is usually an early diastolic murmur at the left sternal border, which is best heard with the patient sitting forward at the end of expiration. Patients are said to have a water-hammer (collapsing) pulse and a wide blood pressure index (i.e. a high systolic and a low diastolic blood pressure). In chronic aortic regurgitation, seen in conditions such as Marfan's syndrome and congenital bicuspid aortic valve, the apex is often displaced laterally due to left ventricular dilatation. Aortic regurgitation is associated with a number of eponymous signs that are often referred to in examinations:

- Corrigan's sign: visible pulsation of the carotid arteries
- de Musset's sign: head bobbing
- Quincke's sign: pulsation of the nail beds
- Traube's phenomenon: pistol shot sound on femoral artery auscultation.

Sir Dominic John Corrigan, Irish physician (1802–80).

Paul de Musset, French author (1804–80). He first described the sign in a biography of his brother, Louis de Musset (a contemporary poet and playwright).

Heinrich Irenaens Quincke, German physician (1842–1922).

Ludwig Traube, German physician (1818–76).

Theme 10: Haematological malignancy

1. A – Acute lymphoblastic leukaemia

Acute lymphoblastic leukaemia (ALL) is the most common leukaemia in children, and is caused by the clonal proliferation of lymphoid precursor (blast) cells that have been arrested at an early stage of development. The blast cells infiltrate the marrow and lymphoid tissue, causing pancytopenia and lymphadenopathy, respectively. The central nervous system (CNS) can also be affected, causing headache, vomiting, meningism, cranial nerve palsies and seizure. The marrow failure and subsequent pancytopenia produce the common features of anaemia, bleeding/bruising and infection. Bone pain is another common presenting symptom. A full blood count confirms anaemia and thrombocytopenia, but demonstrates a high white cell count (due to circulating blast cells). The investigation of choice is bone marrow aspiration, which shows a hypercellular marrow with >20% blasts. Treatment involves the use of chemotherapy, as well as supportive measures such as transfusion and antibiotics. Chemotherapy is traditionally delivered in three main stages: remission induction, consolidation and maintenance (which can be for a number of years). Since patients with ALL are at high risk of neurological disease, they are often given CNS prophylaxis in the form of intrathecal methotrexate and radiotherapy. The prognosis of ALL is good with appropriate treatment.

Allogeneic bone marrow transplantation is curative for some haematological malignancies. Patients are initially 'conditioned' (i.e. have their own bone marrow killed by cyclophosphamide and total body irradiation). Healthy stem cells collected from a donor are then injected into the patient. It takes around 4 weeks for the patient to make enough cells from the transplanted stem cells. There is an upper age limit of 55 years for bone marrow transplantation. Complications include infection, graft-versus-host disease, pneumonitis and secondary malignancy. In some cases, *autologous bone marrow transplantation* is undertaken. In this case, the patient's own marrow is harvested and given back as a 'rescue' after chemotherapy. Autologous marrow transplantation is used only in patients with good remission, as there is a higher risk of relapse.

2. B – Acute myeloid leukaemia

Acute myeloid leukaemia (AML) is caused by the proliferation of myeloid precursor cells. This condition is generally seen in adulthood and is rapidly fatal if untreated. AML is seen as a new disease and in patients with myeloproliferative disorders. Patients with Down's syndrome are at increased risk of both ALL and AML, with the risk of AML being highest in the first 3 years of life. AML is increasingly seen in patients who have received chemotherapy in the past for other malignancies such as lymphoma. The presentation of AML is variable. Many sufferers are asymptomatic and are diagnosed incidentally whereas others become very unwell very quickly. Marrow failure caused by blast infiltration causes anaemia, thrombocytopenia and neutropenia. Investigation usually shows a significantly raised white blood cell count, although it may be normal or even low. Cellular inclusions called Auer rods which are seen on microscopy are pathognomonic of AML. Management of AML involves blood and platelet transfusion, treatment of infections and chemotherapy. In patients less than 55 years of age, stem cell transplantation is considered. The prognosis of AML is worse than that of ALL. Up to 80% of patients can be expected to achieve remission, but most relapse, and the cure rate is only 30%. The prognosis is worse in elderly people and in patients with a history of myeloproliferative disorders.

3. E – Chronic myeloid leukaemia

Chronic myeloid leukaemia (CML) is a myeloproliferative disorder. There is excessive proliferation of myeloid cells in the bone marrow. Patients typically have massive splenomegaly, anaemia, bruising and infection on a background generalized illness. Up to 90% of CML patients have a genetic translocation involving chromosomes 9 and 22 known as the Philadelphia chromosome. A blood film shows myeloblasts (granulocyte precursors) and granulocytosis. Patients with CML but without the Philadelphia chromosome have a worse prognosis than those with the translocation. There are three stages of disease in CML: the chronic phase (responsive to treatment), the accelerated phase (where disease is difficult to control) and the blast crisis phase (where disease progresses into an acute leukaemia, usually AML). The median survival is 5 years. Death usually occurs within months of blast transformation (from bleeding and infection). Chemotherapy is often used, but allogeneic stem cell transplantation is the only hope of cure.

Chronic lymphocytic leukaemia (CLL) accounts for 30% of leukaemias in the over-50s. It is characterized by the accumulation of incompetent CD5+ B cells that fail to secrete antibody (instead secreting light chains). Patients present with anaemia, painless lymphadenopathy, splenomegaly and infection. A blood film reveals a mature lymphocytosis (with anaemia and thrombocytopenia). The median survival is 6 years. CLL can occasionally transform into a high-grade aggressive lymphoma (Richter's transformation).

Hairy cell leukaemia is a rare B-cell disorder with 'hairy' cells in the bone marrow. These cells characteristically express CD25 and CD103.

4. M – Tumour lysis syndrome

Tumour lysis syndrome is usually seen in patients with lymphoproliferative malignancy following chemotherapy. Massive cell death results in the release of potassium, phosphate and uric acid into the circulation. The phosphate binds to serum calcium, causing hypocalcaemia with the clinical features of perioral paraesthesia, tetany, Trousseau's sign (carpal spasm on inflating a blood pressure cuff around the upper limb), Chvostek's sign (twitching of the face when tapping over the facial nerve at the angle of the jaw) and arrhythmia. Patients are also at risk of acute renal failure secondary to the release of nephrotoxic uric acid. Treatment of tumour lysis syndrome is with intravenous fluids, allopurinol, renal support and correction of electrolyte imbalance. In patients known to be at risk of tumour lysis syndrome, intravenous fluids should be prescribed and prophylactic allopurinol or rasburicase given to reduce levels of uric acid.

Armand Trousseau, French physician (1801–67).

Frantisek Chvostek, Austrian physician (1835–84).

5. K – Neutropenic sepsis

Patients with leukaemia are at risk of neutropenia due to marrow infiltration and the cytotoxic effects of chemotherapy on bone marrow. When neutropenic patients encounter pathogens they often become septic. The clinical features of sepsis include pyrexia, hypotension, hypoxia and tachycardia (a fever >38°C for >1 hour in a patient with neutrophils $<1 \times 10^9$/L is indicative of neutropenic sepsis). In severe infection, disseminated intravascular coagulation and multiorgan failure may be seen. A septic screen, including chest X-ray, urinalysis, skin swabs, sputum culture, line cultures and peripheral blood cultures, should be requested, but should not delay treatment. Broad-spectrum intravenous antibiotics should be started empirically before sensitivities are known. Recombinant granulocyte colony-stimulating factor (G-CSF), which stimulates the production and proliferation of neutrophils, is sometimes given prophylactically following chemotherapy to reduce the risk of prolonged neutropenia and sepsis. Despite the availability of such technically advanced measures, good hand hygiene and reverse barrier nursing are the most effective way to prevent sepsis in patients.

Theme 11: Headache 2

1. I – Space-occupying lesions

A constant, dull headache that is worse in the morning (after periods of being supine) and exacerbated by coughing, straining and laughing is typical of an underlying space-occupying lesion. The headache may be accompanied by nausea and vomiting, blurring of vision and focal neurological signs. Fundoscopy may show bilateral papilloedema. This history requires an urgent CT head scan to confirm the presence of a lesion.

2. C – Giant cell arteritis

Giant cell arteritis is an inflammatory vasculitis of the cranial branches of the arteries arising from the aorta. It is most common in the over-50s and twice as frequent in women. Patients present with malaise, fever, temporal headache, scalp tenderness and pain on chewing (jaw claudication). On examination, the temporal artery is tender, enlarged and non-pulsatile. Some cases are associated with polymyalgia rheumatica (proximal muscle pain and stiffness without weakness). Diagnosis is with temporal artery biopsy, which shows patchy granulomatous necrosis with giant cells. Not all of the artery may be affected, so a negative biopsy result does not rule out disease. Furthermore, arteritis of the ophthalmic artery can lead to ischaemic optic neuritis and permanent blindness, so it is important to treat this condition immediately if there is clinical suspicion before performing biopsy. Treatment is with prednisolone.

3. J – Tension headache

Tension headaches are the most common headaches and are experienced by most people at some time. The pain is usually generalized and constant, radiating forward from the occiput, and is worse in the evening. Patients may describe a pressure sensation, like a tight band around the head. Local tenderness may be present. In contrast to migraine, headaches may persist for months and are not associated with vomiting or photophobia. Tension headaches are often unresponsive to analgesia, and excessive use of codeine can worsen them ('analgesia headache'). Reassurance and stress management are often helpful, and low-dose amitriptyline may be effective.

4. H – Sinusitis

Acute sinusitis is inflammation of the paranasal sinuses, which usually occurs following a bacterial upper respiratory tract infection. The pain of acute sinusitis is worse on bending and coughing, and may be accompanied by headache. The site of the pain depends on which sinus is affected. Acute maxillary sinusitis causes pain over the cheek, which may be referred to the teeth. Acute frontal sinusitis causes pain above the eyes. Acute ethmoid and sphenoid sinusitis can result in pain between or behind the eyes. In reality, however, the site of sinusitis may be very difficult to distinguish. In maxillary sinusitis, a skull X-ray may show a fluid level on the affected side. Treatment is with antibiotics (amoxicillin) and analgesia. Vasoconstricting nose drops (1% ephedrine) aid drainage of the sinus.

5. G – Sagittal sinus thrombosis

Cerebral venous sinus thrombosis describes a clot in one of the dural venous sinuses of the brain. The clinical features can depend on the underlying location of the thrombosis. Presentation is generally with a sudden-onset headache, seizures and signs of raised intracranial pressure, e.g. papilloedema, hypertension and bradycardia. More specific symptoms may be seen with cavernous sinus thrombosis (proptosis, ptosis, ophthalmoplegia, reduced sensation in the first division of the trigeminal nerve) and transverse sinus thrombosis (hemiparesis). Risk factors for the development of venous thromboses include contraceptive pill use, pregnancy, nephrotic syndrome and thrombophilias (protein S or C deficiency and antithrombin III deficiency). The diagnosis is confirmed by demonstrating the clot on CT or MRI. In sagittal sinus thrombosis, the 'empty delta sign' may be seen (a triangular area of enhancement within the sagittal sinus with a relatively low-attenuating centre). Management is with anticoagulation.

Coitus-induced headache usually occurs in middle-aged men. It is characterized by a sudden, severe headache at the climax of sex. Headaches persist for 10–15 minutes and there is no vomiting or neck stiffness. An *ice-pick headache* is a sudden, stabbing pain in the head that lasts only a split second. An *ice-cream headache* is a sharp, severe occipital pain lasting 30–60 seconds that is triggered by cold stimuli.

Theme 12: Arterial blood gases

Simple interpretation of arterial blood gases is usually all that is required in final EMQs. The pH value shows if the gas is acidotic (<7.35) or alkalotic (>7.45). Next, you need to find out if the alkalosis or acidosis is due to a metabolic or respiratory cause – this is done by looking at the $P\text{CO}_2$ and bicarbonate levels. There are two things that you need to bear in mind before continuing: (1) carbon dioxide is acidic and bicarbonate is alkaline; and (2) bicarbonate equates to 'metabolic' and $P\text{CO}_2$ means 'respiratory'. An alkalosis can be due to either a high bicarbonate ('metabolic alkalosis') or a low $P\text{CO}_2$ ('respiratory alkalosis'). Conversely, an acidosis can be caused by either a low bicarbonate ('metabolic acidosis') or a high $P\text{CO}_2$ ('respiratory acidosis').

In some cases of blood gas disturbance, the body has time to compensate. In other words, whichever chemical is causing the imbalance is counteracted by the opposite one. For example, if there is a high bicarbonate (metabolic alkalosis), then the $P\text{CO}_2$ starts to increase to raise the acidity and counteract the alkalosis. If compensation is successful, the pH will then return to within the normal range (7.35–7.45), even if the bicarbonate and $P\text{CO}_2$ levels are abnormal. It is important to know that the body can never overcompensate, i.e. if there is an initial acidosis, the body can never make that into an alkalosis, and the pH will always remain on the acidic side of normal (<7.40). Similarly, a compensated alkalosis will always have a pH >7.40, on the alkalotic side of normal.

Respiratory failure is defined as a $P\text{O}_2$ <8.0. Type I respiratory failure occurs when there is hypoxia in the presence of a low or normal $P\text{CO}_2$. Type II respiratory failure is hypoxia in the presence of a high $P\text{CO}_2$.

1. I – Type I respiratory failure

The pH, $P\text{CO}_2$ and bicarbonate levels are normal in this case, so there is no acid–base disorder. However, this man has hypoxia ($P\text{O}_2$ <8 kPa), which denotes respiratory failure. Because the $P\text{CO}_2$ is not high, it is a type I respiratory failure. Hypoxia is a common cause of confusion.

2. E – Metabolic acidosis

This girl's pH is acidotic (<7.35). The low $P\text{CO}_2$ contributes to alkalosis, but the low bicarbonate would cause an acidosis. The acidosis must therefore be due to the bicarbonate, with the carbon dioxide making an attempt to compensate, but not quite managing. This is therefore a partially compensated metabolic acidosis and, along with the patient's presentation, suggests diabetic ketoacidosis.

3. A – Fully compensated metabolic acidosis

This girl has a normal pH but abnormal carbon dioxide and bicarbonate levels. Therefore, there is definitely an acid–base balance, but it has been fully compensated. Because the pH is on the acidic side of normal (<7.40), you can safely say that the original disturbance was an acidosis. The low bicarbonate would cause the acidosis and the low $P\text{CO}_2$ would result in the compensatory alkalosis. Overall, this picture is a fully compensated metabolic acidosis, which could be accounted for by salicylate poisoning.

4. F – Metabolic alkalosis

This man has an abnormal pH of 7.49, which is alkalotic (>7.45). Because the bicarbonate is high, we know that this is a metabolic acidosis. The $P\text{CO}_2$ is within the normal range and the patient is not hypoxic, so overall he has a metabolic alkalosis with no effort at compensation. This blood gas is explained by his vomiting, with loss of gastric acid.

5. G – Respiratory acidosis

The pH is 7.31 (an acidosis). The bicarbonate is normal but the carbon dioxide is high, so it must be this that is contributing to the acid–base imbalance (respiratory acidosis). Since there is no effort at compensation by bicarbonate, this is an uncompensated respiratory acidosis and could be due to an underlying chest infection.

Theme 13: Management of rheumatological disease

1. D – Indometacin

This man is having an episode of acute gout. The management of acute gout is with non-steroidal anti-inflammatory drugs (NSAIDs), such as indometacin. Allopurinol is not given to treat acute attacks – it is only for prophylaxis. In fact, if allopurinol is given within a month of acute gout, there is a risk that it will precipitate another attack.

2. I – Steroids

This woman has temporal arteritis, which needs urgent treatment with steroids to reduce the risk of irreversible visual loss.

3. J – Sulfasalazine

This woman has a classic history of rheumatoid arthritis. Because symptomatic therapy is not working, she will need additional treatment with a disease-modifying antirheumatic drug (DMARD). Examples of DMARDs are ciclosporin, sulfasalazine, methotrexate, azathioprine and hydroxychloroquine. The first-line DMARD used in the UK is sulfasalazine. This patient has a rheumatoid nodule, and should ideally not receive methotrexate (which causes accelerated nodule growth).

4. H – Physiotherapy

This man has ankylosing spondylitis. Initial pain management is with slow-release NSAIDs, such as indometacin. However, this patient has a history of peptic ulcers, so NSAIDs are contraindicated. Physiotherapy is an alternative initial management option that may provide symptomatic relief.

5. C – Heparin

This woman has recurrent venous thromboembolism and miscarriages, suggestive of antiphospholipid syndrome (see 'Connective tissue disease' – Paper 4 Answers, Theme 13). People with antiphospholipid syndrome who have not yet suffered thrombosis are given regular low-dose aspirin. The patient in this scenario has already had two DVTs, and she should already be on warfarin. However, warfarin is teratogenic, and pregnant patients are given heparin instead to ensure viability of the fetus and reduce the risk of miscarriage.

Theme 14: Jaundice

Jaundice is defined as an elevation of serum bilirubin. The metabolism of bilirubin is as follows. The haem components of red blood cells are broken down by macrophages in the spleen and bone marrow to produce unconjugated bilirubin. This unconjugated bilirubin is insoluble and therefore not excretable. The liver then conjugates the bilirubin to make it soluble so that it can be excreted via the biliary tract into the duodenum. Duodenal bilirubin travels to the terminal ileum, where it is converted into urobilinogen. Urobilinogen has three fates: it can be absorbed by the blood and excreted via the kidneys into urine; it can be converted to stercobilinogen and excreted with the faeces; or it can be reabsorbed and re-excreted by the liver.

The causes of jaundice are divided into pre-hepatic, hepatic and post-hepatic, depending on the location of the underlying abnormality. *Pre-hepatic jaundice* results from an increased bile production due to haemolysis. Examples include hereditary spherocytosis and haemolytic transfusion reactions. There is an unconjugated hyperbilirubinaemia (insoluble bilirubin), so none is found in the urine. *Hepatic jaundice* is due to impaired bile conjugation and excretion in the liver, caused, for example, by hepatitis, cirrhosis, drugs or tumours. Here there is a mixed unconjugated and conjugated hyperbilirubinaemia. *Post-hepatic jaundice* is caused by biliary obstruction, e.g. by gallstones, tumour or infection. This results in a conjugated (soluble) hyperbilirubinaemia, with pale stools and dark urine.

1. H – Pancreatic carcinoma

This older man has painless progressive jaundice and weight loss with a palpable gallbladder, features that point strongly to carcinoma of the head of the pancreas. Pancreatic carcinoma is the fifth most common cancer in developed countries, occurring most often in the over-60s. Sixty per cent of tumours are located in the head of the pancreas, and these often obstruct the outflow of bile in the common bile duct. Risk factors for pancreatic carcinoma include diabetes, smoking and excess alcohol consumption. The classic presentation of carcinoma of the pancreas is with painless progressive jaundice. However, some patients complain of a dull epigastric pain that radiates to the back. If the tumour obstructs the common bile duct, there is obstruction of bile flow, resulting in a full, palpable gallbladder. Remember Courvoisier's law: 'If in the presence of jaundice the gallbladder is palpable, then the cause is unlikely to be stones' (i.e. it is likely to be a tumour!). Suspected pancreatic tumours should be delineated with a CT scan. Operative excision of pancreatic carcinomas is by Whipple's procedure. In this procedure, four things are removed: the pancreatic head, which contains the tumour; the common bile duct and gallbladder; the distal stomach; and some of the duodenum. Overall, pancreatic tumours have a very poor prognosis – most people are dead within 6 months.

Ludwig Georg Courvoisier, Swiss surgeon (1843–1918).

2. C – Common bile duct stone

This patient is describing the pain of biliary colic, which is caused by the gallbladder contracting against an obstruction (e.g. a gallstone). She has had several episodes of similar pain in the past that have been triggered by fatty food – a characteristic feature of biliary colic. This exacerbation is likely to have been caused by one of her gallstones moving into her common bile duct, causing biliary colic and jaundice. If this patient had a raised temperature and inflammatory markers, a provisional diagnosis of cholangitis could be made (inflammation of the biliary tree, which is usually secondary to infection of stagnant bile). Investigation of common bile duct stones usually involves an ultrasound scan followed by endoscopic retrograde cholangiopancreatography (ECRP). In ERCP, an endoscope is introduced into the duodenum, and the ampulla of Vater, where the common bile duct enters the duodenum, is identified and cannulated. A radio-opaque dye is then introduced into the common bile duct, allowing X-ray imaging of the biliary tree. ERCP can be used as a diagnostic and therapeutic investigation. If a stone is identified in the common bile duct, an incision can be made at the biliary sphincter of Oddi (sphincterotomy), which allows the stone to pass into the duodenum. In addition, if any stricture is identified in the duct, a stent can be inserted to maintain its patency.

3. F – Hepatic metastases

This patient is likely to have hepatic metastases secondary to a bowel malignancy. He gives a history of altered bowel habit, bleeding per rectum and weight loss, which should always be regarded as 'red flag' symptoms and investigated as soon as possible. The finding of hepatomegaly with an uneven border suggests hepatic metastases. Hepatic metastases can also be diagnosed by ultrasound and CT. The presence of multiple metastases in the liver can disrupt the architecture of the biliary tree and impede drainage into the small intestine. Conjugated bilirubin spills into the circulation, causing a conjugated jaundice. Other features of hepatic metastases include right upper quadrant abdominal pain caused by liver capsule expansion, clotting derangement and liver failure. Tumours that commonly metastasize to the liver include colon, breast, neuroendocrine, pancreatic, lung and gastric tumours, as well as lymphomas. In most situations, the presence of hepatic metastases suggests end-stage disease warranting palliative care. In some cases, resection may be possible.

4. J – Viral hepatitis

The history of general illness, abdominal pain and jaundice associated with high-risk behaviours such as intravenous drug use should always raise the suspicion of viral hepatitis. The most likely pathogen in this case is the hepatitis B virus (HBV), a DNA virus with an incubation period of between 40 and 160 days. Hepatitis B usually begins with a generalized illness, flu-like symptoms and arthralgia. Jaundice develops a little later, and is generally mild compared with that of hepatitis A. In some cases, the patient may develop fulminant liver failure.

There are a number of other viruses that can cause hepatitis. Hepatitis A virus is spread by the faecal–oral route, and usually causes a self-limiting illness that is often associated with the development of profound jaundice. Hepatitis E is similar to hepatitis A, with the distinction that if contracted during pregnancy it is associated with a high mortality. Hepatitis C virus (HCV) is spread by blood products and sexual intercourse, and is associated with a mild/asymptomatic acute infection followed by chronic carriage in up to 85% of those infected. Chronic carriers of HCV are at risk of developing cirrhosis, liver failure and hepatocellular carcinoma. Hepatitis D virus is an incomplete virus that can infect only people who already have HBV infection. When present in HBV-positive individuals, it often results in a more severe disease and an increased likelihood of developing cirrhosis and fulminant liver failure. Other causes of viral hepatitis include cytomegalovirus, Epstein–Barr virus and hepatitis G virus.

5. I – Paracetamol intoxication

This patient has taken a significant overdose of co-codamol, which contains paracetamol in combination with various strengths of codeine. Co-codamol 8/500 contains 500 mg of paracetamol and 8 mg of codeine per tablet. The paracetamol that the patient has ingested has surpassed the liver's ability to detoxify toxic metabolites via glutathione conjugation. The toxic metabolites of paracetamol therefore remain in the liver, causing hepatic necrosis and eventual liver failure. The antidote to paracetamol overdose is *N*-acetylcysteine. This restores the levels of endogenous glutathione, which then conjugates and detoxifies the paracetamol metabolites. A more detailed explanation of the pathophysiology and treatment of paracetamol overdose can be found in 'Overdose and antidotes' (Paper 9 Answers, Theme 11).

Theme 15: Spinal cord lesions

In general, the spinal cord is made up of three tracts on either side. A useful, simplified model of the spinal cord is as follows. The spinothalamic tract makes up the anterior third of the spinal cord, and provides pain and temperature fibres to the contralateral side. The corticospinal tract is the middle third of the spinal cord, and provides motor fibres to the ipsilateral side. Finally, the dorsal columns are found along the posterior length of the spinal cord, and provide vibration sense and proprioception to the ipsilateral side.

1. B – Brown-Séquard syndrome

Brown-Séquard syndrome describes the features of unilateral transection (hemisection) of the spinal cord. Affected patients suffer ipsilateral loss of motor function, with impaired joint position and vibration sense (dorsal column dysfunction). There is also a contralateral sensory loss for pain and temperature. Brown-Séquard syndrome has the best prognosis of all spinal cord lesions.

Charles-Edouard Brown-Séquard, British neurologist (1817–94).

2. F – Syringomyelia

Syringomyelia describes the presence of a longitudinal fluid cavity (syrinx) within the spinal cord. These cavities are usually in the cervical segments, and disrupt the spinothalamic tracts. Patients present in their 20s or 30s with a segmental dissociated loss of spinothalamic function (i.e. spinothalamic function above and below the lesion is preserved). Dorsal column and motor function remain intact. When a syrinx affects the brain stem, the condition is called syringobulbia. Diagnosis of syringomyelia is by MRI, and management is by surgical decompression of the syrinx.

Syringomyelia may be associated with an Arnold–Chiari malformation, congenital herniation of the cerebellar tonsils through the foramen magnum at the base of the skull. Syringomyelia may also be caused by tumours of, or trauma to, the spinal cord.

Syrinx from Greek (*syrinx* = tube). The word 'syringe' also derives from this.

Julius Arnold, German pathologist (1835–1915).

Hans Chiari, German pathologist (1851–1916).

3. D – Central cord syndrome

Central cord syndrome is the most common spinal cord lesion. It occurs in older people with cervical spondylosis who sustain a hyperextension injury. There is flaccid weakness of the arms, but motor and sensory fibres to the lower limb are comparatively preserved, as these are located more peripherally in the spinal cord. Central cord lesions have a fair prognosis.

4. C – Cauda equina syndrome

The spinal cord ends around the level of the junction between L1 and L2. Beyond this lies a bundle-like structure of spinal nerve roots known as the cauda equina. If narrowing of the spinal canal occurs below the level of L2 (e.g. in central cord prolapse or from compression by a tumour), then the spinal nerve roots are compromised and cauda equina syndrome results. Features of cauda equina syndrome include a triad of bowel/bladder disturbance (retention or incontinence), bilateral leg pain and weakness, and loss of sensation in the saddle area (around the perineum). Cauda equina syndrome is considered an emergency and requires urgent decompression either medically or surgically.

Cauda equina, from Latin *cauda* = tail + *equus* = horse.

5. E – Posterior cord syndrome

Hyperextension injuries can result in loss of dorsal column function (posterior cord syndrome). These injuries are very rare, and motor and sensory function is preserved. Gait is impaired due to impaired proprioception. The prognosis of posterior cord lesions is good.

Anterior cord syndrome occurs secondary to a flexion–compression injury. There is loss of neurological function of the anterior two-thirds of the spinal cord, namely the spinothalamic (pain and temperature) and corticospinal (motor) tracts. There is greater motor loss in the legs than in the arms. Anterior cord syndrome has the worst prognosis of all spinal cord lesions.

Practice Paper 6: Questions

Theme 1: Central nervous system infections

Options

A. Cerebral abscess
B. Kuru
C. Meningitis
D. Poliomyelitis
E. Rabies
F. Subacute sclerosing panencephalitis
G. Tetanus

For each of the following scenarios, select the most likely underlying infection. Each option may be used once, more than once or not at all.

1. A 14-year-old boy is brought to the GP with weakness in his left leg. This started 2 days ago and was preceded by a flu-like illness. On examination, the left leg is markedly weaker than the right. There is no evidence of cognitive impairment.

2. An 18-year-old man attends the emergency department with a 12-hour history of worsening headache and vomiting. He was previously well. On examination, neck flexion causes severe pain. There is no evidence of cognitive impairment.

3. A 34-year-old woman is brought to the emergency department by her husband. Over the last 2 days, she has become extremely anxious and has started hallucinating. She is refusing to eat or drink, saying that it causes severe pain in her stomach.

4. A 28-year-old woman presents to the emergency department with a 3-day history of worsening headache, fever and drowsiness. Examination is unremarkable, but there is no evidence of cognitive impairment. While you are taking blood from her, she has a seizure.

5. A 12-year-old boy is brought to the GP by his mother. She is worried that his performance at school has deteriorated markedly this term and that he does not seem himself anymore. He was previously well, but had measles as a child. Examination is unremarkable, but there is evidence of cognitive impairment.

Theme 2: Cutaneous malignancies

Options

A. Acral lentiginous melanoma
B. Actinic keratosis
C. Amelanotic melanoma
D. Basal cell carcinoma
E. Bowen's disease
F. Keratoacanthoma
G. Lentigo maligna melanoma
H. Nodular melanoma
I. Squamous cell carcinoma
J. Superficial spreading malignant melanoma

For each of the following people presenting with skin lesions, select the most likely diagnosis. Each option may be used once, more than once or not at all.

1. A 49-year-old man presents with a lesion on his arm that first appeared last month but has grown rapidly since. On examination, there is a 2 cm nodule with a central necrotic plug.

2. A 65-year-old man presents with a lesion on his upper ear that has been present for months but that has now begun to ulcerate. On examination, there is a non-pigmented, hyperkeratotic, crusty lesion with raised everted edges on the pinna.

3. A 37-year-old woman presents with a flat, irregular, pigmented lesion on her leg. This has grown in size in the past month, and occasionally bleeds.

4. A 64-year old woman presents with a large pinkish-brown lesion on her lower leg. On examination, the lesion is 4 cm, flat and scaly, with an irregular border.

5. A 78-year-old woman has had a large pigmented lesion on her left cheek for some years. She presents to her GP because a thickened, pigmented, irregular lesion is growing on the edge of the previous one.

Theme 3: Investigation of dyspnoea

Options

A. Bronchoscopy and biopsy
B. Chest X-ray
C. CT pulmonary angiography
D. D-dimers
E. Lung function tests
F. Kveim–Siltzbach test
G. Mantoux test
H. No investigation required
I. Pleural biopsy
J. Sputum culture
K. Sweat test
L. Ventilation–perfusion scan

For each of the following scenarios, select the next most appropriate investigation. Each option may be used once, more than once or not at all.

1. A 42-year-old woman presents with sudden-onset shortness of breath and a sharp chest pain on the right side. She is obviously distressed. Auscultation of the chest reveals no abnormality and there is no hyper-resonance to percussion.

2. A 42-year-old woman presents with sudden-onset shortness of breath and a sharp chest pain on the right side. She is obviously distressed. Auscultation of the chest reveals no abnormality and there is no hyper-resonance to percussion. A chest X-ray shows clear lung fields.

3. A 42-year-old woman presents with sudden-onset shortness of breath and a sharp chest pain on the right side. She is obviously distressed. Auscultation of the chest reveals no abnormality and there is no hyper-resonance to percussion. A chest X-ray shows occasional patchy shadowing.

4. A 42-year-old woman presents with sudden-onset shortness of breath and a sharp chest pain on the right side. She is obviously distressed and is coughing up large amounts of green sputum. Auscultation of the chest reveals crackles at the right lower zone. A chest X-ray confirms right lower lobe consolidation.

5. A 42-year-old woman presents with sudden-onset shortness of breath and a sharp chest pain on the right side. She is obviously distressed. Auscultation of the chest reveals hyper-resonance to percussion over the right side. The trachea is deviated to the left.

Theme 4: Platelet disorders

Options

A. Aplastic anaemia
B. Disseminated intravascular coagulation
C. Essential thrombocythaemia
D. Haemophilia A
E. Haemophilia B
F. Heparin-induced thrombocytopenia
G. Idiopathic thrombocytopenic purpura
H. Pancytopenia secondary to bone marrow infiltration
I. Post-transfusion thrombocytopenia
J. Reactive thrombocytosis
K. Vitamin K deficiency
L. Von Willebrand disease

For each of the following scenarios, select the most likely underlying platelet disorder. Each option may be used once, more than once or not at all.

1. A 12-year-old boy presents to the GP 2 weeks after contracting chickenpox. He has a non-blanching, palpable, purple rash all over his body and is bleeding from his gums. The full blood count shows a haemoglobin concentration of 14 g/dL, a platelet count of 40×10^9/L and a white cell count of 7×10^9/L. A clotting screen shows a normal PT and a normal APTT.

2. A 50-year-old woman is found to have a platelet count of 80×10^9/L 3 days after starting treatment for a deep vein thrombosis. She is not actively bleeding and has no other symptoms.

3. A 75-year-old man presents with a severe chest infection. He is known to have advanced myeloma. His full blood count shows a haemoglobin concentration of 5.5 g/dL, a mean cell volume of 100 fL, a platelet count of 30×10^9/L, a white cell count of 0.7×10^9/L and a neutrophil count of 0.1×10^9/L.

4. A 23-year-old woman presents to her GP complaining of easy bruising and heavy periods. Investigation reveals a mild iron-deficiency anaemia, a normal platelet count and a normal PT. The APTT is 50 s (normal 35–45 s). The bleeding time is 15 s (normal <7 s). Her father suffered from a bleeding disorder.

5. A 60-year-old woman is noticed to have a platelet count of 1200×10^9/L while being investigated for chronic headaches. Apart from occasional abdominal discomfort, she is fit and well. A bone marrow biopsy is taken, and shows a hypercellular marrow with increased numbers of megakaryocytes.

Theme 5: Cranial nerve function

Options

A. Abducens
B. Accessory
C. Facial
D. Glossopharyngeal
E. Hypoglossal
F. Oculomotor
G. Olfactory
H. Optic
I. Trigeminal
J. Trochlear
K. Vagus
L. Vestibulocochlear

For each of the following functions, select the most appropriate cranial nerve. Each option may be used once, more than once or not at all.

1. This nerve supplies the muscles of the tongue.

2. This nerve supplies the muscle that moves the eye laterally.

3. This nerve supplies the sternocleidomastoid muscle.

4. This nerve supplies the muscles of mastication.

5. This nerve supplies taste sensation to the anterior two-thirds of the tongue.

Theme 6: Hyperglycaemia

Options

A. Acromegaly
B. Acute pancreatitis
C. Corticosteroid therapy
D. Cushing's syndrome
E. Liver cirrhosis
F. Polycystic ovarian syndrome
G. Ramipril
H. Thiazide diuretics
I. Viral hepatitis

For each of the following scenarios, select the most likely cause of hyperglycaemia. Each option may be used once, more than once or not at all.

1. A 34-year-old man is being treated for acute cellular rejection of his transplanted kidney with high-dose methylprednisolone. He feels well and has not complained of any new symptoms. A random plasma glucose is 11.9 mmol/L.

2. A 45-year-old man with alcohol dependence is being managed on a surgical ward. He presented with severe epigastric pain in association with a significantly raised serum amylase. A random plasma glucose is 13.2 mmol/L.

3. A 65-year-old woman has a small cell lung carcinoma. She develops purple striae on her abdomen and has a blood pressure of 156/104 mmHg. A random plasma glucose is 12.5 mmol/L.

4. A 48-year-old man presents to his GP with a long history of general lethargy and depression. On examination, he has large hands and paraesthesiae in the first three fingers of the left hand. A random capillary blood glucose is 14.2 mmol/L.

5. A 65-year-old man attends the GP for lifestyle advice. He is being treated for high blood pressure but is otherwise well. A random capillary blood glucose is 13.0 mmol/L.

Theme 7: Signs of liver disease

Options

A. Asterixis
B. Caput medusae
C. Cirrhosis
D. Constructional apraxia
E. Dupuytren's contracture
F. Hepatomegaly
G. Jaundice
H. Kaiser–Fleischer rings
I. Leukonychia
J. Palmar erythema
K. Spider naevi
L. Xanthelasma

For each of the following scenarios, select the most appropriate physical sign. Each option may be used once, more than once or not at all.

1. A 64-year-old woman with a long history of alcohol abuse presents to her GP because she cannot fully extend the ring and little fingers on her left hand. Since her fingers are permanently partially flexed, she can no longer place her hand flat on a flat surface.

2. A 55-year-old man with cirrhosis secondary to alcoholic liver disease presents to the emergency department in a confused state. When asked to hold his arms outstretched with his hands cocked back, his wrists begin to jerk in a flexion–extension motion.

3. A 34-year-old man who is being investigated for jaundice is shown to have a smooth mass in his right upper quadrant. The mass is palpable 4 cm below the costal margin and moves down with respiration.

4. A 12-year-old girl being investigated for cirrhosis and behavioural changes is shown to have a green–yellow discoloration around her iris on slit-lamp examination.

5. A 57-year-old man with ascites and cirrhosis of the liver is noted to have distended veins around his umbilicus.

Theme 8: Acute renal failure

Options

A. Acute tubular necrosis
B. Analgesia nephropathy
C. Haemolytic uraemic syndrome
D. Idiopathic thrombocytopenic purpura
E. Interstitial renal failure secondary to glomerular nephritis
F. Interstitial renal failure secondary to non-steroidal anti-inflammatory drugs
G. Interstitial renal failure secondary to nephrotoxic antibiotics
H. Post-renal acute renal failure secondary to prostatic hypertrophy
I. Post-renal acute renal failure secondary to renal calculi
J. Pre-renal acute renal failure secondary to cardiac failure
K. Pre-renal acute renal failure secondary to coarctation of the aorta
L. Pre-renal acute renal failure secondary to hypovolaemia
M. Pre-renal acute renal failure secondary to renal artery stenosis

For each of the following scenarios, select the most likely cause of acute renal failure. Each option may be used once, more than once or not at all.

1. A 34-year-old man has lost a significant amount of blood following a motorbike accident. His blood test results include a serum urea of 20.2 mmol/L, a creatinine of 220 μmol/L, a potassium of 5.7 mmol/L and a sodium of 137 mmol/L. Urine electrolytes and osmolarity are normal. A CT scan confirms that there was no damage to the kidneys during the accident.

2. A 14-year-old boy has a 3-day history of diarrhoea and vomiting. Blood tests show a serum urea of 23.1 mmol/L, a creatinine of 400 μmol/L, a potassium of 5.9 mmol/L and a sodium of 134 mmol/L. The full blood count and blood film show a normocytic anaemia with fractionated red blood cells. A stool sample later confirms the presence of *Escherichia coli* O157.

3. A 76-year-old man presents to the emergency department unable to pass urine. This has been preceded by a 1-month history of difficulty passing water. His bladder is palpable up to the umbilicus. Blood tests show a urea of 16 mmol/L and a creatinine of 130 μmol/L.

4. An 87-year-old woman had seen her GP after straining her back while lifting a heavy box. She was prescribed a course of diclofenac. Five days later, she presents to the emergency department feeling generally unwell and slightly confused. Blood tests confirm that she is in acute renal failure.

5. A 68-year-old man becomes generally unwell after being started on ramipril for hypertension. He has a history of ischaemic heart disease. On examination, there are bilateral renal bruits. Blood tests show a serum urea of 22.8 mmol/L, a creatinine of 340 μmol/L, a potassium of 5.9 mmol/L and a sodium of 145 mmol/L.

Theme 9: Infective gastroenteritis

Options

A. *Bacillus cereus*
B. *Campylobacter jejuni*
C. *Clostridium botulinum*
D. *Clostridium difficile*
E. *Escherichia coli*
F. Rotavirus
G. *Staphylococcus aureus*
H. *Shigella sonnei*

For each of the following scenarios, select the most likely underlying pathogen. Each option may be used once, more than once or not at all.

1. A 67-year-old woman is in hospital being treated for a severe chest infection with intravenous antibiotics. On day 5, she develops severe watery diarrhoea. Examination is unremarkable.

2. A 35-year-old woman presents to her GP with profuse bloody diarrhoea and vomiting. On questioning, she admits to attending a barbecue 2 days ago, where she ate chicken burgers.

3. A 55-year-old man develops severe vomiting and watery diarrhoea 3 hours after eating fried rice from a late-night takeaway. Immediately before this, he was well.

4. A 16-year-old boy presents to his GP with vomiting that developed hours after eating a rewarmed rare steak. He denies diarrhoea.

5. A 3-year-old boy develops diarrhoea and vomiting the week before Christmas. A number of the other children at his nursery and his older sister are affected by a similar illness.

Theme 10: Seizures

Options

A. Anoxic seizure
B. Complex partial seizure
C. Febrile convulsion
D. Narcolepsy
E. Partial motor seizure
F. Partial sensory seizure
G. Pseudo-seizure
H. Status epilepticus
I. Tonic–clonic seizure
J. Tonic seizure
K. Versive seizure

For each of the following scenarios, select the most appropriate description. Each option may be used once, more than once or not at all.

1. A 14-year-old boy is playing football at school when he suddenly falls to the floor. Soon after, his friends notice him jerking around and unresponsive. During the episode, he is incontinent of urine and starts bleeding from his mouth. When the boy finally regains consciousness, he is confused and sleepy.

2. A 36-year-old woman is found on the street having a fit by passers-by. They stand close until she finishes fitting, and then try to rouse her. Before she regains consciousness, she starts having another seizure. By the time the ambulance arrives 10 minutes later, she is still fitting.

3. A 19-year-old man attends the university GP with sleep problems. He finds that he falls asleep multiple times during the day, including during small group seminars. On two occasions, he also experienced sudden collapses – both when he was laughing. His friends say that he was not incontinent during these episodes, nor did he bite his tongue.

4. A 21-year-old woman is sitting in the pub with friends. At one point, her friends notice that she is staring blankly into space, licking her lips. She remains sitting in her chair, and at no point does she begin fitting. After a few minutes, she returns to normal. She denies being aware of what happened.

5. A 3-year-old girl is brought to the emergency department after having a fit. She has no history of epilepsy and is on no medication. The seizure lasted 5 minutes. She is very hot to touch, and on examination you notice an inflamed left ear drum. Her father says that she has been pulling at her ear all day.

Theme 11: Side-effects of cardiovascular medication

Options

A. Amiodarone
B. Aspirin
C. Atenolol
D. Candesartan
E. Daltaparin
F. Digoxin
G. Furosemide
H. Glyceryl trinitrate
I. Ramipril
J. Sando-K
K. Simvastatin
L. Spironolactone
M. Streptokinase
N. Verapamil

For each of the following scenarios, select the most likely offending drug. Each option may be used once, more than once or not at all.

1. A 64-year-old man develops a dry cough about 1 week after starting a new blood pressure medication.

2. A 58-year-old woman develops bilateral swelling of her ankles 2 weeks after her GP has prescribed an antihypertensive drug.

3. A 74-year-old man is being treated for left ventricular failure as an inpatient. He is noticed to have U-waves on a routine ECG.

4. A 56-year-old woman presents to her GP with profound muscular pain, weakness and fever 5 days after beginning a course of an unknown 'heart tablet'.

5. A 55-year-old man who is being treated for ST-elevation myocardial infarction in the emergency department resuscitation room suddenly becomes hypotensive.

Theme 12: Drugs used during cardiac arrest

Options

A. Adrenaline
B. Amiodarone
C. Atropine
D. Calcium gluconate
E. Digoxin
F. Dopamine
G. Magnesium sulphate
H. Naloxone
I. Salbutamol

For each of the following descriptions, select the most appropriate drug. Each option may be used once, more than once or not at all.

1. This drug is used during cardiac arrest to increase coronary perfusion pressure.

2. This anti-arrhythmic drug is used in the standard management of ventricular fibrillation and pulseless ventricular tachycardia.

3. This drug, in addition to adrenaline, is specifically indicated in the management of asystole and pulseless electrical activity with a heart rate of less than 60 beats/min.

4. This drug can be used to treat ventricular fibrillation that is refractory to defibrillation when adrenaline and amiodarone have failed.

5. This drug should be considered for use in cardiac arrest secondary to hyperkalaemia.

Theme 13: Investigation of rheumatological disease

Options

A. Angiography
B. Anti-U1-RNP
C. cANCA
D. Joint aspiration and culture
E. Joint aspiration and microscopy
F. Muscle biopsy
G. Rheumatoid factor
H. Schirmer's test
I. Schober's test
J. Spine X-ray
K. Temporal artery biopsy

For each of the following scenarios, select the next most appropriate investigation. Each option may be used once, more than once or not at all.

1. A 47-year-old woman presents with a 2-month history of hip and shoulder weakness. She is finding it especially difficult to climb stairs. On examination, you notice a pink, scaly lesion on her knuckles.

2. A 22-year-old woman presents with a long history of dry, itchy eyes and a dry mouth. She denies having any problems with her vision. There is no abnormality on examination.

3. A 29-year-old woman presents with a 3-month history of general malaise, fever and weight loss. Over the last week, she has developed an intermittent cramping pain in her right arm. On examination, the upper limbs appear normal, but the radial pulses are not palpable.

4. A 61-year-old man presents with sudden-onset, severe pain in his left toe, which occurred at rest. He is otherwise well. On examination, the small joint of the great toe is swollen, red and tender.

5. A 57-year-old woman presents to the emergency department with malaise and a left-sided headache that has been getting worse over the last 24 hours. She also complains of some pain in her shoulders. On examination, she is tender over the left side of her head. Fundoscopy is unremarkable.

Theme 14: Diagnosis of thyroid disease 2

Options

A. Anaplastic carcinoma
B. De Quervain's thyroiditis
C. Follicular carcinoma
D. Graves' disease
E. Hashimoto's thyroiditis
F. Haemorrhage into a cyst
G. Medullary carcinoma
H. Myxoedema coma
I. Primary myxoedema
J. Thyroid storm
K. Toxic multinodular goitre

For each of the following people with thyroid disease, select the most likely diagnosis. Each option may be used once, more than once or not at all.

1. A 50-year-old woman attends her GP complaining of low mood and lethargy. She has had this for a few months and has had much time off work. On further questioning, she admits to being constipated and to having gained weight. On examination, no abnormality is apparent in the neck and no lymphadenopathy is palpable.

2. A 28-year-old woman goes to her GP following a sudden, sharp pain in her neck earlier in the day. Since then, she has found it difficult to breathe. On examination, you find a swelling on the right side of her neck. The patient tells you that this swelling has been there for some time and has never previously caused her any trouble.

3. A 32-year-old woman presents with a 5-week history of resting tremor and diarrhoea. She mentions that just before these symptoms occurred she had some time off work with a cough and cold. On examination, her pulse is 96/min and regular. The thyroid gland in generally enlarged, soft and tender to the touch. No cervical lymph nodes are palpable.

4. An anxious 22-year-old woman presents to her GP with a month's history of worsening diarrhoea. On further questioning, she admits losing 10 pounds (4.5 kg) over the last few weeks, despite having a good appetite. On examination, you notice a slight tremor, and her pulse is 110/min and irregular. Examination of the neck demonstrates no deformity or palpable nodes, although a bruit is heard over the thyroid.

5. A 62-year-old woman is brought by her husband to the emergency department with reduced consciousness. On examination, she has a temperature of 30°C and her pulse is 48/min. Her husband tells you that she has a history of depression and has recently been refusing to take her regular medications.

Theme 15: Diagnosis of chest pain

Options

A. Acute myocardial infarction
B. Aortic dissection
C. Boerhaave's syndrome
D. Decubitus angina
E. Gastro-oesophageal reflux disease
F. Herpes zoster
G. Mitral valve prolapse
H. Oesophageal spasm
I. Pericarditis
J. Pulmonary oedema
K. Pulmonary embolism
L. Stable angina
M. Tietze's syndrome

For each of the following scenarios, select the most likely diagnosis. Each option may be used once, more than once or not at all.

1. A 60-year-man with known hypertension presents to the emergency department with a 2-hour history of central chest pain and interscapular back pain. Over the next 30 minutes, he develops slurred speech and reduced power and sensation on his left side.

2. A 30-year-old woman with a known congenital heart defect presents to her GP with a 4-week history of left-sided chest pain and palpitations that are worse on exertion. The pain does not radiate, has no other associated symptoms and is not worse on inspiration. On examination, there is a mid-systolic click best heard at the apex on auscultation of the heart.

3. A 70-year-old man presents to his GP following an episode of central crushing chest pain that started 30 minutes after going to bed. The pain did not radiate and there were no associated symptoms. Following two puffs of sublingual glyceryl trinitrate spray, his chest pain resolved. The ECG shows no abnormalities. This is the third time in the last 2 weeks that these symptoms have occurred on going to bed.

4. A 36-year-old man with alcohol dependence presents to the emergency department with a 5-hour history of vomiting followed by chest pain. On examination, his heart sounds are normal. There is reduced air entry at the left lung base, which is also dull to percussion. You also notice a cracking sensation on your fingertips when you palpate his carotid arteries. The ECG shows sinus tachycardia.

5. A 70-year-old man presents to the emergency department with retrosternal chest pain that is crushing in nature. This has happened on several occasions previously, and usually occurs after drinking hot fluids. Despite there being no ECG changes, he is given glyceryl trinitrate, which partially relieves the pain. After 30 minutes, the pain relieves spontaneously.

Practice Paper 6: Answers

Theme 1: Central nervous system infections

1. D – Poliomyelitis

Poliomyelitis is caused by the poliovirus. Infection occurs through the nasopharynx and is more common in developing countries. The virus infects the grey matter of the nervous system, especially the anterior horn cells in the lumbar region. Initial infection causes a mild fever and headache, progressing to aseptic meningitis. Weakness then starts in one muscle group and can progress to widespread paresis. Respiratory failure occurs if the intercostal muscles are affected. Diagnosis is confirmed by culturing poliovirus from cerebrospinal fluid (CSF) or stool. Management is with bed rest (as exercise worsens or precipitates paralysis) and ventilation if required. Any muscle weakness that remains after 1 month of initial infection is likely to remain permanent. Prevention of poliomyelitis is with immunization by a live vaccine.

Poliomyelitis, from Greek *polio* = grey + *myelon* = marrow (indicating spinal cord).

2. C – Meningitis

Meningitis is inflammation of the lining of the brain. Common clinical features are headache, photophobia, severe vomiting and neck stiffness. The characteristic purpuric rash is seen only with meningococcal septicaemia (*Neisseria meningitidis*). Examination findings in meningitis include Kernig's sign (pain on knee extension when the hips are flexed) and Brudzinski's sign (pain on passive neck flexion). There are many underlying causes of meningitis.

Viral meningitis is the most common cause, and is usually benign and self-limiting. There is an acute onset of headache and rapid development of meningism, without focal neurology. CSF demonstrates high lymphocytes, normal glucose and normal protein. (For a summary of CSF results in meningitis, see 'Interpretation of cerebrospinal fluid results' – Paper 1 Answers, Theme 7.) Treatment is symptomatic.

Bacterial meningitis has a number of causes, depending on age: neonates (*Escherichia coli*, group B streptococci and *Listeria monocytogenes*), young children (*Haemophilus influenzae, N. meningitidis* and *Streptococcus pneumoniae*) and older people (*N. meningitidis, S. pneumoniae*). *N. meningitidis* is the most common cause, and is spread by airborne droplets. Apart from the usual features of meningitis, complications of meningococcal septicaemia include a purpuric rash, shock, disseminated intravascular coagulation, renal failure, gangrene, arthritis and pericarditis. Management is with immediate empirical antibiotics, e.g. benzylpenicillin or cefotaxime. A lumbar puncture is mandatory if there is no contraindication. A CT of the head should be done before this to exclude any causes of raised intracranial pressure, which would cause coning of the brain-stem through the foramen magnum during lumbar puncture. All contacts of patients with bacterial meningitis are given prophylaxis e.g. rifampicin.

Tuberculous meningitis has a slower onset of symptoms, with headache, vomiting, low-grade fever and confusion. Typical meningism may be absent, but patients often have focal neurological signs. The CSF in tuberculous meningitis is clear, but, if allowed to stand, it forms a fine clot (spider's web). Treatment is with anti-tuberculous drugs for at least 12 months.

Other causes of meningitis include fungal infections (*Cryptococcus neoformans* in immunocompromised individuals), prions (Creutzfeldt–Jakob disease and kuru), protozoa (malaria and toxoplasmosis), malignant invasion and aseptic meningitis (systemic lupus erythematosus, sarcoidosis and Mollaret's syndrome). Mollaret's syndrome describes recurrent aseptic meningitis characterized by epithelioid cells in the CSF.

3. E – Rabies

Rabies is caused by a rhabdovirus that infects the central nervous tissue and salivary glands. It is transmitted by saliva through bites and licks, and humans are usually infected by dogs. A few weeks after infection, fever and paraesthesiae at the site of the bite develop. There may be a prodrome of anxiety and hydrophobia (attempts at drinking provoke violent spasm of the diaphragm and other inspiratory muscles). Delusions, hallucinations, spitting, biting, mania and hyperpyrexia develop, and death occurs within a week of onset of symptoms. Diagnosis is clinical and management is palliative, as very few survive. The only people who have survived rabies are those who managed to gain timely post-exposure prophylaxis with antirabies antiserum. Rabies can be avoided with a vaccine.

Rabies, from Latin *rabies* = rage.

4. A – Cerebral abscess

Bacteria can enter the cerebrum either via the blood or directly (from the paranasal sinuses or the middle ear). Features of cerebral abscesses include fever, headache, meningism and drowsiness. An abscess can also present chronically as a mass lesion (with seizures, focal neurological signs and raised intracranial pressure). A CT scan will demonstrate an abscess as an area of low density surrounded by a capsule. Treatment is with antibiotics, although a burr-hole aspiration may be needed. The mortality rate is 20%.

Viral encephalitis presents with acute-onset headache, focal neurology, seizures and impaired consciousness. The most common cause in Europe is herpes simplex virus (HSV). A CT head scan shows low-density lesions (representing inflammation of the cortex). A lumbar puncture yields excess lymphocytes, a normal glucose and elevated protein. Management is with aciclovir (for the HSV), anticonvulsants (for seizures) and dexamethasone (to alleviate the raised intracranial pressure).

5. F – Subacute sclerosing panencephalitis

Subacute sclerosing panencephalitis is a fatal disorder caused by the measles virus. It begins many years after the original measles infection with insidious intellectual deterioration, apathy, myoclonic jerks, rigidity and dementia. The

EEG is distinctive (showing periodic bursts of triphasic waves). There is no effective treatment, and death occurs within years.

Tetanus is caused by the Gram-positive bacillus *Clostridium tetani*, a commensal of human and animal guts and found in the soil. Infection enters the body through wounds. The bacterium secretes an exotoxin that causes trismus (painless masseter spasm) and contraction of the muscles of the face, neck and trunk. Patients eventually die of exhaustion, asphyxia or aspiration pneumonia. Management is with intravenous tetanus antitoxin and benzylpenicillin.

Theme 2: Cutaneous malignancies

1. F – Keratoacanthoma

A keratoacanthoma (or molluscum sebaceum) is a benign tumour of hair follicle cells. It occurs on sun-exposed sites (e.g. the face and arms), and is more common in elderly people. Keratoacanthomas grow rapidly over 6–8 weeks, and are characterized by a rolled edge with a central keratin plug, which can fall out and leave a crater. Spontaneous resolution occurs, but takes several months and leaves a deep scar. Keratoacanthomas are usually excised, as there is a small risk of transformation to squamous cell carcinoma. Squamous cell carcinomas differ from keratoacanthomas in that they grow slowly, there is no central core and they gradually ulcerate.

Keratoacanthoma, from Greek *kerat* = horn + *akantha* = thorn; a thorn of horn.

2. I – Squamous cell carcinoma

Squamous cell carcinoma (SCC) is a malignant tumour of keratinocytes that occurs in those aged over 50 in sun-damaged sites. Predisposing factors for their development include X-ray exposure, smoking, human papillomavirus and a genetic susceptibility. SCCs typically have raised everted edges with a central scab. Management is by surgical excision, with lymph node dissection or radiotherapy if there is evidence of spread.

An *actinic keratosis* (also known as a solar keratosis) is a hyperkeratotic, yellow–brown crusty lesion that occurs on sun-damaged sites. Although these lesions are benign, they are premalignant to SCC. For this reason, actinic keratoses should be removed, e.g. by excision, shaving or cryotherapy.

3. J – Superficial spreading malignant melanoma

Malignant melanoma is a malignant tumour of melanocytes and is the most lethal of skin tumours. It is most common in white people living near the equator, and is twice as common in women. Risk factors include repeated ultraviolet exposure, previous malignant melanoma, multiple melanocytic naevi and having a large congenital naevus. Primary treatment is by surgical excision. Prognosis is related to tumour depth (Breslow score).

Superficial spreading malignant melanoma is the most common type of malignant melanoma. It occurs most often in younger females on the leg. The tumour is macular with an irregular edge, and may itch or bleed.

4. E – Bowen's disease

Bowen's disease (squamous cell carcinoma in situ) is a premalignant intraepidermal carcinoma with atypical keratinocytes. It typically occurs on the legs of older women. Bowen's disease presents as large pink or brown flat lesions with a superficial crust that may look like eczema. Previous exposure to arsenic can predispose to the condition. A small percentage of cases can progress to SCC. Treatment is by excision. *Erythroplasia of Queyrat* is Bowen's disease of the glans penis. It appears as a red, velvety lesion.

John Templeton Bowen, American dermatologist (1857–1941).

Louis Queyrat, French dermatologist (1872–1933).

5. G – Lentigo maligna melanoma

The original lesion that this woman has on her cheek is a lentigo maligna (or Hutchinson's malignant freckle) – a large irregular pigmented area that occurs most often in elderly people on sun-exposed skin. Lentigo maligna is associated with malignant transformation to melanoma (lentigo maligna melanoma). Thickening, darkening or ulceration within a lentigo maligna signals the onset of malignancy.

Lentigo, from Latin *lentigo* = lentil; the word was originally used to describe freckles.

Sir Jonathan Hutchinson, English surgeon and pathologist (1828–1913).

Other forms of malignant melanoma include nodular, acral lentiginous and amelanotic types. *Nodular melanomas* present as thick, protruding, smooth, sharply defined lesions that grow in a vertical direction and may bleed and ulcerate. They are the most aggressive of all melanomas. Nodular melanomas need not be pigmented (amelanotic melanomas) – these are associated with a poorer prognosis, as the lesions are not as noticeable. *Acral lentiginous melanomas* (or subungual melanomas) present as expanding pigmented lesions on the palms, soles and nail beds. This is the most common presentation in African-Caribbean people.

Theme 3: Investigation of dyspnoea

1. B – Chest X-ray

This woman presents with a history highly suggestive of a pulmonary embolism (PE). A chest X-ray should be performed first, and this will help dictate further management and rule out other pathology.

2. L – Ventilation–perfusion scan

This woman has a history suggestive of PE and a clear chest X-ray. Because the X-ray is clear, she is suitable for a ventilation–perfusion ($\dot{V}/\dot{Q}$) scan in the first instance.

3. C – CT pulmonary angiography

This woman has a history suggestive of PE, together with shadowing on the chest X-ray. A $\dot{V}/\dot{Q}$ scan is likely to produce results that are difficult to interpret, given the underlying lung disease. CT pulmonary angiography is therefore the best investigation in this case.

4. J – Sputum culture

This patient has pneumonia, as shown on X-ray. A sputum culture should be sent off to help determine the underlying cause and dictate future therapy.

5. H – No investigation required

This woman has a tension pneumothorax. Instead of wasting time confirming this by chest X-ray, the pressure should be relieved using a cannula inserted into the second intercostal space at the midclavicular line.

Theme 4: Platelet disorders

1. G – Idiopathic thrombocytopenic purpura

In idiopathic thrombocytopenic purpura (ITP), autoantibodies are formed against platelets, resulting in their premature destruction. This condition, which is usually seen shortly after a viral illness such as varicella-zoster infection, causes the platelet count to fall rapidly. The patient usually develops a purpuric rash and experiences bleeding from the skin and mucous membranes. In very severe cases, there may be more significant bleeding, including intracranial haemorrhage. Investigation shows a normal prothrombin time (PT) and a normal activated partial thromboplastin time (APTT), since the clotting factors and clotting cascade are unaffected. The bleeding time is prolonged, as the thrombocytopenia reduces the rate of platelet activation and aggregation at the site of injury. The disease is usually self-limiting and requires no specific management. In severe disease, corticosteroids or immunoglobulin may be used.

2. F – Heparin-induced thrombocytopenia

Thrombocytopenia can be induced by a number of drugs. In this case, the responsible drug is likely to be a low-molecular-weight heparin (LMWH), e.g. enoxaparin. LMWH is commonly prescribed in hospital for the prevention and treatment of deep vein thrombosis and PE. Type I heparin-induced thrombocytopenia (HIT) is a non-immune, transient, asymptomatic thrombocytopenia that is seen in up to 10% of patients given heparin. Platelet levels usually remain above 80 × 10^9/L, and no treatment is required. The platelet count improves spontaneously, even when heparin is continued. Type II HIT is a rare but serious condition that may result in multi-organ failure and death secondary to an autoimmune process. There is a mild thrombocytopenia associated with idiosyncratic arterial and venous thrombus formation. Type II HIT is seen in approximately 3–5% of patients who are prescribed unfractionated heparin, but is much less common with LMWH. If type II HIT is suspected, heparin must be stopped immediately and an alternative treatment instigated. Thrombolytic agents such as streptokinase may be needed to treat significant thrombosis.

3. H – Pancytopenia secondary to bone marrow infiltration

This patient is anaemic, thrombocytopenic and neutropenic – collectively referred to as pancytopenia. The most likely cause in this case is bone marrow infiltration secondary to multiple myeloma. Such patients are at significant risk of anaemia, bleeding and infection. Other causes of pancytopenia include severe megaloblastic anaemia, aplastic anaemia and hypersplenism. Treatment of this condition is supportive with blood and platelet transfusion, strict infection control and intravenous antibiotics for infection.

4. L – Von Willebrand disease

In von Willebrand's disease, there is a quantitative or qualitative deficiency of von Willebrand factor (vWF), which is a protein that promotes platelet adhesion to the vascular wall and subsequent aggregation. It also plays a role in the transport of factor VIII and in preventing its premature destruction. There are three main types of von Willebrand disease. In type 1 disease, there are reduced levels of normal vWF. Type 2 disease is due to the production of defective vWF. In type 3 disease, there is a total lack of vWF production and a significantly reduced level of factor VIII. Types 1 and 2 disease are autosomal dominant conditions. Type 3 disease is autosomal recessive. Types 1 and 2 disease are usually mild, with patients complaining of bruising, epistaxis and menorrhagia. Type 3 disease is more severe, and may cause bleeding into joints and soft tissues (haemarthrosis). Investigation of vWF shows a normal platelet level and a normal PT. APTT may be slightly prolonged due to reduced levels of factor VIII in severe disease. The bleeding time is increased, as platelets fail to adhere to the vessel wall and aggregate.

Mild disease requires no treatment. In moderate disease, the antifibrinolytic drug tranexamic acid can be given to reduce bleeding. Desmopressin (DDAVP), a vasopressin analogue, is able to release vWF and factor VIII from internal stores, and is sometimes used in moderate type 1 disease. (The inability to produce functioning vWF in type 2 disease and the absolute lack of vWF in type 3 disease means that DDAVP is not effective in these cases.) In severe disease, vWF and factor VIII can be replaced with factor VIII concentrate, fresh frozen plasma and cryoprecipitate (e.g. prior to surgery or in acute bleeding episodes).

Erik Adolf von Willebrand, Swedish physician (1870–1949).

5. C – Essential thrombocythaemia

Essential thrombocythaemia (ET) is a myeloproliferative disorder characterized by excessive production of defective platelets derived from abnormal megakaryocytes in the bone marrow. The main complications of ET are due to the formation of thrombi within the microcirculation. Symptoms include headache, digital ischaemia and abdominal pain secondary to splenic infarction. Many patients also suffer from erythromelalgia, i.e. aching and burning of the hands and feet secondary to ischaemia. Occasionally, there is paradoxical bleeding from the mucous membranes, such as the gastrointestinal tract and uterus. Investigation usually shows a platelet count in excess of 1000×10^9/L. The haemoglobin concentration and haematocrit are normal (unless there is significant blood loss, in which case there may be a microcytic anaemia). Definitive diagnosis requires bone marrow aspiration, which typically shows a hypercellular marrow with large numbers of megakaryocytes. Asymptomatic disease often requires no intervention. Severe and symptomatic disease can be treated with chemotherapy, usually with hydroxyurea or interferon-β, and low-dose aspirin.

Theme 5: Cranial nerve function

1. E – Hypoglossal

2. A – Abducens

3. B – Accessory

4. I – Trigeminal

5. C – Facial

The cranial nerves and their functions can be summarized as follows:

I (olfactory):	Smell
II (optic):	Visual acuity and visual fields Afferent arm of pupillary light and accommodation reflexes
III (oculomotor):	Eye muscles (inferior oblique, medial/superior/inferior rectus) Levator palpabrae muscles (upper eyelid) Efferent arm of pupillary light reflex
IV (trochlear):	Superior oblique muscle (moves eye inferomedially)
V (trigeminal):	Sensation of face Muscle of mastication and jaw jerk Afferent arm of corneal reflex
VI (abducens):	Lateral rectus muscle (moves eye laterally)
VII (facial):	Muscles of facial expression Taste to anterior two-thirds of tongue Nerve to stapedius (which dampens loud sounds) Sensation around skin of ear Efferent arm of corneal reflex
VIII (vestibulocochlear):	Ear and vestibular system
IX (glossopharyngeal):	Taste to posterior third of tongue Afferent arm of gag reflex
X (vagus):	Muscles of pharynx and larynx Efferent arm of gag reflex
XI (accessory):	Trapezius and sternocleidomastoid muscles
XII (hypoglossal):	Muscles of the tongue

Theme 6: Hyperglycaemia

1. C – Corticosteroid therapy

Methylprednisolone is an intravenous synthetic corticosteroid used for the prevention of acute cellular rejection of transplanted organs and for the treatment of inflammatory disorders. Corticosteroid therapy is associated with a number of short- and long-term complications, including hyperglycaemia, diabetes, sodium retention, fluid retention and hypertension. The prolonged use of glucocorticoids may result in the development of Cushing's syndrome, causing osteoporosis, adrenal suppression, weight gain, glaucoma and an increased risk of cardiovascular disease.

2. B – Acute pancreatitis

Acute pancreatitis is a serious condition in which the pancreas becomes inflamed and necrotized. In the developed world, the most common causes of pancreatitis are alcohol excess and gallstones. Other causes include trauma, steroids, hyperlipidaemia, autoimmune disease and some drugs. The inflammatory process can damage the islets of Langerhans, resulting in reduced insulin secretion and subsequent hyperglycaemia. Treatment of pancreatitis is usually conservative with fluid therapy, glucose control and analgesia.

3. D – Cushing's syndrome

Cushing's syndrome is a multisystem disease caused by excessive levels of circulating corticosteroids. It can be iatrogenic secondary to long-term corticosteroid therapy or caused by the excessive secretion of adrenocorticotropic hormone (ACTH, corticotropin). When ACTH is secreted autonomously, e.g. from a pituitary adenoma or small cell carcinoma, it is not under the control of negative feedback. The result is unregulated secretion of cortisol and other hormones from the adrenal cortex, causing hypertension, central weight gain, moon face, poor-quality skin, bruising, poor wound healing, hirsutism, acne, striae, oligomenorrhoea, osteoporosis, hyperglycaemia, polyuria, polydipsia, myopathy, depression and psychosis. Treatment of corticosteroid excess involves correcting the underlying cause (e.g. stopping corticosteroid therapy, tumour resection or radiotherapy) and managing complications such as hypertension and hyperglycaemia. In cases where surgery or radiotherapy is contraindicated (e.g. metastatic disease), ketoconazole may be trialled.

4. A – Acromegaly

This patient has acromegaly caused by the excessive secretion of growth hormone (GH) from a pituitary adenoma. In adults, the symptoms of GH excess often have an insidious onset, and include general illness, lethargy, headache and proximal limb weakness. Other features that may be found on examination include large 'spade-like' hands, hepatomegaly, splenomegaly, cardiomegaly, carpal tunnel syndrome and bilateral hemianopia caused by compression of the optic chiasm. GH is mainly anabolic and opposes the action of insulin, resulting in hyperglycaemia and diabetes. Patients with acromegaly often develop cardiovascular disease. Insulin-like growth factor 1 (IGF-1) is secreted in response to GH and is responsible for many of its actions. IGF-1 is more consistently elevated compared with GH and is more reliable as a diagnostic tool. In addition, the failure of GH levels to be suppressed by a 75 g oral bolus of glucose indicates GH excess. CT or MRI of the brain is indicated to identify the tumour, and is useful when planning surgery. Trans-sphenoidal removal of the adenoma is the treatment of choice, with or without pituitary radiotherapy and pharmacotherapy. The drugs used in the management of acromegaly include octreotide and bromocriptine. Octreotide is a somatostatin analogue that inhibits the production of GH. Bromocriptine is a dopamine agonist that reduces GH secretion.

5. H – Thiazide diuretics

Thiazide diuretics, such as bendroflumethiazide, are known to trigger hyperglycaemia and exacerbate diabetes. The risk is more prominent in patients taking higher doses. Other classes of drug that may induce diabetes include β-blockers, antipsychotics and steroids.

Theme 7: Signs of liver disease

1. E – Dupuytren's contracture

Dupuytren's contracture is a progressive fibroplasia of the palmar facia that results in a flexion contracture of the fingers. It is most common in the ring and little fingers. Risk factors include male sex, a family history, diabetes mellitus, alcoholic cirrhosis, phenytoin use, trauma, AIDS, Peyronie's disease (idiopathic fibrosis of the corpus cavernosum) and Ledderhose's disease (fibrosis of the plantar fascia, resulting in a similar deformity). On examination, the thickened palmar aponeurosis can be felt. Treatment is by excision of the thickened part of the aponeurosis.

Guillaume Dupuytren, French surgeon (1777–1835).

2. A – Asterixis

Asterixis describes a jerking flexion–extension movement of the hand seen when the arms are placed in an outstretched position with the wrists cocked back. It is associated with hepatic encephalopathy, and should be tested for in all patients with liver disease who present with an acute deterioration of disease, worsening ascites, confusion, agitation, reversal of sleeping pattern and stupor. Patients with hepatic encephalopathy may also find it difficult to perform certain motor tasks, such as drawing a five-pointed star. This is known as constructional apraxia.

3. F – Hepatomegaly

Hepatomegaly describes enlargement of the liver. It is detected clinically by palpating the right upper quadrant during inspiration. As the patient inspires, the liver is displaced inferiorly by the lungs onto the examiner's hand. The liver should not be palpable in normal individuals, with the exception of children and very thin patients. The presence of hepatomegaly is usually described in terms of size, e.g. number of finger-breadths below the costal margin. The texture of the liver edge should also be documented, i.e. whether it is smooth or craggy. Conditions that cause hepatomegaly with a smooth margin include viral hepatitis, biliary tract obstruction, hepatic vein thrombosis (Budd–Chiari syndrome), right heart failure and myeloproliferative disease. Hepatomegaly with a craggy border is usually associated with hepatic metastatic disease, polycystic disease and occasionally cirrhosis (although this usually causes the liver to contract and shrink).

4. H – Kaiser–Fleischer rings

Kaiser–Fleischer rings are seen in Wilson's disease, in which copper is deposited in vital organs due to an error in metabolism that prevents its secretion into the bile. Kaiser–Fleischer rings are due to the deposition of copper in Descemet's membrane, which is located between the corneal stroma and endothelium in the eye. They appear as brown–green rings around the iris, and are seen in up to 90% of patients with Wilson's disease. In most patients, they can be seen only using a slit-lamp examination, although they may be visible with the naked eye in patients with light-blue eyes and in those with advanced disease.

5. B – Caput medusae

In portal hypertension secondary to cirrhosis, the high pressure within the portal vein results in portosystemic shunting, i.e. flow of blood under high pressure into collateral veins such as the submucosal oesophageal veins, rectal veins and umbilical veins. Under higher than normal pressure, these veins become dilated, engorged and tortuous. Caput medusae is a sign of portal hypertension in which the umbilical veins become dilated and engorged and are seen to radiate from the umbilicus. A similar sign is also seen in inferior vena caval obstruction, and is differentiated from caput medusae by determining the flow of blood. In inferior vena caval obstruction, the blood flows towards the head in an attempt to bypass the blocked vessel. In caput medusae, the blood flows towards the legs. Portosystemic shunting is also responsible for the development of rectal varices and oesophageal varices in patients with portal hypertension.

Caput medusae, from Latin = head of Medusa; Medusa was a mythological creature who had snakes for hair and would turn those who looked at her into stone.

Theme 8: Acute renal failure

1. L – Pre-renal acute renal failure secondary to hypovolaemia

Acute renal failure can be defined as the deterioration of renal function over hours or days. By far the most common cause of acute renal failure is hypoperfusion of the kidney, referred to as pre-renal acute renal failure. This is usually seen with hypovolaemia secondary to conditions such as acute blood loss, vomiting, diarrhoea and burns. It may also occur in normovolaemic patients with sepsis, cardiac failure or renal artery stenosis. Investigation demonstrates high serum urea, creatinine and potassium concentrations, and a poor urine output. Pre-renal acute renal failure is treated by correcting the underlying condition and restoring the patient's circulating volume with intravenous fluids. If the kidneys are hypoperfused for a significant amount of time, autoregulatory mechanisms within the renal vasculature fail, causing tubular cell damage and death. This condition is known as acute tubular necrosis (ATN) and results in failure of active sodium reabsorption and failure to concentrate the urine. The urine produced in ATN typically has a high sodium concentration, a low osmolarity, a low urine: serum urea ratio and a low urine:plasma osmolarity ratio. ATN usually resolves if the underlying cause is corrected and appropriate fluid therapy is delivered, although recovery may take weeks. During recovery, there is an oliguric phase (when both glomerular filtration and tubular function are compromised), followed by a diuretic phase (when glomerular filtration recovers before tubular function is regained).

2. C – Haemolytic uraemic syndrome

In haemolytic uraemic syndrome (HUS), there is acute renal failure, microangiopathic haemolytic anaemia and thrombocytopenia. This condition is classically seen in childhood following gastroenteritis caused by *Escherichia coli* O157, which produces nephrotoxic verotoxins. Other gastrointestinal and respiratory tract pathogens may also cause HUS, but are seen less frequently. The haemolytic anaemia and thrombocytopenia are due to erythrocyte and platelet destruction within fibrin meshes that are deposited on affected endothelial membranes. Other features of HUS include haematuria, proteinuria, purpuric rash and central nervous system complications. Treatment of HUS is supportive. Some patients require temporary peritoneal dialysis or haemodialysis. Occasionally, renal function is permanently compromised, necessitating long-term renal replacement therapy and renal transplantation.

3. H – Post-renal acute renal failure secondary to prostatic hypertrophy

Acute renal failure secondary to urinary tract obstruction is referred to as post-renal acute renal failure. Urinary tract obstruction may be caused by prostatic hypertrophy, urinary tract calculi, renal tract malignancy, constipation or retroperitoneal fibrosis. In this case, the patient presented with urinary retention secondary to prostatic disease. The obstruction causes urine to accumulate under high pressure in the renal pelvis, resulting in a deterioration in renal function. In cases of urinary retention secondary to prostate pathology, a urinary catheter should be inserted to bypass the obstruction until a more definitive treatment can be organized, e.g. transurethral resection of the prostate (TURP).

4. F – Interstitial renal failure secondary to non-steroidal anti-inflammatory drugs

Diclofenac is a strong non-steroidal anti-inflammatory drug (NSAID) that is usually prescribed for muscular injury and renal colic. NSAIDs inhibit the production of prostaglandins, which are essential in maintaining renal perfusion. NSAIDs are therefore nephrotoxic and should be avoided in patients with known renal disease and in those at risk of renal disease, e.g. elderly people. Long-term use of NSAIDs may lead to analgesic nephropathy and chronic renal failure.

5. M – Pre-renal acute renal failure secondary to renal artery stenosis

Renal artery stenosis is typically seen in patients with atherosclerotic disease or fibromuscular dysplasia. The arterial stenosis results in renal hypoperfusion, which in turn stimulates the secretion of renin from the juxtaglomerular cells of the kidney. Renin converts angiotensinogen into angiotensin. Angiotensin is converted to angiotensin II by angiotensin-converting enzyme (ACE). In patients with renal artery stenosis, angiotensin II is responsible for maintaining the glomerular filtration pressure by constricting the efferent arterioles in the nephron. If patients with bilateral renal stenosis are prescribed ACE inhibitors such as ramipril, the reduced synthesis of angiotensin II means that the efferent arterioles can no longer constrict, which results in loss of glomerular filtration pressure and the development of acute renal failure. For this reason, ACE inhibitors and angiotensin II receptor blockers are contraindicated in patients with known renal artery stenosis.

Theme 9: Infective gastroenteritis

1. D – *Clostridium difficile*

Clostridium difficile is a Gram-positive commensal bacterium of the gastrointestinal tract that can proliferate when the intestinal flora is disturbed by the use of broad-spectrum antibiotics. *C. difficile* produces two enterotoxins (A and B), which cause severe inflammation of the intestinal mucosa and the formation of thick fibrous bands (pseudomembranes) in the intestine, which can harbour large numbers of bacteria. The patient often has significant diarrhoea, which can lead to rapid dehydration, electrolyte imbalance and death. *C. difficile* is treated by managing the patient's fluid and electrolyte balance and prescribing a course of metronidazole or vancomycin. Much effort is being put into in the prevention of clostridial infection by promoting the correct use of broad-spectrum antibiotics and educating hospital staff and visitors regarding the importance of hand washing. It should be noted that the spores of *C. difficile* are not destroyed by alcohol hand gel – meaning that soap and water must be used every time!

2. B – *Campylobacter jejuni*

Campylobacter jejuni infection is one of the most common causes of bacterial gastroenteritis in the UK. It is contracted by the ingestion of contaminated food and unpasteurised milk. There is an incubation period of 2–5 days, after which the patient develops profuse and bloody diarrhoea that often contains pus. The infection usually lasts less than a week before spontaneous recovery. It can usually be managed supportively, but occasionally requires a course of erythromycin. Recovery is usually complete, although *C. jejuni* infection is very rarely associated with the development of Reiter's syndrome or Guillain–Barré syndrome.

3. A – *Bacillus cereus*

Bacillus cereus is a spore-producing bacterium that can induce diarrhoea and vomiting within hours of ingestion. Infection is usually due to consuming rewarmed rice that has been contaminated with spores, e.g. rice that has been boiled and left several hours before frying (hence the term 'Chinese fried rice syndrome'). It is usually a relatively short-lived infection and clears up within 24 hours. Antibiotics are not indicated.

4. G – *Staphylococcus aureus*

Staphylococcus aureus food poisoning is caused by heat-resistant enterotoxins that interact with the vagus nerve, causing vomiting within hours of ingestion. Diarrhoea is not usually a feature. The illness is self-limiting and requires symptomatic treatment only.

5. F – Rotavirus

Rotavirus infection commonly occurs in children and hospitalized patients during the winter period. It spreads readily from person to person and has an incubation period of 2 days. The patient may have a prodrome of upper respiratory tract illness followed by development of diarrhoea and vomiting. The illness is self-limiting and usually requires no treatment other than supportive measures. Some children and frail adults require intravenous fluids to treat dehydration and electrolyte imbalance that is not responding to oral rehydration.

Theme 10: Seizures

A seizure is an abnormal event due to electrical discharge in the brain. Epilepsy is the tendency to have seizures. Seizures can be partial (in one part of the brain) or generalized (both hemispheres). Partial seizures can spread to the rest of the brain (secondary generalization). Seizures can be precipitated by SLIDE (**S**leep deprivation, **L**ight flickering, **I**nfection, **D**rugs/alcohol and **E**xhaustion).

After a first seizure, an MRI or CT scan is performed to investigate an underlying cause. Anticonvulsants are considered after a second seizure. Examples of anticonvulsants are sodium valproate, carbamazepine, phenytoin and gabapentin. Side-effects of these drugs include ataxia, nystagmus and dysarthria. Specific side-effects of phenytoin are gum hypertrophy, hypertrichosis, folate deficiency and neuropathy.

1. I – Tonic–clonic seizure

Tonic–clonic seizures may be preceded by an aura. The patient initially goes rigid and unconscious (with or without central cyanosis). The rigidity is periodically relaxed, resulting in clonic jerks. This may be accompanied by incontinence and tongue-biting. (A severely bitten, bleeding tongue after loss of consciousness is pathognomonic of a seizure.) Eventually, the rigidity is replaced by a flaccid state of deep coma. When patients regain consciousness, they are confused and want to sleep.

Pseudo-seizures are attacks resembling seizures that are psychogenic in origin. Cyanosis and tongue-biting are rare, but incontinence may occur. Pseudo-seizures may be accompanied by a dramatic flailing of limbs and back arching. They are most common in women with a history of abuse during childhood.

2. H – Status epilepticus

Status epilepticus is defined as a series of seizures occurring without the patient regaining awareness between attacks, and may last longer than 30 minutes. This usually involves recurrent tonic–clonic seizures and is life threatening. Status epilepticus may be precipitated by abrupt drug withdrawal and metabolic disturbances. Management is initially with intravenous benzodiazepines (e.g. lorazepam or diazepam). If seizures do not terminate, an intravenous phenytoin infusion is commenced.

3. D – Narcolepsy

Narcolepsy is a neurological condition caused by a loss of inhibition of rapid eye movement sleep. It has four main features: irresistible attacks of sleep at inappropriate times, cataplexy (sudden loss of muscle tone when intense emotion occurs, leading to collapse), hypnagogic/hypnopompic hallucinations (hallucinations that occur on falling asleep and waking, respectively) and sleep paralysis. Factors that suggest narcolepsy are a short duration of sleep (10–20 minutes), an inability to control sleep attacks and interrupted night-time sleep, as well as the four main features. Treatment is with central nervous system stimulants, e.g. amphetamines.

4. B – Complex partial seizure

A simple partial seizure is one where consciousness is preserved. In complex partial seizures, consciousness is affected. Patients having a complex partial seizure stop what they are doing, stare blankly and may display automatisms (e.g. lip smacking). This may be preceded by complex hallucinations. After a few minutes, consciousness returns and the patient is drowsy.

5. C – Febrile convulsion

Febrile convulsions occur in 3% of children, most commonly between the ages of 6 months and 3 years. Seizures are usually generalized tonic–clonic. Management includes looking for an underlying infection and the use of antipyretics.

Partial motor seizures arise in the pre-central gyrus. They are characterized by jerking and spasm of the contralateral motor areas and may spread to one side of the whole body. Attacks that begin in one area and spread gradually are known as a jacksonian march. These seizures can last hours, and prolonged episodes may result in post-seizure paralysis (Todd's paresis). *Partial sensory seizures* arise in the sensory cortex and cause tingling and electric sensations in the contralateral face and limbs. *Versive seizures* occur with frontal lobe epilepsy and are characterized by forced deviation of the eyes to the opposite side of the seizure.

Transient global amnesia is an abrupt, discrete reversible loss of short-term memory that lasts a few hours. During this time, patients know who they are and can perform motor acts, but act bemused. There is retrograde amnesia for the last few weeks. After 4–6 hours, memory returns to normal. Episodes tend not to recur, and once epilepsy has been excluded further investigation is not required.

Reflex anoxic seizures occur after a fainting episode in children secondary to transient cerebral hypoxia. The child becomes pale and unresponsive, followed by tonic–clonic activity. Attacks last 30–60 seconds and recovery is rapid.

Theme 11: Side-effects of cardiovascular medication

1. I – Ramipril

Ramipril is an example of an ACE inhibitor. Other examples include perindopril, lisinopril and enalapril. A dry cough is a relatively common class side-effect of ACE inhibitors. Under normal circumstances, the enzyme angiotensin II metabolizes bradykinin in the lungs. The blockade of this enzyme by ACE inhibitors leads to a build-up of bradykinin, which stimulates coughing. In some individuals, the cough is persistent and intolerable. In such cases, an angiotensin II receptor antagonist, such as candesartan, may be used as an alternative. This class of drug blocks angiotensin AT_1-receptors and therefore has no effect on the metabolism of bradykinin.

2. N – Verapamil

Verapamil is a calcium channel blocker that is used in the management of hypertension, angina and arrhythmias. Bilateral ankle oedema is a well known side-effect of calcium channel blockers. Other side-effects include dizziness, headaches and facial flushing.

3. G – Furosemide

Furosemide is a loop diuretic that inhibits reabsorption of sodium and potassium at the ascending loop of Henle. Patients taking furosemide are therefore at risk of hypokalaemia and hyponatraemia. ECG findings in hypokalaemia include flattened T-waves, tall U-waves (a positive deflection seen after the T-wave), ST-segment depression and a prolonged QT interval. Patients are at risk of atrial and ventricular arrhythmia. Mild-to-moderate hypokalaemia can be managed by reducing or stopping the offending drug and prescribing a potassium supplement such as Sando-K. In severe cases, the patient should be placed on a cardiac monitor and receive intravenous potassium in 0.9% saline at a concentration no higher than 40 mmol/L and at a rate no higher than 20 mmol/h.

4. K – Simvastatin

Statins are used to actively lower cholesterol in the primary and secondary prevention of cardiovascular disease. They reduce cholesterol synthesis and increase low-density lipoprotein (LDL) metabolism in the liver. Acute myositis is a rare but potentially serious side-effect of statin pharmacotherapy. Myositis usually presents with fatigue, fever, muscular pain and weakness, and in its most serious form may proceed to rhabdomyositis and acute renal failure. If serum creatine kinase (CK), a biochemical marker for muscular damage, is above five times the upper limit of normal in the presence of the above symptoms, the drug should be stopped. The patient is at increased risk of myositis when a combination of lipid-lowering drugs is prescribed, e.g. a statin plus nicotinic acid. Statins are also known to cause hepatotoxicity, and therefore should be avoided in patients with active liver disease and deranged liver function tests.

5. M – Streptokinase

Streptokinase is a thrombolytic agent commonly used to treat ST-elevation myocardial infarction in the acute setting. Streptokinase has many adverse effects, including haemorrhagic stroke, gastrointestinal bleeding, reperfusion arrhythmia, allergic reaction and anaphylaxis. The most common adverse effect of streptokinase is hypotension. Provided that all other observations are normal and there is no sign of bleeding, the infusion is slowed. In addition, the patient should be nursed head-down and receive intravenous fluids.

Theme 12: Drugs used during cardiac arrest

1. A – Adrenaline

Adrenaline (epinephrine) interacts with α- and β-adrenergic receptors to cause peripheral and splanchnic vasoconstriction, which diverts blood away from the skin and gastrointestinal tract to the heart and brain. The net effect is an increase in coronary and cerebral perfusion pressures. Current resuscitation protocols advise that, in shockable arrhythmias (i.e. ventricular fibrillation and pulseless ventricular tachycardia), adrenaline be given as a 1 mg intravenous dose of 1:10 000 solution prior to the third shock and every 3–5 minutes thereafter. In non-shockable arrhythmias (e.g. asystole and pulseless electrical activity), adrenaline should be given at the start of the resuscitation attempt and every 3–5 minutes thereafter. Adrenaline is also available in a 1:1000 solution (where 1 mg = 1 mL). This solution should not be given intravenously, and is reserved for use in anaphylaxis, when it is given intramuscularly.

2. B – Amiodarone

Amiodarone is a membrane-stabilizing drug that increases the refractory period of the cardiac cycle. It is given as a 300 mg intravenous bolus before the fourth shock in shockable arrhythmias. It is not part of the non-shockable arrhythmia protocols. Amiodarone is also used in non-cardiac arrest situations to treat ventricular tachycardia, supraventricular tachycardia and atrial fibrillation.

3. C – Atropine

Atropine is an antimuscarinic drug that blocks the vagus nerve, thus increasing the rate of sinoatrial node and atrioventricular node depolarization. It is given as a one-off 3 mg intravenous dose in patients with asystole or pulseless electrical activity with a heart rate of less than 60 beats/min. It can also be given in 500 μg increments (up to 3 mg) in patients with symptomatic heart block.

4. G – Magnesium sulphate

Magnesium sulphate can be given as a 2 g (8 mmol) intravenous bolus in ventricular fibrillation refractory to defibrillation. It can also be given in cardiac arrest when the arrhythmia may be secondary to, or is compounded by, hypomagnesaemia. Other uses of magnesium sulphate include the treatment of torsades de pointes, atrial fibrillation and life-threatening asthma.

5. D – Calcium gluconate

Hyperkalaemia is a common cause of ventricular arrhythmia and cardiac arrest. If hyperkalaemia is suspected as the cause of cardiac arrest, a 10 mL dose of 10% calcium gluconate should be given as a slow intravenous bolus. This should be followed by a large saline flush, as calcium is venotoxic and may lead to loss of intravenous access. Calcium gluconate stabilizes the myocardium against the toxic actions of potassium, but has no effect on the overall serum potassium concentration.

Theme 13: Investigation of rheumatological disease

1. F – Muscle biopsy

This woman has dermatomyositis, a connective tissue disease characterized by proximal muscle weakness (hips and shoulders) with characteristic skin lesions (a purple rash on the eyelids and scaly pink papules on the knuckles). The best investigation is a muscle biopsy, which demonstrates inflammation and necrosis. For more information on dermatomyositis, see 'Connective tissue disease' (Paper 4 Answers, Theme 13).

2. H – Schirmer's test

This woman has Sjögren's syndrome, characterized by dry eyes (keratoconjunctivitis sicca) and a dry mouth (xerostoma). Diagnosis is with Schirmer's test. A 35 mm-long piece of filter paper is placed under the lower eyelid for 5 minutes – if less than 10 mm becomes moist, this indicates Sjögren's syndrome.

3. A – Angiography

This woman has Takayasu's arteritis, a vasculitis of the aorta and the other major arteries. Inflammation causes stenosis of the arteries, which leads to absence of distal pulses and limb claudication. Angiography will demonstrate stenosis of the affected vessels. For more information on Takayasu's arteritis, see 'Vasculitis' (Paper 1 Answers, Theme 12).

4. E – Joint aspiration and microscopy

The likely diagnosis in this man is acute gout. The diagnosis can be confirmed by performing a joint aspiration and sending for microscopy. The presence of negatively birefringent, needle-shaped crystals is indicative of gout. In practice, you would send some joint fluid for culture anyway to rule out septic arthritis. For more information on gout, see 'Diagnosis of joint pain 2' (Paper 3 Answers, Theme 6).

5. K – Temporal artery biopsy

This woman has features highly suspicious of temporal arteritis (with associated polymyalgia rheumatica). Because of the risk of irreversible blindness, suspected temporal arteritis should be treated immediately with steroids. The diagnosis should be confirmed using a temporal artery biopsy. It should be noted that only segments of the temporal artery are affected by temporal arteritis, so, while a positive biopsy result confirms disease, a negative one cannot rule it out. More information on temporal arteritis and polymyalgia rheumatic can be found in 'Vasculitis' (Paper 1 Answers, Theme 12).

Theme 14: Diagnosis of thyroid disease 2

1. I – Primary myxoedema

This woman presents with some classic features of an underactive thyroid. Along with the lack of goitre, this makes primary myxoedema the best answer. Primary myxoedema (from Greek *myxa* = slime + *oedema* = swelling) is also known as spontaneous atrophic hypothyroidism. It is characterized by an idiopathic reduction in the production of thyroid hormones. Features of hypothyroidism include a hoarse voice, constipation, feeling cold, weight gain, low mood, lethargy, coarse hair and dysmenorrhoea. The diagnosis of primary hypothyroidism is made by demonstrating a low thyroxine (T_4) despite a high thyroid-stimulating hormone (TSH). Hypothyroidism is treated with daily thyroxine, which is taken for life.

2. F – Haemorrhage into a cyst

This woman has a history of a thyroid cyst. The acute presentation of neck pain and growth of the lesion suggest haemorrhage into the cyst. Haemorrhage can result in tracheal compression and stridor. If possible, aspiration of the cyst contents should be performed to alleviate tracheal compression and maintain airway patency. If aspiration is not possible, surgical intervention may be required.

3. B – De Quervain's thyroiditis

De Quervain's thyroiditis ('subacute thyroiditis') is usually precipitated by a viral infection, such influenza, Coxsackie virus or mumps. There is inflammation of the thyroid gland, with subsequent release of thyroid hormones, resulting in a transient mild hyperthyroidism (hence the tremor and diarrhoea in this patient). Patients present with pain in the thyroid region, neck, jaw and ears that is worse with swallowing and neck movement. Eventually, thyroid function returns to normal, although some patients become mildly hypothyroid for up to 6 months. De Quervain's thyroiditis requires no specific treatment, but non-steroidal anti-inflammatories can be given for pain.

4. D – Graves' disease

This woman demonstrates features of thyrotoxicosis (anxiety, diarrhoea, tremor and weight loss despite a good appetite) with a thyroid bruit. The presence of hyperthyroidism with a bruit indicates a likely diagnosis of Graves' disease. Graves' disease is an autoimmune condition resulting in over-activity of the thyroid. The hyperthyroidism is due to the presence of antibodies that stimulate the TSH receptor, resulting in a high secretion of thyroid hormones. Apart from the generic features of thyrotoxicosis (e.g. diarrhoea, feeling warm, weight loss despite a good appetite and tremor), patients with Graves' disease may also demonstrate a thyroid bruit, pretibial myxoedema and ophthalmoplegia. Specific examples of eye disease in Graves' disease are lid retraction and proptosis (a 'bulging' appearance of the eyes due to myxoedematous infiltration of the muscles behind the eye). Treatment options for hyperthyroidism include carbimazole, iodine-131 and subtotal thyroidectomy. β-Blockers, such as propranolol, help diminish the symptoms of thyrotoxicosis, but do not affect the underlying disease.

5. H – Myxoedema coma

Older patients with undiagnosed hypothyroidism, or those who do not take their medications, can present with features of severe hypothyroidism, or a myxoedema coma. These include an impaired consciousness, hypothermia, bradycardia and hypoglycaemia. The woman in this scenario has this presentation, and it could be that her regular medication included thyroxine for hypothyroidism (which could have caused her depression). Patients with a myxoedema coma should be transferred to intensive care for fluids, gentle rewarming and intravenous thyroid hormones. The mortality rate is 50%.

The opposite condition, where there is a sudden large concentration of circulating thyroid hormones, is called a 'thyroid storm'. It can be precipitated by infection or stress. Patients present with fever, tachycardia, agitation, atrial fibrillation and heart failure. Treatment is again in intensive care with fluids, gentle cooling and intravenous β-blockers (propranolol). Sodium iopodate (which inhibits thyroxine release) and carbimazole (inhibits synthesis of thyroxine) are also administered. The mortality rate is around 10%.

Theme 15: Diagnosis of chest pain

1. B – Aortic dissection

This is a classic history of aortic dissection. Risk factors associated with aortic dissection include hypertension, generalized atherosclerosis and connective tissue disorders such as Marfan's syndrome and Ehlers–Danlos syndrome. The pain tends to be severe and tearing in nature, and is associated with shortness of breath and autonomic symptoms. When aortic dissection occurs, the blood breaks through the intimal layer of the vessel and creates a false lumen that tracks through the media. The false lumen may reconnect with the original lumen distally, in which case the patient usually remains stable. If this does not occur, the dissection can occlude the major branches of the aorta, causing hemiplegia (carotid arteries), acute limb ischaemia (subclavian arteries), ischaemic bowel (mesenteric arteries) and acute renal failure (renal arteries). It is this pathological process that causes patients with dissection to present with neurological defects and uneven radial pulses and brachial blood pressures. If the dissection tracks proximately towards the heart, it may cause acute aortic valve regurgitation, inferior myocardial infarction and cardiac tamponade.

There are two types of aortic dissection. Type B dissection involves the descending aorta only (distal to left subclavian artery), and is usually treated conservatively by controlling high blood pressure with antihypertensive medications and nitrates. Type A dissection involves the ascending aorta, and nearly always requires surgical correction.

2. G – Mitral valve prolapse

Mitral valve prolapse is a relatively common condition that tends to affect young women and those with a history of congenital heart disease such as atrial septal defect and patent ductus arteriosus. Many people with mitral valve prolapse are asymptomatic. Those who experience symptoms tend to complain of atypical chest pain and palpitations that are exacerbated by exercise. Less common complications include postural hypotension, syncope, bacterial endocarditis, cerebral and systemic emboli, and ventricular arrhythmia. On auscultation, there may be a midsystolic click, which is sometimes associated with a late-systolic murmur. Diagnosis is by echocardiography. Treatment is mainly symptomatic with 'pill in the pocket' β-blockers that are taken during episodes of pain and palpitations. Due to the increased risk of bacterial endocarditis, patients with mitral valve prolapse should receive antibiotic prophylaxis prior to invasive procedures.

3. D – Decubitus angina

Decubitus angina describes typical angina pain on lying flat at night time. The reabsorption of peripheral fluid into the venous circulation that occurs while lying flat places additional strain on the heart. The diseased coronary arteries are unable to deliver adequate blood to supply the increased myocardial oxygen demand. Decubitus angina occurs when anti-angina therapy is suboptimal and when coronary artery disease is severe.

Decubitus, from Latin *decumbere* 'to lie down', related to *cubitum* 'elbow'.

4. C – Boerhaave's syndrome

Boerhaave's syndrome describes transmural rupture of a normal oesophagus, which usually occurs secondary to prolonged and forceful vomiting. Patients often present intoxicated, with lower chest and epigastric pain. They are often peripherally shut down and shocked. Other features include shortness of breath, pulmonary effusion and subcutaneous emphysema in the neck (which is felt as 'bubble-wrap' on palpating the skin). Boerhaave's syndrome is definitively diagnosed by a gastrografin (water-soluble contrast) swallow or CT scan. Chest X-ray may show a pulmonary effusion and subcutaneous emphysema. Patients require fluid resuscitation, broad-spectrum antibiotics to prevent mediastinitis and surgery to repair larger defects.

Herman Boerhaave, Dutch physician (1668–1738).

5. H – Oesophageal spasm

Oesophageal spasm is rare, and is often confused with angina. It classically presents with retrosternal chest pain, with or without dysphagia. It is caused by abnormal peristaltic contraction in the distal half of the oesophagus, which may occur spontaneously or secondary to precipitating factors such as hot food. The pain is very similar to angina and is classically partially relieved by nitrates and calcium channel blockers. Twenty-four-hour oesophageal manometry may show paroxysmal oesophageal contractions. Barium swallow may demonstrate a 'corkscrew oesophagus' caused by the abnormal peristalsis, although this is seen only during active spasm. Conservative treatment is with nitrates or calcium channel blockers. In severe disease, botulinum toxin may be injected into the oesophagus to provide temporary relief. Surgical treatment is indicated in disabling disease.

Practice Paper 7: Questions

Theme 1: The multidisciplinary team

Options

A. Chiropodist
B. Community midwife
C. Community psychiatric nurse
D. Dietician
E. District nurse
F. Health visitor
G. Occupational therapist
H. Orthotist
I. Practice receptionist
J. Social worker

For each of the following scenarios, select the most appropriate member of the multidisciplinary team. Each option may be used once, more than once or not at all.

1. A 34-year-old man has difficulty walking after a motorcycle accident. He is unable to dorsiflex his right foot, and therefore has to excessively lift his right knee when walking to prevent his foot from catching the ground.

2. A 72-year-old man is due to be discharged after a left hip replacement. He is still having some difficulty walking up and down stairs, and needs a rail fitted at home to allow him better access to his bathroom on the first floor.

3. An 84-year-old woman is discharged from hospital following an emergency operation for bowel obstruction. She needs someone to help change her wound dressing regularly; however, she is immobile and lives alone.

4. A 27-year-old man is ready to be discharged after emergency surgery. He is of no fixed abode and needs assistance regarding accommodation.

5. A 22-year-old woman gave birth 2 months ago. She wants someone to provide her with advice on immunization schedules for her baby.

Theme 2: Abnormalities of movement

Options

A. Akathisia
B. Asterixis
C. Athetosis
D. Chorea
E. Dystonia
F. Essential tremor
G. Hemiballismus
H. Intention tremor
I. Physiological tremor
J. Resting tremor
K. Rubral tremor
L. Tardive dyskinesia

For each of the following descriptions, select the most appropriate movement abnormality. Each option may be used once, more than once or not at all.

1. A 40-year-old woman has a long history of shaking in her hands. She finds that it is worse with writing, and this is interfering with her job. Alcohol relieves the tremor, and she is worried that she may develop alcohol dependence.

2. A 65-year-old man has been taking haloperidol for many years. On examination, he has unusual facial movements which look as though he is chewing or sucking his tongue.

3. A 25-year-old man is developing twitching, jerky movements in his upper and lower limbs. He is worried, as his father died of movement problems when he was young.

4. A 43-year-old woman with multiple sclerosis has started to get involuntary, violent tremors in her hands for no reason. These can come on at any time and are socially disabling, as they often result in dropping or spilling whatever she is holding.

5. A 22-year-old man suddenly develops spasm in the right side of his neck, causing his head to turn to this side. The spasm is relieved after a few minutes.

Theme 3: Treatment of liver disease

Options

A. Aciclovir
B. Cholestyramine
C. ERCP
D. Interferon-α
E. Intravenous antibiotics
F. Liver transplantation
G. Penicillamine
H. Supportive care
I. Ursodeoxycholic acid
J. Venesection

For each of the following scenarios, select the most appropriate management. Each option may be used once, more than once or not at all.

1. A 12-year-old girl being investigated for cirrhosis and behavioural changes is shown to have a green–yellow discoloration around her iris on slit-lamp examination.

2. A 32-year-old man has recently returned from holiday in India, where he stayed with locals and dined with them. Two weeks later, he presents with jaundice and lethargy. Liver function tests reveal a massively raised alanine transaminase and a significantly raised bilirubin.

3. A 34-year-old man presents with a 1-month history of vague upper abdominal pain. He is on insulin for diabetes, but is otherwise well. On examination, there appears to be a bronzed tan to the skin, although the patient denies having been on holiday.

4. A 28-year-old woman presents to the emergency department with a 2-month history of lethargy, abdominal pain and jaundice. On further questioning, she admits to using intravenous drugs. Blood tests reveal the presence of hepatitis C infection.

5. A 42-year-old woman presents with a 4-week history of generalized itching. She has developed yellow lesions in the skin around her eyes. Blood tests reveal deranged liver function tests.

Theme 4: Management of respiratory disease 1

Options

A. Amoxicillin
B. Cannula into second intercostal space midclavicular line
C. Cannula into sixth intercostal space midclavicular line
D. Chemotherapy
E. Co-trimoxazole
F. Erythromycin
G. Inhaled anticholinergic
H. Inhaled β-agonist
I. Low-molecular-weight heparin
J. Metronidazole
K. No management required
L. Radiotherapy
M. Rifampicin and isoniazid
N. Steroids
O. Warfarin

For each of the following scenarios, select the most appropriate management. Each option may be used once, more than once or not at all.

1. A 47-year-old man presents with a 2-day history of feeling generally unwell and short of breath. Today, he started coughing up thick green sputum. Auscultation reveals bronchial breathing at the right base. He is allergic to penicillin.

2. A 67-year-old woman has viral gastroenteritis. During the illness, she accidently aspirates some of her vomit. A few days later, she develops a cough with productive sputum. A chest X-ray confirms right middle lobe consolidation.

3. A 38-year-old woman has a 2-month history of worsening shortness of breath and a dry cough. She also complains of night sweats. On examination, her oxygen saturations are 89%. She has no other symptoms and no history of respiratory disease, but is known to have HIV infection.

4. A 49-year-old man presents to the GP with worsening shortness of breath and a cough productive of bloody sputum. He has lost a stone (6 kg) in weight over the last month. A chest X-ray shows consolidation at the both apices.

5. A 68-year-old man has a 3-week history of haemoptysis. He has lost a stone (6 kg) in weight over this period of time. A biopsy taken at bronchoscopy confirms a non-small cell lung tumour. A CT scan shows that the disease is not surgically resectable.

Theme 5: Complications of treatment of rheumatoid arthritis

Options

A. Azathioprine
B. Chloroquine
C. Diclofenac
D. *d*-Penicillamine
E. Gold
F. Leflunomide
G. Methotrexate
H. Steroids
I. Sulfasalazine

For each of the following descriptions, select the most likely offending drug. Each option may be used once, more than once or not at all.

1. A 41-year-old man is having treatment for rheumatoid arthritis. He is admitted to the emergency department after passing black, tarry stools. An endoscopy confirms the presence of gastric ulceration.

2. A 41-year-old man is having treatment for rheumatoid arthritis. He and his wife have been trying for a baby but have been unable to conceive. Tests at the fertility clinic have shown him to be subfertile.

3. A 41-year-old man is having treatment for rheumatoid arthritis. Over the last few days, he has developed a yellow tinge to his skin and eyes, associated with pain in his right upper abdomen.

4. A 41-year-old man is having treatment for rheumatoid arthritis. He has gained a significant amount of weight in the last year, predominantly around his waist and on his face. He has also been feeling low in mood.

5. A 41-year-old man is having treatment for rheumatoid arthritis. Over the last 3 months, he has become progressively shorter of breath and now feels out of breath on minimal exertion. Auscultation of his lungs reveals fine end-inspiratory crackles.

Theme 6: Diseases of calcium and the parathyroid axis

Options

A. Bone metastases
B. Ectopic parathyroid hormone secretion
C. Hypomagnesaemia
D. Hypoparathyroidism
E. Hypothyroidism
F. Iatrogenic calcium overdose
G. Parathyroid gland malignancy
H. Parathyroid hormone-related protein secretion
I. Primary hyperparathyroidism
J. Pseudohypoparathyroidism
K. Pseudo-pseudohypoparathyroidism
L. Secondary hyperparathyroidism
M. Tertiary hyperparathyroidism

For each of the following scenarios, select the most appropriate diagnosis. Each option may be used once, more than once or not at all.

1. A 56-year-old man presents to the GP with a 2-month history of excessive urine production, constipation and general lethargy. A set of blood tests is requested, and shows a corrected calcium of 2.8 mmol/L (reference range 2.2–2.6 mmol/L) and a significantly raised parathyroid hormone.

2. A 7-year-old girl with chronic renal failure secondary to autosomal recessive polycystic kidney disease is found to have a corrected calcium of 1.90 mmol/L, a phosphate of 2.4 mmol/L (reference range 0.7–1.4 mmol/L) and a significantly raised parathyroid hormone.

3. A 37-year-old woman who underwent a thyroidectomy yesterday complains to the nurses that she has a tingling sensation around her lips and feels generally weak. A set of routine blood test is requested, and shows a normal full blood count, a normal renal function, a normal albumin and a corrected calcium of 1.8 mmol/L.

4. A 74-year-old man with known small cell lung cancer is found to have a corrected calcium of 2.8 mmol/L and a low parathyroid hormone.

5. A 26-year-old woman with chronic renal failure secondary to renal dysplasia has a corrected calcium of 2.6 mmol/L, a phosphate of 2.1 mmol/L and a significantly raised parathyroid hormone.

Theme 7: Diseases of the myocardium and pericardium

Options

A. Arrhythmogenic right ventricular cardiomyopathy
B. Atrial myxoma
C. Cardiac tamponade
D. Constrictive cardiomyopathy
E. Dilated cardiomyopathy
F. Hypertrophic obstructive cardiomyopathy
G. Myocarditis
H. Non-ST-elevation myocardial infarction
I. Restrictive cardiomyopathy
J. Subacute bacterial endocarditis
K. Uraemic pericarditis
L. Viral pericarditis

For each of the following scenarios, select the most likely diagnosis. Each option may be used once, more than once or not at all.

1. A 23-year-old amateur footballer collapses and dies while training. Witnesses say that there was no contact from other players. His only past medical history is two previous episodes of syncope while at the gym, but no cause was identified.

2. A 46-year-old man presents to the GP with a history of shortness of breath that occurs on exertion and when lying down at night. On general inspection, he notices multiple spider naevi on his chest and face. On examination of his heart, the apex beat is displaced laterally and there is a pansystolic murmur that is difficult to identify since the heartbeat is irregularly irregular.

3. A 64-year-old woman is referred for echocardiography following a history of weight loss, low-grade fever, non-specific chest pain and palpitations. While performing the echocardiogram, the technician notices a polypoid mass attached to the septal wall in the left atrium.

4. A 45-year-old man presents to the emergency department with central chest pain that is stabbing in nature and is exacerbated by lying down at night. Blood tests show a potassium of 5.4 mmol/L, a sodium of 145 mmol/L, a urea of 15 mmol/L and a creatinine of 540 μmol/L.

5. A 46-year-old woman presents to the emergency department with a short history of worsening shortness of breath and a reduced exercise tolerance. She has been suffering with lethargy, muscle aches, fever and palpitations for 2 weeks. Routine blood tests show a raised white blood cell count and a raised C-reactive protein. A plasma troponin returns at 1.2 ng/mL.

Theme 8: Visual defects 1

Options

A. Abducens nerve palsy
B. Oculomotor nerve palsy
C. Optic chiasm lesion
D. Optic nerve lesion
E. Optic tract lesion
F. Parietal lobe lesion
G. Temporal lobe lesion
H. Trochlear nerve palsy

For each of the following scenarios, select the most likely visual defect. Each option may be used once, more than once or not at all.

1. A 38-year-old woman complains of a 6-week history of worsening headaches. This morning, she noticed that she was occasionally getting double vision, which was most noticeable when she looked towards the left side.

2. A 42-year-old woman presents to the GP with headaches that are worse in the morning. She has also noticed a gradual change in her appearance, citing growth in her chin, nose and hands. She mentions recent trouble with her vision. On examination, she is blind in the temporal visual fields of both eyes.

3. A 28-year-old man presents with a short history of blurred vision. He has no other symptoms. On examination, his right eye is looking downwards and laterally, and he is unable to move it from this position. The pupil on the right side is smaller than that on the left.

4. A 59-year-old man presents with problems with his vision. Over the last few weeks, he has had near-misses on the motorway where he almost hit other vehicles when pulling into the fast lane. On examination, he is blind in the lateral half of his right eye and the medial half of his left eye.

5. A 67-year-old woman has noticed some problems with her vision. Over the last few days, when her pet parrot has flown down towards her from the right side, she has not noticed him. On examination, she is blind in the upper right quadrants of the visual field in both eyes.

Theme 9: Signs in gastrointestinal disease

Options

A. Angular stomatitis
B. Dermatitis herpetiformis
C. Episcleritis
D. Erythema multiform
E. Erythema nodosum
F. Leukoplakia
G. Pyoderma gangrenosum
H. Sister Joseph nodule
I. Virchow's node

For each of the following scenarios, select the most appropriate physical sign. Each option may be used once, more than once or not at all.

1. A 65-year-old woman with a history of dyspepsia and significant weight loss is noticed to have a 2 cm mass above her left clavicle.

2. A 17-year-old man with Crohn's disease presents to his GP with a lesion on his left shin. It began as a pustule, which became erythematous and ulcerated with time. The ulcer is deep, and the edges are well demarcated and have a blue tinge.

3. A 34-year-old man with active ulcerative colitis presents to his GP complaining of several painful red lesions on his shins. On examination, there are multiple, purple, tender, macular lesions on both shins.

4. A 56-year-old woman who is being investigated for a gastrointestinal cause of iron-deficiency anaemia is noticed to have fissures in each corner of her mouth.

5. A 37-year-old woman with coeliac disease develops an intensely itchy blistering rash on her wrists and forearms.

Theme 10: Complications of renal replacement therapy

A. Acute organ rejection
B. Anaemia
C. Aneurysm formation
D. Amyloidosis
E. Chronic organ rejection
F. Exit-site infection of line
G. Hypocalcaemia
H. Hyperacute organ rejection
I. Hypertension
J. Hypotension
K. Ischaemic heart disease
L. Peritonitis
M. Renal cysts
N. Vascular steal syndrome

For each of the following scenarios, select the most appropriate complication. Each option may be used once, more than once or not at all.

1. During a haemodialysis session, a 14-year-old boy complains of light-headedness. He looks pale and slightly sweaty. His blood pressure is measured at 70/30 mmHg.

2. A 13-year-old girl who is receiving peritoneal dialysis for end-stage renal failure presents to the emergency department with abdominal pain and fever. Her peritoneal dialysis fluid is cloudy. On examination, her abdomen is rigid and she displays involuntary guarding.

3. A 45-year-old man who received a cadaveric renal transplant 3 months ago begins to complain of fever and pain around the transplanted kidney. Blood tests show a steady rise in serum urea and creatinine, despite the patient being appropriately hydrated.

4. A 47-year-old man has been receiving haemodialysis for several years since he was diagnosed with adult polycystic disease. He is starting to develop episodic chest pain on exertion.

5. A 34-year-old woman with a recently fashioned radiocephalic arteriovenous fistula for haemodialysis presents to her GP with a blue–grey discoloration of her hand and cramping in her fingers.

Theme 11: Ulcers

Options

A. Arterial ulcer
B. Curling's ulcer
C. Cushing's ulcer
D. Marjolin's ulcer
E. Martorell's ulcer
F. Necrobiosis lipoidica
G. Neuropathic ulcer
H. Pyoderma gangrenosum
I. Rodent ulcer
J. Syphilitic ulcer
K. Venous ulcer

For each of the following scenarios, select the most likely ulcer. Each option may be used once, more than once or not at all.

1. A 52-year-old woman presents to her GP with a raised, pink papule on her left arm. On examination, you note that the lesion is painless and firm and arises from an underlying scar. She mentions that the scar was from a burn injury that happened 20 years ago.

2. An 18-year-old man was cycling home without a helmet when he was knocked over by a car. He suffered a severe blow to his head. On admission to the emergency department, the patient had a massive haematemesis and was booked for an urgent endoscopy.

3. A 67-year-old man attends his GP with a cramping pain in his buttocks that occurs on walking. When he develops the cramp, he has to rest until it disappears. On examination, it is difficult to feel his distal lower limb pulses. On the dorsal left foot there is a deep, sharply defined ulcer that the patient finds painful.

4. A 23-year-old woman presents with a history of diarrhoea associated with the passage of blood and mucus. She claims to feel unwell and tired and to have lost weight in the recent months. On examination, you notice a deep, necrotic ulcer on her leg with dark-red edges.

5. A 37-year-old woman attends her regular diabetes clinic with an ulcer on the sole of her right foot. On examination, the foot is warm and peripheral pulses are palpable. The ulcer itself is deep and painless, and you find that she has sensory loss below the ankles bilaterally.

Theme 12: Tachycardias and tachyarrhythmias

Options

A. Atrioventricular node re-entry tachycardia
B. Chronic atrial fibrillation
C. Multifocal atrial tachycardia
D. Paroxysmal atrial fibrillation
E. Sick sinus syndrome
F. Sinus tachycardia
G. Torsades de pointes
H. Ventricular extrasystoles
I. Ventricular fibrillation
J. Wolff–Parkinson–White syndrome

For each of the following scenarios, select the most likely tachycardia or tachyarrhythmia. Each option may be used once, more than once or not at all.

1. A 76-year-old man with known ischaemic heart disease is referred for a 24-hour ECG tape after suffering occasional palpitations. The tape shows periods of sinus bradycardia followed by episodes of sinus tachycardia.

2. A 55-year-old man is noticed to have a heart rate of 110 beats/min while on the high-dependency unit following abdominal surgery. His other observations include blood pressure 146/92 mmHg, respiratory rate 14/min and oxygen saturations 99% on 2 L of oxygen via nasal cannulae. His epidural analgesia was stopped that morning, and he is complaining of abdominal pain with a severity of 8/10.

3. A 75-year-old woman who suffers occasional episodes of palpitations presents to the emergency department with a painful left leg. She was previously fit and well. The leg is pale, cold and slightly mottled at presentation. The ankle–brachial pulse index is 0.3 on the left and 0.9 on the right. An ECG performed by the nursing staff is normal.

4. A 55-year-old man is brought to the emergency department following a sudden collapse while gardening. He is unconscious and unresponsive. He has no palpable pulse or respiratory effort. A heart monitor shows a disorganized, broad, complex, irregular rhythm with a fluctuating baseline.

5. A 36-year-old woman presents to the emergency department with chest pain and a sensation of feeling her heart pounding. Apart from a history of schizophrenia, she has no medical problems. A heart monitor is attached and shows a broad complex tachycardia with a rate of 210 beats/min on a variable axis.

Theme 13: Oncological emergencies

Options

A. Addisonian crisis
B. Anaphylaxis
C. Chemotherapy complication
D. Hypercalcaemia
E. Hyperkalaemia
F. Hypocalcaemia
G. Intracerebral bleed
H. Meningitis
I. Raised intracranial pressure
J. Spinal cord compression
K. Superior vena caval obstruction
L. Syndrome of inappropriate ADH secretion
M. Tumour lysis syndrome

For each of the following scenarios, select the most likely underlying problem. Each option may be used once, more than once or not at all.

1. A 75-year-old man with lung cancer presents to his GP with a swollen face, headache and worsening shortness of breath. On examination, there are engorged veins on his face and chest.

2. A 54-year-old woman with metastatic breast cancer presents to the emergency department feeling generally unwell and confused. Her daughter mentions that she has a poor appetite and has been vomiting.

3. A 62-year-old man with known metastatic prostate carcinoma presents to the emergency department with sudden-onset leg weakness. On examination, he has significantly reduced power in both legs, bilateral brisk knee and ankle reflexes, and bilateral upgoing plantar reflexes.

4. A 65-year-old woman presents to the emergency department complaining of a severe headache that has been getting worse over the last 3 months. It is worse in the morning and on leaning forward, and is not relieved by paracetamol.

5. A 67-year-old man with a known small cell lung carcinoma is brought to the emergency department following a seizure. On questioning, he does not recall any details surrounding the event. Blood tests show a sodium of 112 mmol/L, a potassium of 4.6 mmol/L, a urea of 5 mmol/L and a creatinine of 110 µmol/L. His urine is very concentrated.

Theme 14: Management of endocrine disease

Options

A. Iodine-131
B. Carbimazole
C. Desmopressin
D. Hydrocortisone and fludrocortisone
E. Octreotide
F. Spironolactone
G. Surgical resection and radiotherapy
H. Thyroxine alone
I. Total thyroidectomy and thyroxine

For each of the following presentations of endocrine disease select the best management option. Each option may be used once, more than once or not at all.

1. A 72-year-old woman presents with worsening difficulty in swallowing food. Because of this, she is finding it hard to eat. On examination, you note a large, hard, irregular mass in the neck that is attached to the overlying skin. She tells you that the lump has been present for a month and has been growing rapidly.

2. A 32-year-old woman presents to her GP with a 1-month history of worsening diarrhoea and heat intolerance. On examination, she has a mild tremor and 'bulging' eyes. She would like treatment for her condition, but warns you that she is pregnant.

3. A 26-year-old man attends his first outpatient clinic following a head injury that resulted in hospitalization last month. He complains of recent polyuria and polydipsia, but no other symptoms. His blood pressure is 120/85 mmHg and his heart rate is 72 beats/min.

4. An 18-year-old woman attends her GP with a lump in her neck that has been present for a few weeks. On examination, the lump is smooth and non-tender, and moves up with swallowing but not on tongue protrusion. Cervical lymphadenopathy is also noted.

5. A 14-year-old girl attends the paediatric outpatient clinic following meningococcal septicaemia a few weeks previously. She complains of feeling tired and weak and having a poor appetite. She feels dizzy when standing up from a sitting position. Her blood tests show sodium 127 mmol/L and potassium 5.4 mmol/L.

Theme 15: Management of neurological conditions 2

Options

A. Amphetamines
B. Aspirin
C. Benzylpenicillin
D. Carbamazepine
E. Chlordiazepoxide
F. Donepezil
G. Levodopa
H. Lorazepam
I. Metronidazole
J. Reassurance
K. Rifampicin and isoniazid

For each of the following scenarios, select the most appropriate management. Each option may be used once, more than once or not at all.

1. A 62-year-old man has a 6-month history of tremor that occurs at rest. He finds it especially difficult to perform fine movements with his hands, such as writing. On examination, his right arm is rigid.

2. A 48-year-old woman has intermittent facial pain. She says that it is specifically on the left side, is burning and stabbing in nature, and is worse when touching the area. Examination is unremarkable.

3. A 27-year-old woman has a 10-hour history of severe headache, vomiting and malaise. She was previously well. Examination reveals pain on neck flexion and a dark-red rash on her legs that does not blanch.

4. An 18-year-old man is found on the street having a seizure. By the time the ambulance arrives 20 minutes later, he is still fitting.

5. A 62-year-old man has sudden-onset weakness of the left side of his face and difficulty speaking. A CT head scan is performed, and shows no evidence of haemorrhage.

Practice Paper 7: Answers

Theme 1: The multidisciplinary team

Thanks to the General Medical Council's *Good Medical Practice* guidelines, these kinds of questions are more likely to crop up in examinations. And yes, the practice receptionist is part of the multidisciplinary team!

1. H – Orthotist

An orthotist is someone who measures, designs and fits orthoses (external devices that can be applied to correct a deformity, rather like splints). This patient has a right-sided foot drop and so will need an orthosis to prevent the ankle from dropping and impeding walking. Physiotherapy will also be required.

Orthotics, from Greek *ortho* = straighten.

2. G – Occupational therapist

Occupational therapists help people perform their activities of daily living, ranging from mobility within the home to cooking, dressing and eating.

3. E – District nurse

District nurses provide care within the community. Their workload includes looking after housebound and recently discharged patients, helping them manage wound dressings and monitor medications.

4. J – Social worker

Social workers look after individuals and their contacts from a social perspective (e.g. families and friends). They also liaise with other organizations, including schools, the NHS, housing agencies and charitable organizations, to plan packages of care and support for the individual.

5. F – Health visitor

Community midwives look after mother and baby during the first 10 days after birth (although this can be extended to 28 days if necessary). After this point, the health visitor (a qualified nurse) takes over care. Health visitors also run health promotion and smoking cessation clinics.

Theme 2: Abnormalities of movement

1. F – Essential tremor

Tremors are rhythmic oscillating movements of a limb, part of a limb or the head. Essential tremors are slow, are often familial, and may be made more obvious during certain actions such as writing. Essential tremors are characteristically improved with alcohol. β-Blockers can be used to improve such tremors.

Physiological tremors are seen in normal people, and have a frequency of 8–15 Hz. Physiological tremors can be exaggerated with anxiety, fatigue, fever and alcohol withdrawal. The *resting tremor* is pathognomonic of Parkinson's disease and has a frequency of 4–6 Hz. It is characteristically pill-rolling and is usually asymmetrical. An *intention tremor* is a feature of cerebellar disease. There is a slow broad tremor that occurs at the end of a purposeful movement, such as trying to press a button. It is caused by a breakdown of feedback control of targeted movements. *Asterixis* results from failure of the parietal mechanisms required to maintain posture. For example, when the hands are extended at the wrist, the posture is periodically dropped, allowing the hands to drop briefly before the posture is taken up again. Asterixis is caused by renal failure, liver failure, hypercapnia and drug toxicity (phenytoin). Unilateral asterixis can be seen with focal parietal or thalamic lesions.

Hertz (Hz) is the unit of frequency ('cycles per second'), describing periodic phenomena. It is named after Heinrich Hertz (1857–94), the German physicist who first demonstrated the existence of electromagnetic waves

Asterixis, from Greek *a* = without + *sterixis* = fixed position.

2. L – Tardive dyskinesia

Haloperidol is a typical antipsychotic, which blocks dopamine D_2-receptors in the central nervous system in various pathways, including the nigrostriatal pathway. This results in a number of side-effects, including: parkinsonism (rigidity, bradykinesia and tremor, which can begin within 1 month and are treated with anticholinergics, e.g. procyclidine); acute dystonias (occur within 72 hours of treatment and include trismus, tongue protrusion, spasmodic torticollis, opisthotonus, oculogyric crisis and grimacing); akathisia (occurs within 60 days and features a subjective feeling of inner tension and restless leg syndrome, but can be treated with β-blockers and benzodiazepines); and tardive dyskinesia (affects 20% in the long term and presents with chewing, grimacing, sucking and a darting tongue).

3. D – Chorea

This man has Huntington's disease, an autosomal dominant disorder characterized by choreiform movements. Chorea describes jerky, small-amplitude, involuntary movements, such as fidgety movements of the limbs and grimacing of the face. Other causes of chorea include Wilson's disease, cerebral trauma and rheumatic fever.

Athetoses are slow, writing movements of the limbs. *Hemiballismus* describes drastic movements of the limbs unilaterally.

Chorea, from Greek *choreia* = dance.

Hemiballismus, from Greek *ballein* = to throw.

4. K – Rubral tremor

Lesions in the superior cerebellar peduncle cause a rubral tremor – a violent, large-amplitude, postural tremor that worsens as the target is approached. It is common in advanced multiple sclerosis and can be disabling.

5. E – Dystonia

Dystonia is when a limb or the head involuntarily takes up an abnormal posture. Examples of dystonias include spasmodic torticollis (spasm of neck muscles, causing the head to rotate to one side), blepharospasm (closure of the eyelid) and oculogyric crisis (forced upward deviation of the eye).

Myoclonus is a brief, isolated, non-purposeful jerk of limb muscles. Myoclonic jerks are normal at the onset of sleep (hypnic jerks) and are a component of the normal startle response. They also occur in epileptic seizures. *Tics* are repetitive, semipurposeful movements, such as blinking, winking and grinning. They are distinguished from other involuntary movements by the ability of the patient to voluntarily suppress them, at least for a short time. Gilles de la Tourette syndrome is the tendency to multiple complex motor and vocal tics.

Georges Gilles de la Tourette, French neurologist (1857–1904).

Theme 3: Treatment of liver disease

1. G – Penicillamine

Wilson's disease is caused by an error in metabolism that prevents copper from being excreted in the bile. Copper builds up in the serum and is deposited in vital organs such as the liver, kidney and basal ganglia of the brain. Penicillamine is the first-line treatment of Wilson's disease. It is a product of penicillin that acts as a chelating agent by forming complexes with copper in the serum which are then excreted in the urine. Penicillamine has a significant side-effect profile, which includes hypersensitivity reactions, rash, mouth ulcers, thrombocytopenia, glomerulonephritis and agranulocytosis. Interestingly, adverse reactions to penicillamine are less common in patients with Wilson's disease compared with those without the condition. Patients with Wilson's disease should be advised to avoid foods with high copper content, such as chocolate, and to take zinc supplements, which reduce intestinal copper absorption.

2. H – Supportive care

Hepatitis A is usually a self-limiting illness that requires supportive care only until the acute stage has passed. In the acute stages of infection, patients should be advised to avoid fatty foods and alcohol, as these may worsen symptoms. Some patients will go on to develop fulminant liver failure and require liver transplantation.

3. J – Venesection

Hereditary haemochromatosis is a common genetic condition in which the patient absorbs too much iron from the intestinal tract; this iron is then deposited in the liver, myocardium, skin and endocrine organs, resulting in multisystem disease. The first-line treatment of this condition is venesection. The patient should be bled on a regular basis (e.g. 1 unit/week until their haemoglobin is less than 10 g/dL, at which point the frequency should be reduced to once every 2 months or so). In certain situations when venesection cannot be tolerated by the patient, an iron-chelating agent such as desferrioxamine can be used. Patients with hereditary haemochromatosis should avoid food and medications with high levels of iron and should be screened for diabetes caused by pancreatic iron deposition.

4. D – Interferon-α

Interferons are endogenous proteins secreted by the immune system that inhibit viral replication. Interferon-α (IFN-α) is known to have activity against the hepatitis C RNA virus, and is often used in the management of chronic hepatitis C. The majority of patients have a good initial response to IFN-α, but only 25% derive a sustained benefit. It has recently been shown that the combination of IFN-α and the antiviral drug ribavarin is more effective than IFN-α alone in the management of hepatitis C. Therefore, it is now recommended that these drugs be used in conjunction in moderate-to-severe hepatitis C infection.

5. F – Liver transplantation

In primary biliary cirrhosis, an autoimmune reaction causes granulomatous inflammation of the interlobular bile ducts, resulting in jaundice, cirrhosis and liver failure. If untreated, the majority of patients die within 2 years of developing jaundice. Liver transplantation is therefore indicated in most patients with a persistent bilirubin level over 100 μmol/L. Intractable pruritis is also considered by many practitioners to be an indication for transplantation. Symptomatic treatments used in primary biliary cirrhosis include cholestyramine and ursodeoxycholic acid. Cholestyramine is used to treat pruritis; it works by irreversibly binding bile in the intestine and preventing its reabsorption. Ursodeoxycholic acid is a bile acid that reduces cholesterol absorption; it is usually used to dissolve cholesterol gallstones and to treat hypercholesterolaemia associated with disorders of lipid metabolism. In primary biliary cirrhosis, ursodeoxycholic acid has been shown to improve symptoms and quality of life, but does not have any influence on survival.

Theme 4: Management of respiratory disease 1

1. F – Erythromycin

This man has a community-acquired pneumonia. The first-line management of uncomplicated pneumonia is oral amoxicillin. Patients who are allergic to penicillins are given erythromycin instead.

2. J – Metronidazole

This woman has developed an aspiration pneumonia, the treatment of which should include metronidazole to cover for anaerobic bacteria.

3. E – Co-trimoxazole

Pneumocystis pneumonia is associated with HIV infection. Treatment is with co-trimoxazole (trimethoprim and sulfamethoxazole).

4. M – Rifampicin and isoniazid

This man has tuberculosis. This should be treated with antituberculous drugs for 6 months: rifampicin, isoniazid, pyrazinamide and ethambutol for 4 months, followed by rifampicin and isoniazid alone for a further 2 months.

5. L – Radiotherapy

Non-small cell lung tumours that cannot be resected are responsive to radiotherapy. Small cell lung tumours are given chemotherapy.

Theme 5: Complications of treatment of rheumatoid arthritis

1. C – Diclofenac

2. I – Sulfasalazine

3. F – Leflunomide

4. H – Steroids

5. G – Methotrexate

The medical management of rheumatoid arthritis can be split into the use of symptom-modifying drugs and the use of disease-modifying drugs.

Symptom-modifying drugs reduce pain, stiffness and swelling, but have no effect on disease progression. Such medications include non-steroidal anti-inflammatory drugs (NSAIDs, e.g. diclofenac) and corticosteroids. Corticosteroid injections are used to relieve joint pain. Injections are limited to four per year, as frequent injections accelerate joint damage. Side-effects of NSAIDs include peptic ulceration and renal impairment. Excessive steroids can result in Cushing's syndrome (with moon face, plethora, central obesity, buffalo hump, abdominal striae, acne, depression and hirsutism).

Disease-modifying antirheumatic drugs (DMARDs) alleviate symptoms, dampen inflammation and slow disease progression, but can be prescribed only by a rheumatologist. For this reason, DMARDs should be started early to prevent the irreversible effects of long-term joint inflammation. These drugs can take up to 6 months to reach full effect, but more than one drug can be used in combination. Extra-articular features of rheumatoid arthritis are not affected by DMARDs, although rheumatoid nodules may regress. In the UK, sulfasalazine is the first-line DMARD, followed by methotrexate. The main DMARDs can be remembered using the mnemonic 'CALM GASP'. These drugs and their side-effects are as follows:

Cyclophosphamide: risk of malignancy, bone marrow suppression
Azathioprine: gastrointestinal upset, bone marrow suppression
Leflunomide: hepatitis, hypertension
Methotrexate: worsening of rheumatoid nodules, liver/lung fibrosis
Gold: rash, proteinuria, bone marrow suppression
Antimalarials: retinal damage
Sulfasalazine: infertility in males, bone marrow suppression
Penicillamine: rash, bone marrow suppression.

Biological therapies are used when DMARDs have failed (defined as failure of disease to respond to methotrexate and at least one other DMARD). Examples are tumour necrosis factor α (TNF-α) blockers (infliximab, adalimumab and etanercept) and interleukin-1 (IL-1) blockers (anakinra). The onset of action of biological therapies is rapid (usually 2 weeks). Adverse effects of biological therapies are immunosuppression (leading to severe infections), worsening of heart failure and demyelination.

Fifty per cent of people with rheumatoid arthritis are unable to work 10 years after the initial diagnosis. Poor prognostic features include the presence of rheumatoid nodules, HLA-DR4, extra-articular features and female sex.

Theme 6: Diseases of calcium and the parathyroid axis

1. I – Primary hyperparathyroidism

Primary hyperparathyroidism is one of the most common causes of non-malignant hypercalcaemia. The symptoms of hypercalcaemia include lethargy, polyuria, polydipsia, peptic ulcer disease, stone formation and depression. Patients with very high serum calcium levels are at risk of cardiac arrest. In health, calcium metabolism is largely regulated by parathyroid hormone (PTH), which is secreted from the parathyroid glands. PTH increases serum calcium concentration by promoting bone resorption, renal phosphate excretion and vitamin D synthesis. The net effect of PTH is a rise in serum calcium and a fall in serum phosphate. Primary hyperparathyroidism is usually due to a single parathyroid adenoma that autonomously secretes excessive amounts of PTH. It is diagnosed by identifying hypercalcaemia in the presence of raised PTH levels. Treatment is by parathyroidectomy. Significant hypercalcaemia should be treated with fluid resuscitation and bisphosphonates.

2. L – Secondary hyperparathyroidism

In chronic renal failure, the combination of hyperphosphataemia and reduced synthesis of vitamin D can result in chronic hypocalcaemia. Since the normal physiological response to hypocalcaemia is to secrete PTH from the parathyroid glands, patients with chronic hypocalcaemia often have persistently elevated PTH levels. This is referred to as secondary hyperparathyroidism and is a normal physiological response. The high levels of circulating PTH in secondary hypothyroidism promote the resorption of bone in an attempt to mobilize calcium stores and correct the underlying hypocalcaemia. If this continues for a prolonged period, the patient will develop osteodystrophy, which can manifest as bone pain, osteomalacia and pathological fracture. Treatment of secondary hypocalcaemia requires a vitamin D analogue, such as alfacalcidol, which will increase serum calcium levels and in turn suppress PTH secretion. Hyperphosphataemia can usually be treated using phosphate binders such as calcium carbonate, which reduce its bioavailability.

3. D – Hypoparathyroidism

Hypoparathyroidism is a relatively common, and transient, complication of subtotal thyroidectomy. Reduced levels of PTH result in high phosphate levels and low calcium levels. The symptoms of hypocalcaemia include perioral paraesthesiae, muscular cramping and depression. Signs of hypocalcaemia include carpopedal spasm when a blood pressure cuff is inflated over the brachial artery (Trousseau's sign) and facial twitching when the facial nerve is excited by tapping above the parotid gland (Chvostek's sign). If the patient is stable and only suffering mild symptoms, the condition can be corrected using oral calcium supplementation. If the patient is very symptomatic, a 10 mL intravenous dose of 10% calcium gluconate can be administered. Approximately 1% of patients will develop permanent hypoparathyroidism following subtotal thyroidectomy.

Pseudohypoparathyroidism is an autosomal dominant condition characterized by end-organ resistance to PTH. Features include learning difficulties, short statute and short fouth and fifth metacarpals, accompanied by a low PTH, low calcium and high phosphate. *Pseudo-pseudohypoparathyroidism* describes the condition where all the phenotypic features of pseudohypoparathyroidism are present, in conjunction with a normal biochemistry.

4. H – Parathyroid hormone-related protein secretion

Ectopic PTH-related protein mimics the action of PTH. It is often secreted from small cell malignant tumours and is a common cause of hypercalcaemia in malignancy. This condition is usually treated with fluid therapy and bisphosphonates. Calcitonin can be used in refractory disease.

5. M – Tertiary hyperparathyroidism

Tertiary hyperparathyroidism occurs following a prolonged period of secondary hyperparathyroidism. The parathyroid glands hypertrophy and begin to secrete PTH autonomously, i.e. this is no longer a physiological response to negative feedback (see Case 2 above). The patient will usually have a high serum calcium level and a high PTH level. It is best to avoid the development of tertiary hyperparathyroidism by the correct and early management of secondary hyperparathyroidism. In severe disease, it is possible to remove the majority of the parathyroid tissue to reduce hormone levels.

Theme 7: Diseases of the myocardium and pericardium

1. F – Hypertrophic obstructive cardiomyopathy

Hypertrophic obstructive cardiomyopathy (HOCM) is an autosomal dominant disease that results in hypertrophy of the myocardium, usually localized to the interventricular septum. It is the most common cardiomyopathy. Patients are often asymptomatic and diagnosed as part of family screening programmes. When symptoms are present, they include exertional dyspnoea, syncope, palpitations and angina. Patients are at risk of potentially fatal atrial and ventricular arrhythmias. The risk of arrhythmia and subsequent sudden cardiac death is higher during and shortly after exertion. Those with HOCM are therefore advised to avoid sporting activities. Findings on examination include a forceful double apex beat, jerky carotid artery pulsation and an ejection systolic murmur due to aortic outflow obstruction. Diagnosis is usually confirmed by echocardiography. Treatment options include β-blockade to reduce myocardial oxygen demand, calcium channel blockers and anti-arrhythmic agents such as amiodarone. Cardiac pacing and internal cardiac defibrillators are available to those individuals who have experienced dangerous ventricular arrhythmias. Debulking ablation of the myocardium, surgery and cardiac transplantation are used for refractive and end-stage disease.

2. E – Dilated cardiomyopathy

In dilated cardiomyopathy, the left ventricle becomes dilated and inefficient, placing the patient at risk of arrhythmia (particularly atrial fibrillation), embolic disease and heart failure. The condition is occasionally familial, but is usually acquired and often secondary to excess alcohol consumption, ischaemic heart disease, metabolic disease, myocarditis and primary muscular diseases, including muscular dystrophy. Treatment is largely symptomatic, with arrhythmias and heart failure being treated as usual. Patients with dilated cardiomyopathy require anticoagulation to reduce the risk of embolic disease. Those who are known to experience dangerous ventricular arrhythmia require an internal cardiac defibrillator. Cardiac transplantation is a last resort for disease that is refractory to maximum medical therapy.

3. B – Atrial myxoma

Atrial myxoma, despite being relatively rare, is the most common tumour of the heart. It is a benign gelatinous neoplasm and is predominantly found attached to the septal wall of the left atrium by a pedicle. Symptoms include chest pain, dyspnoea, fever, lethargy and weight loss. Auscultation my reveal a loud first heart sound and a diastolic 'plop' due to prolapse of the tumour through the mitral valve. The presentation is similar to infective endocarditis and can cause diagnostic difficulties. Atrial myxomas can often embolize (with typical embolic consequences), but they do not metastasize. Echocardiography is the investigation of choice, and usually identifies a cystic polypoid mass. Treatment is by surgical excision. If removal is not complete, myxoma may recur.

The Carney complex is an autosomal dominant condition characterized by atrial and cutaneous myxomas, spotty skin hyperpigmentation and endocrine overactivity. It is associated with around 10% of cases of atrial myxoma.

J Aidan Carney, American pathologist (b1934).

4. K – Uraemic pericarditis

This is a classic history for pericarditis. In this case, the patient has a significantly elevated serum urea (possibly due to chronic renal impairment), which irritates the pericardium, leading to an inflammatory response. Other causes of pericarditis include viral infection (Coxsackie virus), autoimmune disease, myocardial infarction, tuberculosis, malignancy, amyloidosis and sarcoidosis. Patients present with retrosternal stabbing pain that may radiate to the shoulder/neck and is worse on movement, inspiration and lying flat. The pain characteristically improves on leaning forward. Patients may have a low-grade fever, and a pericardial rub (high-pitched scratching sound) may be heard on auscultation. ECG may demonstrate saddle-shaped ST elevation and T inversion in random leads. Treatment involves management of the underlying cause and regular non-steroidal anti-inflammatory drugs for symptomatic relief.

5. G – Myocarditis

Myocarditis is most commonly due to viral infection with Coxsackie B virus. Other causes include autoimmune disease, rheumatic fever, diphtheria, and a multitude of other viral, bacterial and fungal pathogens. Presentation is usually with a period of general illness, lethargy, fever and palpitations, followed by symptoms of left ventricular failure. Definitive diagnosis is often difficult, as evidence of infection is rarely found. Plasma troponin and cardiac enzymes are elevated in proportion to the extent of damage. Endomyocardial biopsy is sometimes employed to aid diagnosis. Treatment is predominantly symptomatic, including management of congestive cardiac failure and arrhythmias. Patients are advised to avoid exertion during the illness, as this may precipitate fatal ventricular arrhythmias. Some people recover fully, while others have a prolonged illness resulting in dilated cardiomyopathy. A number of patients die in the acute stages due to arrhythmias, congestive cardiac failure and refractory cardiogenic shock.

Theme 8: Visual defects 1

Innervation of the eye Each eye is innervated by its own optic nerve. The fibres of the nasal (medial) retina communicate information regarding the lateral visual field. Conversely, the fibres of the temporal (lateral) retina carry information regarding the medial visual field. The optic nerve fibres from each eye intersect at the optic chiasm, which lies a few millimetres above the pituitary gland. At the chiasm, the fibres from the nasal retina swap sides, while the temporal fibres remain on the ipsilateral side. On each side, fibres of the ipsilateral temporal retina and contralateral nasal retina continue as the optic tract to the lateral geniculate body. The upper fibres then pass through the temporal lobe and the lower fibres through the parietal lobe.

Muscles controlling the eye The trochlear nerve (cranial nerve IV) innervates the superior oblique muscle, which moves the eye down and out. The abducens nerve (cranial nerve VI) innervates the lateral rectus, which abducts the eye. The oculomotor nerve (cranial nerve III) innervates all the remaining ocular muscles, the levator palpebrae (upper eyelid) and the ciliary body (required for pupil constriction). The phrase 'LR6, SO4' can be used to remember that lateral rectus is innervated by cranial nerve VI and the superior oblique by cranial nerve IV.

Chiasm, from Greek *chiasma* = crossing.

Trochlear, from Latin *trochlea* = pulley.

1. A – Abducens nerve palsy

This woman may have a brain tumour. The consequent raised intracranial pressure can result in compression of the abducens nerve on the temporal bone. The abducens nerve innervates the lateral rectus, the muscle that abducts the eye. A palsy of this nerve results in diplopia on gazing laterally towards the side of the lesion, since there is no abduction of the eye on this side. In this scenario, the patient experiences diplopia on left lateral gaze, signifying a left abducens nerve palsy.

2. C – Optic chiasm lesion

This woman has acromegaly, a pituitary tumour. Because the pituitary gland lies just below the optic chiasm, tumours in this gland can compress here. At the optic chiasm, the nasal retinal fibres (which supply the temporal visual fields) cross sides. Compression at the chiasm will therefore cause bilateral loss of temporal visual fields. This is known as a bitemporal hemianopia.

3. B – Oculomotor nerve palsy

The oculomotor nerve innervates all the extraocular muscles (except the lateral rectus and superior oblique), the ciliary body and the levator palpebrae muscle. An oculomotor nerve palsy will therefore result in unopposed action of the lateral rectus and superior oblique (the eye looks down and out), ptosis (drooping of the eyelid) and mydriasis (dilated pupil).

Because the trochlear nerve supplies the superior oblique, which moves the eye down and out, *trochlear nerve palsy* will result in vertical diplopia (double vision when looking down).

4. E – Optic tract lesion

The optic tract describes the fibres that continue from the optic chiasm towards the brain. Each optic tract contains fibres from the ipsilateral temporal retina (supplying the ipsilateral nasal visual field) and the contralateral nasal retina (supplying the contralateral temporal visual field). A lesion of the optic tract will therefore cause blindness in the contralateral half of the visual field in each eye. In other words, a lesion of the left optic tract results in blindness in the right side of the visual field in both eyes (and vice versa). This is known as contralateral homonymous hemianopia.

The optic nerve innervates the whole eye. A *lesion of the optic nerve* will therefore result in blindness of one eye.

5. G – Temporal lobe lesion

The upper fibres from the optic tract travel through the temporal lobe and the lower fibres pass through the parietal lobe. Whereas lesions in the optic tract cause a contralateral homonymous hemianopia (see above), a lesion in the temporal lobe will result in a contralateral homonymous upper quadrantopia (loss of the upper quarter of the visual field on the same side in both eyes). Similarly, *parietal lobe lesions* cause a contralateral homonymous lower quadrantopia. *Occipital lobe lesions* result in a homonymous hemianopia, often with macular sparing.

Theme 9: Signs in gastrointestinal disease

1. I – Virchow's node

Virchow's node, also known as Troisier's sign, is an enlarged palpable left-sided supraclavicular lymph node that is associated with metastatic gastrointestinal malignancy. In this case, it is likely that the patient has a gastric malignancy.

2. G – Pyoderma gangrenosum

Pyoderma gangrenosum is a necrotizing dermatological condition associated with systemic disease, including inflammatory bowel disease, rheumatoid arthritis and haematological malignancy. It usually begins with a small red pustule that gradually increases in size and ulcerates over time. The edges of the lesion classically have a blue–purple discoloration. The patient may also experience general lethargy, fever and myalgia. The treatment of pyoderma gangrenosum requires management of the underlying condition and the use of topical or systemic steroids. In more severe disease, immune system modulators such as azathioprine or sulfasalazine may be indicated.

3. E – Erythema nodosum

Erythema nodosum is a dermatological condition caused by inflammation of subcutaneous adipose tissue (panniculitis). It usually presents with a number of raised, painful, reddish-purple lesions on the shins. The patient may also suffer from lethargy, fever and myalgia. Erythema nodosum is associated with a number of conditions, including ulcerative colitis, Crohn's disease, streptococcal pharyngitis, chlamydial urethritis, tuberculosis and sarcoidosis, as well as with the use of certain medications (e.g. the oral contraceptive pill). The lesions tend to resolve over 2–6 weeks without treatment.

4. A – Angular stomatitis

Angular stomatitis describes erythema and fissuring at the corners of the mouth secondary to iron-deficiency anaemia. Other signs of iron-deficiency anaemia include koilonychia (spoon-shaped nails), palmar crease pallor, conjunctival pallor and tachycardia. The presence of iron-deficiency anaemia without an obvious cause should be investigated thoroughly to exclude gastrointestinal causes such as malignancy, coeliac disease and Crohn's disease.

5. B – Dermatitis herpetiformis

Dermatitis herpetiformis is an intensely itchy, blistering rash that is associated with coeliac disease. It is usually found on the extensor surfaces of the elbows and knees, but can also be found on the back, buttocks and forehead. Treatment usually involves the implementation of a gluten-free diet in combination with oral dapsone and topical corticosteroids.

Theme 10: Complications of renal replacement therapy

1. J – Hypotension

Hypotension is perhaps the most common complication of haemodialysis. As well as removing waste products such as urea and potassium from the circulation, haemodialysis can be tailored to remove excess fluid from fluid-overloaded patients. This process is called ultrafiltration. If the ultrafiltration is excessive or inappropriate, it may deplete the patient's intravascular fluid volume, causing them to become hypotensive. Hypotension during dialysis is more common in patients with cardiovascular disease, heart failure and autonomic disease, as their ability to respond to hypotension is diminished.

2. L – Peritonitis

Infection is one of the most common complications of peritoneal dialysis. Peritonitis in peritoneal dialysis patients is usually due to poor technique or to equipment/connection failure, which allows bacteria to enter the peritoneum. Patients present with abdominal pain, fever, rigors and a cloudy dialysis fluid. A sample of dialysis fluid should be sent for white cell count, differential count, and microscopy, culture and sensitivity. The most common pathogen found is *Staphylococcus epidermidis* (a skin commensal). A more serious infection is caused by *Staphylococcus aureus* infection. The treatment of peritoneal dialysis-associated peritonitis is with intraperitoneal broad-spectrum antibiotics, e.g. vancomycin 25 mg/L and ceftazidime 125 mg/L for at least 2 weeks.

3. A – Acute organ rejection

Acute rejection occurs within 6 months of transplantation and is due to a T-cell-mediated response to protein antigens on the donor kidney. Despite the use of immunosuppressants such as tacrolimus and ciclosporin, acute rejection is seen in up to 70% of patients following renal transplantation. It is treated by a course of methylprednisolone. Unresponsive cases are given antithymocyte globulin (ATG). ATG is an antibody derived from rabbits that destroys human T cells, reducing the patient's ability to raise an immune response against the donor kidney. The two other main types of organ rejection are hyperacute rejection and chronic rejection. *Hyperacute rejection* occurs within hours of transplantation, and is mediated by the complement system. It is caused by the presence of antibodies to antigens within the donor kidney, and necessitates immediate removal of the kidney to prevent a potentially fatal systemic inflammatory response. *Chronic rejection* takes place 6 months after transplantation and is usually discovered by increasing serum creatinine levels. It is mediated by a chronic immune response against the donor kidney. There is also an element of vascular fibrosis, which is not treatable by immunosuppression. Patients confirmed to have chronic rejection should be considered for a second donor organ.

4. K – Ischaemic heart disease

This patient has angina caused by coronary artery disease. Cardiovascular disease is the most common cause of death in patients receiving haemodialysis. The pathogenic mechanism is complicated, and is likely to involve accelerated atheroma formation, hypertension, vascular calcification and chronic left ventricular failure secondary to fluid overload.

5. N – Vascular steal syndrome

An arteriovenous fistula is formed when a surgical anastomosis is formed between a vein and a neighbouring artery. The fistula provides easy access to high flow rates amenable to haemodialysis. During haemodialysis, two needles are inserted into the fistula. One needle removes blood from the circulation and delivers it to the dialysis machine, while the other returns the dialysed blood to the patient. Steal syndrome occurs when too much blood enters the fistula at the expense of distal tissues, i.e. the hand and fingers in radiocephalic fistulas. The diminished arterial blood supply to the hand causes discoloration, pain, cramps and paraesthesiae, with tissue ischaemia and necrosis in severe cases. In addition, the patient will have a weak radial pulse and a low brachial–wrist pulse index. Other complications involving arteriovenous fistulas include thrombosis and aneurysm formation.

Theme 11: Ulcers

1. D – Marjolin's ulcer

Marjolin's ulcer is the development of a squamous cell carcinoma occurring in an area of scarred or traumatized skin, such as a burn injury, chronic wound or venous ulcer. Lesions appear as raised, fleshy, firm papules that grow slowly. Treatment is by wide local excision.

Jean Nicholas Marjolin (1780–1850), French surgeon. He described the condition in 1828.

2. C – Cushing's ulcer

Cushing's ulcer (also known as Rokitansky–Cushing syndrome) is the association of peptic ulceration and/or haemorrhage with intracranial injury or a raised intracranial pressure.

Curling's ulcer is an acute ulcer of the duodenum that occurs a few days severe burns. It occurs because the reduced plasma volume results in necrosis of the gastric mucosa, with ensuing ulceration and perforation.

Karl von Rokitansky, Austrian pathologist (1804–78).

Thomas Blizard Curling, British surgeon (1811–88).

3. A – Arterial ulcer

This man has features of intermittent claudication (cramping in the lower limbs on exertion). This is due to underlying ischaemia (from arterial disease). Other features of ischaemia include cold feet, hair loss, toenail dystrophy, dusky cyanosis and ischaemic ulceration. Arterial ulcers are deep, painful and sharply defined, and usually occur on the shin or foot. The peripheral pulses may be reduced or absent on examination. Contrast angiography will help define arterial lesions, which may be improved by angioplasty or vascular reconstruction.

Venous ulcers occur most often in women after middle age. They occur over a background of deep venous insufficiency. There are many stages of skin changes in venous disease, beginning with oedema and a brown discoloration of the skin. The brown colour comes from haemosiderin deposits, which occur secondary to extravasation of red cells from leaky capillaries. The next stages are an eczema-like appearance, with hardening and constriction of the skin around the ankle (lipodermatosclerosis). The tightening of the skin around the ankle that occurs with lipodermatosclerosis, along with the oedema of the leg proximal to this, results in an 'inverted champagne bottle' appearance. Ulceration of the affected skin often follows trauma and usually affects the medial gaiter area (the gaiter area stretches from the ankle to the proximal calf, much like the gaiters used in hiking to prevent muddy water from getting into boots).

4. H – Pyoderma gangrenosum

Pyoderma gangrenosum is a skin condition that is associated with inflammatory bowel disease (as in this patient), rheumatoid arthritis and myeloid blood dyscrasias (e.g. acute and chronic myeloid leukaemias). It initially appears as purple papules, which enlarge and break down to become deep, necrotic ulcers with a dark-red border. Pyoderma gangrenosum is most common on the legs, but can develop anywhere.

5. G – Neuropathic ulcer

This woman with diabetes has developed sensory loss from the ankles distally – in a 'glove-and-stocking' distribution. As a result of this diabetic neuropathy, patients can cause severe damage to their feet without noticing, and ulcers can develop from trivial traumas. For this reason, people with diabetes should have their peripheral sensation checked regularly, keep their toenails short and avoid walking around barefoot. Neuropathic ulcers often occur on the sole of the foot over areas of pressure (e.g. beneath the metatarsal heads).

A *rodent ulcer*, or basal cell carcinoma, is a malignant tumour of the basal keratinocytes of the epidermis. It is the most common form of skin cancer, found typically on the face of middle-aged and older patients with fair skin. Risk factors for the development of rodent ulcers include ultraviolet light exposure, X-ray exposure, chronic scarring, a genetic predisposition and male sex. Lesions classically present as small, skin-coloured papules with telangiectasia and a pearly edge with central necrosis. These tumours grow slowly but relentlessly, and are locally invasive, destroying soft tissue, cartilage and bone. Metastasis is very rare. Management is by surgical excision.

Syphilitic ulcers present as multiple, painless, maculopapular ulcers with lymphadenopathy, following a primary painless genital ulcer. Syphilis is a sexually transmitted infection caused by *Treponema pallidum*. The primary lesion is a single painless ulcer with a clean base (or chancre) that occurs at the site of inoculation (i.e. the penis, scrotum, vagina or rectum). A few weeks later, secondary syphilis develops (as above). In some cases, the maculopapular lesions of secondary syphilis can coalesce to form large fleshy masses known as condylomata lata.

Martorell's ulcer is an ischaemic ulcer of the leg above the ankle that occurs secondary to hypertension.

Syphilis, from Greek *su* = pig + *philos* = love; pig lover.

Fernando Martorell Otzet, Spanish cardiologist (1906–84).

Theme 12: Tachycardias and tachyarrhythmias

1. E – Sick sinus syndrome

Sick sinus syndrome is caused by a dysfunctional sinoatrial node, usually secondary to age-related fibrosis. It is often diagnosed using a 24-hour ECG tracing requested for patients experiencing palpitations or symptomatic bradycardia such as dizzy spells and syncope. The tracing usually shows sinus bradycardia, atrioventricular block or asystole interspersed with periods of supraventricular tachycardia, such as junctional tachycardias or atrial fibrillation. There is no specific treatment. Although pacemaker insertion may be indicated in cases with severe symptoms, this does not affect prognosis. Anticoagulation is recommended in patients at risk of thromboembolic disease.

2. F – Sinus tachycardia

In this case, the patient is experiencing sinus tachycardia secondary to pain and anxiety. It is important to search for external stimuli such as pain, anxiety and recent exercise that may cause a patient to become tachycardic. Sinus tachycardia is usually a benign condition; however, prolonged periods of tachycardia in patients with significant heart disease may lead to cardiac decomposition and left ventricular failure. As such it is important to manage these patients promptly and appropriately. The treatment in the above case is to prescribe regular and breakthrough analgesia, using the pain ladder, which should be titrated to the patient's pain score.

3. D – Paroxysmal atrial fibrillation

Patients with paroxysmal (intermittent) atrial fibrillation are at significant risk of thromboembolic disease. A thrombus can form during an episode of atrial fibrillation due to the accumulation of stagnant blood in the inefficient atrium. The sudden effective contractions of the atria that occur when the patient reverts to sinus rhythm may cause thrombus disruption and the formation of emboli that enter the systemic circulation. Such emboli may cause stroke, mesenteric infarction, splenic infarction and acute limb ischaemia, as in this case. Patients with paroxysmal atrial fibrillation should be considered for anticoagulation (warfarin) in addition to management of the underlying arrhythmia (β-blockers or amiodarone). Treatment options for the ischaemic limb include heparin infusion, embolectomy, open surgery or amputation. In patients with a poor quality of life and multiple comorbidities it is sometimes more appropriate to manage acute limb ischaemia symptomatically with analgesia.

4. I – Ventricular fibrillation

In ventricular fibrillation, the ventricles contract ineffectively at a rate of 300–600 beats/min. The ECG tracing shows a rapid, irregular rhythm with a fibrillating baseline. The speed and haphazard nature of ventricular contraction means that no cardiac output is possible, and vital organs, including the brain, are not perfused, resulting in rapid death. The only treatment is DC cardioversion according to the Advanced Life Support Guidelines. Adjuncts to treatment include basic life support, intravenous adrenaline (epinephrine) and intravenous amiodarone.

5. G – Torsades de pointes

Torsades de pointes, a specific form of ventricular tachycardia, is a broad complex ventricular arrhythmia caused by prolonged ventricular repolarization, which is seen on ECG as an extended QT interval. A prolonged QT interval may be congenital or acquired. Long-QT syndromes, such as Romano–Ward syndrome, are congenital diseases caused by ion channel abnormalities, and are commonly associated with torsades de pointes. Acquired disease is usually secondary to electrolyte imbalance or drug side-effects. Patients with hypomagnesaemia and hypokalaemia are at particular risk of torsades de pointes. Drugs that are known to trigger torsades de pointes include class Ia antiarrhythmic agents (disopyramide and procainamide), tricyclic antidepressants (amitriptyline and imipramine), phenothiazine antipsychotics (chlorpromazine and prochlorperazine) and non-sedating antihistamines (loratidine).

Torsades de pointes is seen on ECG as a regular broad complex tachycardia with a varying axis whereby the QRS complexes repeatedly switch from an upright to a horizontal position. The patient often experiences palpitations, dizziness, chest pain and syncope. The rhythm usually aborts spontaneously, but has the potential to degenerate into ventricular fibrillation. Prolonged episodes of torsades de pointes that are associated with haemodynamic instability require urgent DC cardioversion. Long-term management includes β-blockade (not in acquired disease, as it may trigger torsades de pointes), permanent pacemakers in severe symptomatic disease and implantable cardioverter–defibrillators (ICDs) in patients at high risk of sudden cardiac death. In cases of acquired disease, any electrolyte imbalance must be corrected and offending drugs stopped.

Cesarino Romano, Italian paediatrician (b1923).

Owen Conor Ward, Irish paediatrician (b1923).

Torsades de pointes, French 'twisting of the points', was first described by François Dessertenne in 1966 (*Arch Mal Coeur Vaiss* 1966; **59**: 263–72).

Theme 13: Oncological emergencies

1. K – Superior vena caval obstruction

Superior vena caval obstruction occurs when the flow along the superior vena cava is obstructed by local pressure from a tumour or thrombosis. It most commonly occurs in association with bronchial carcinoma, mediastinal carcinoma, lymphoma and neoplastic lymphadenopathy. The main features of superior vena caval obstruction are due to venous congestion, and include facial swelling, distended face, neck and chest veins, stridor and dyspnoea. Treatment usually involves immediate dexamethasone and urgent radiotherapy to reduce the tumour size. Tumours that are especially responsive to cytotoxic agents, such as lymphomas, should be referred for urgent chemotherapy.

2. D – Hypercalcaemia

Hypercalcaemia of malignancy is usually due to the ectopic production of parathyroid hormone-related protein, which mimics the action of parathyroid hormone and mobilizes calcium into the bloodstream. Hypercalcaemia may also be due to lytic bone metastases or the activation of osteoclasts, as seen in breast cancer and myeloma, respectively. Acute hypercalcaemia usually presents with confusion, polyuria, polydipsia, constipation and mood changes, and is ultimately diagnosed by measuring serum calcium. Treatment should begin with intravenous fluid hydration, aiming for 3–6 L of 0.9% saline over 24 hours. In severe cases, the patient should receive an intravenous bisphosphonate (e.g. pamidronate), which reduces bone resorption. Calcitonin may be given in hypercalcaemia refractory to hydration and bisphosphonate therapy.

3. J – Spinal cord compression

It is likely that this patient's spinal cord is being compressed by an extradural metastatic lesion of the spine. The presentation of spinal cord compression is variable, and is dependent on the site of the lesion. Typically, the patient has lower motor neuron signs at the level of the lesion and upper motor neuron signs below the lesion. The exception is if the lesion is below the L1–L2 border, where the spinal cord ends and is replaced by the cauda equina. In this situation, only lower motor neurons are affected, producing saddle anaesthesia, leg weakness, reduced reflexes, normal (downgoing) plantar reflexes and urinary retention. Upper motor neuron signs, caused by compression above the L1–L2 border, include leg weakness and eventual hypertonia, brisk reflexes, upgoing plantar reflexes and urinary incontinence. If spinal cord compression is suspected, the patient should be referred for urgent MRI. The treatment options include high-dose steroids, radiotherapy and surgery. If not recognized quickly and treated appropriately, the neurological damage will become permanent.

4. I – Raised intracranial pressure

Raised intracranial pressure in malignancy is usually secondary to a primary brain tumour or brain metastases. It usually presents with a headache that is worse in the mornings and on straining. In more serious disease, the patient may have visual disturbance, papilloedema and seizures. If raised intracranial pressure is suspected, an urgent CT scan should be organized. Treatment is with immediate high-dose steroids (dexamethasone). An urgent referral should be made to an oncologist for possible radiotherapy or neurosurgery.

5. L – Syndrome of inappropriate ADH secretion

Syndrome of inappropriate ADH secretion in malignancy is usually due to ectopic ADH secretion from tumour cells. The most common tumour causing this condition is small cell lung carcinoma. The water retention caused by the excessive production of ADH results in a dilutional hyponatraemia, which, when severe, can cause seizures and permanent neurological damage. In addition to a low serum sodium concentration, the patient will also have raised urine osmolality and high urine sodium concentration. Treatment requires fluid restriction, usually of 1 L/day. If intravenous fluids are required, only 0.9% saline should be used, to prevent a rapid increase in serum sodium. If the sodium is corrected too quickly, the patient may develop central pontine myelinolysis, which can cause severe and permanent neurological complications that can be fatal. Therefore, correction must occur over days, with regular assessment of serum sodium.

Theme 14: Management of endocrine disease

1. G – Surgical resection and radiotherapy

The older woman who presents with dysphagia associated with a large, irregular, hard mass probably has anaplastic carcinoma of the thyroid gland. This tumour has a poor prognosis, despite surgery, chemotherapy or radiotherapy. However, in cases where there are symptomatic issues, such as dysphagia, palliative surgery and radiotherapy can be used to relieve the obstruction.

2. B – Carbimazole

This young pregnant woman presents with thyrotoxicosis and ophthalmoplegia, features typical of Graves' disease. The first-line treatment in the under-40s is carbimazole, a drug that inhibits the production of thyroid hormones. Iodine-131 should be avoided in women who are pregnant or who are around children, due to the risk of radioactivity-induced teratogenicity.

3. C – Desmopressin

Polyuria and polydipsia has many causes, but, when no other symptoms are apparent, you should consider diabetes insipidus (DI). This is characterized by the excretion of excessive quantities of dilute urine with thirst, and is mediated by a lack of active ADH. ADH is secreted by the posterior pituitary gland and has the function of increasing water reabsorption in the kidney. There are two types of DI: cranial DI (which is due to a lack of ADH secretion from the pituitary) and nephrogenic DI (which results from a lack of response of the kidneys to circulating ADH). Causes of cranial DI include head injury (as in this patient), surgery, sarcoidosis and the DIDMOAD syndrome (characterized by **D**iabetes **I**nsipidus, **D**iabetes **M**ellitus, **O**ptic **A**trophy and **D**eafness). Nephrogenic DI can be due to metabolic abnormalities (hypokalaemia or hypercalcaemia), drugs (lithium or demeclocycline), genetic defects and heavy metal poisoning.

Patients with DI may pass up to 20 L of water in a day. The diagnosis of DI is confirmed using the water deprivation test. The patient is deprived of water, and the urine and plasma osmolalities are measured every 2 hours. If there is a raised plasma osmolality (>300 mol/kg) in the presence of urine that is not maximally concentrated (i.e. <660 mol/kg), then the patient has DI. At this point in the test, the patient is given an intramuscular dose of desmopressin (a synthetic analogue of ADH). If the patient now starts concentrating their urine they have cranial DI. If the urine osmolality remains <660 mol/kg nephrogenic DI is confirmed.

Treatment of cranial DI is with desmopressin. Nephrogenic DI is improved by thiazide diuretics.

4. I – Total thyroidectomy and thyroxine

This woman has an enlarging asymptomatic thyroid lump with lymphadenopathy. It is most likely that she has a papillary thyroid cancer. This is managed by total thyroidectomy followed by daily thyroxine to help prevent recurrence of the tumour.

5. D – Hydrocortisone and fludrocortisone

The features that this young girl has are typical of adrenal insufficiency. This, along with the recent meningococcal septicaemia, points to an underlying diagnosis of Waterhouse–Friderichsen syndrome, i.e. bilateral haemorrhage into the adrenal glands caused by meningococcal septicaemia. Management of adrenal insufficiency is by replacement of glucocorticoids (by hydrocortisone) and mineralocorticoids (by fludrocortisone).

Rupert Waterhouse, English physician (1873–1958).

Carl Friderichsen (1886–1979).

Theme 15: Management of neurological conditions 2

1. G – Levodopa

This man has Parkinson's disease, caused by a depletion of dopaminergic neurons in the substantia nigra of the basal ganglia. Presentation is often unilateral with resting tremor in the upper limb. The classic triad of features is tremor, rigidity and bradykinesia (slowness of movement). Other symptoms are tiredness, aching limbs, depression, small handwriting (micrographia), a flexed posture, no expression ('poker face') and cognitive impairment. Examination reveals cogwheel rigidity in the upper limbs and lead-pipe rigidity in the lower limbs. Patients are said to have a festinant gait – where the steps start slowly and hesitantly, but gradually speed up uncontrollably. Diagnosis is clinical. Various drugs are used to manage Parkinson's disease, including levodopa (a dopamine precursor). This is often given with carbidopa – a decarboxylase inhibitor that prevents levodopa being converted to dopamine before it reaches the blood–brain barrier. Other medications are bromocriptine and amantidine.

Because of side-effects, including dystonias, tardive dyskinesia and postural hypotension, drug therapy is often delayed until there is significant disability. There is a reduced lifespan associated with Parkinson's disease – but only due to the increased risk of falls.

James Parkinson, English physician (1755–1824).

2. D – Carbamazepine

This woman has typical features of trigeminal neuralgia. Neuropathic pain such as this is often relieved by some non-conventional analgesics such as carbamazepine, gabapentin and amitriptyline.

3. C – Benzylpenicillin

This woman has meningitis. The presence of a purpuric rash points to meningococcal septicaemia (caused by *Neisseria meningitidis*). The best treatment is benzylpenicillin.

4. H – Lorazepam

This man is in status epilepticus, and needs intravenous lorazepam.

5. B – Aspirin

The patient has had a stroke. Because the CT scan has ruled out underlying haemorrhage, it is safe to administer aspirin.

Practice Paper 8: Questions

Theme 1: Complications of HIV infection 1

Options

A. Candidiasis
B. Cryptococcus infection
C. Cryptosporidiosis
D. Cytomegalovirus infection
E. HIV dementia
F. HIV wasting syndrome
G. Kaposi's sarcoma
H. Lichen planus
I. Pneumocystis infection
J. Seroconversion
K. Stevens–Johnson syndrome
L. Toxoplasmosis

For each of the following people with HIV infection, select the most likely complication. Each option may be used once, more than once or not at all.

1. A 37-year-old man presents to the GP complaining of worsening headaches and vomiting. He also complains of neck stiffness and some blurring of vision. He is known to have HIV infection.

2. A 42-year-old woman has a 2-month history of worsening shortness of breath and a dry cough. She also complains of night sweats. On examination, her oxygen saturations are 89%. She has no other symptoms and no history of respiratory disease, but is known to have HIV infection.

3. A 31-year-old man presents feeling unwell. He complains of malaise, generalized muscle aches and headaches. More recently, he has suffered some blurring of vision and pain in his eyes. He is known to have HIV infection.

4. A 42-year-old woman presents with a 3-week history of difficult and painful swallowing, and she is losing weight as a result of not eating. She otherwise feels well. On examination, the mucous membranes of her mouth are sore and red. She is known to have HIV infection.

5. A 27-year-old man comes to hospital after developing a widespread red rash. On examination, there is blistering of the oral mucosa. He has recently started medication for HIV infection.

Theme 2: Scoring systems in medicine

Options

A. Abbreviated Mental Test Score
B. Breslow Score
C. Curb Score
D. Geriatric Depression Score
E. Glasgow Coma Scale
F. Mini-Mental Test Score
G. Ranson's Criteria
H. Rockall Score
I. Waterlow Score

For each of the following descriptions, select the most appropriate scoring system. Each option may be used once, more than once or not at all.

1. This scoring system should be used to assess a patient's consciousness following head trauma.

2. This scoring system should be used as a quick guide to an elderly patient's cognitive state.

3. This scoring system can be used to assess the risk of an adverse outcome following an upper gastrointestinal bleed.

4. This scoring system helps predict the clinical outcome of a patient with acute pancreatitis.

5. This scoring system should be used to assess a patient's risk of developing a pressure score.

Theme 3: Fainting

Options

A. Carotid sinus sensitivity
B. Epilepsy
C. Hyperventilation
D. Hypoglycaemia
E. Ménière's disease
F. Micturition syncope
G. Postural hypotension
H. Stokes–Adams attack
I. Vasovagal attack
J. Vertebrobasilar insufficiency

For each of the following scenarios, select the most likely cause of collapse. Each option may be used once, more than once or not at all.

1. A 34-year-old woman faints during her daughter's school play. Her husband says that she turned slightly pale and slumped over while still seated. She did not jerk or lose urinary continence. She denies chest pain, shortness of breath or palpitations. She recovered spontaneously after 30 seconds and now feels back to her usual self.

2. A 67-year-old woman is standing in a queue at the post office when she suddenly collapses. Her face becomes extremely pale, and her body starts twitching after 20 seconds. Very soon after, she fully regains consciousness and her face is flushed.

3. A 76-year-old woman is hanging up her laundry on the washing line outside. While reaching up to peg on the last towel, she suddenly becomes dizzy and collapses on the ground. She does not lose consciousness, but takes a few moments to recover.

4. A 55-year-old woman collapses when standing up after watching a film. She denies any chest pain or palpitations. She was unresponsive for a minute, but soon recovered fully. This has happened on several previous occasions when standing up from a lying or sitting position.

5. A 45-year-old man collapses while urinating in a restaurant toilet. He briefly loses consciousness, but soon recovers fully.

Theme 4: Management of respiratory disease 2

Options

A. Amoxicillin
B. Cannula into second intercostal space, midclavicular line
C. Cannula into sixth intercostal space, midclavicular line
D. Chemotherapy
E. Co-trimoxazole
F. Erythromycin
G. Inhaled anticholinergic
H. Inhaled β-agonist
I. Low-molecular-weight heparin
J. Metronidazole
K. No management required
L. Radiotherapy
M. Rifampicin and isoniazid
N. Steroids
O. Warfarin

For each of the following scenarios, select the most appropriate management. Each option may be used once, more than once or not at all.

1. A 38-year-old woman presents with sudden-onset shortness of breath and chest pain. Examination is unremarkable. A chest X-ray is clear, but the diagnosis is eventually confirmed on a ventilation–perfusion scan.

2. A 21-year-old woman is involved in a road traffic accident. When the paramedics arrive, she has a heart rate of 122 beats/min, a respiratory rate of 32/min and a blood pressure of 86/42 mmHg. On examination, breath sounds are absent and there is hyper-resonance to percussion on the left side. The trachea is deviated to the right.

3. A 68-year-old man has a 3-week history of haemoptysis. He has lost a stone (6 kg) in weight over this period of time. A biopsy taken at bronchoscopy confirms a small cell lung tumour. A CT scan shows that the disease is not surgically resectable.

4. An 11-year-old boy presents to his GP with a 6-month history of night cough and intermittent wheeze. He has previously been well. On examination, he is small for his age and has mild eczema on his upper limbs.

5. A 53-year-old man is admitted to hospital after breaking his left arm. An X-ray of the affected limb shows part of the lung fields. On the lungs, holly-shaped white lesions can be seen that cross the lobar boundaries. The patient feels well and auscultation reveals no abnormality.

Theme 5: Non-infective diarrhoea

Options

A. Coeliac disease
B. Irritable bowel syndrome
C. Laxative abuse
D. Medication side-effect
E. Overflow diarrhoea
F. Pancreatitis
G. Thyrotoxicosis
H. Ulcerative colitis
I. Zollinger–Ellison syndrome

For each of the following scenarios, select the most likely diagnosis. Each option may be used once, more than once or not at all.

1. A 19-year-old woman presents to the GP with a 4-week history of diarrhoea. She also mentions that she is constantly hot and experiences occasional palpitations. She has unintentionally lost half a stone (3 kg) in weight in the last month.

2. A 46-year-old man presents with a history of sudden-onset diarrhoea, abdominal pain and fever. The patient says that his stool was very loose and mixed with significant amounts of frank blood.

3. A 14-year-old girl is brought to the GP by her mother, who says that her daughter has been 'going to the toilet' up to six times per day over the last month. On examination, the girl is underweight for her height and has downy hair on her face and arms. There are scratches on the knuckles of her right hand.

4. A 27-year-old woman presents to her GP complaining of a long history of abdominal cramps associated with alternating diarrhoea and constipation. Abdominal examination is unremarkable.

5. An 80-year-old woman who is cared for in a nursing home is noticed to be passing watery diarrhoea despite the fact that she is known to be chronically constipated and faecally impacted.

Theme 6: Signs in endocrinological disease

Options

A. Acanthosis nigricans
B. Hyperpigmentation
C. Irregularly irregular pulse
D. Necrobiosis lipoidica
E. Ophthalmoplegia
F. Pretibial myxoedema
G. Slow to relax reflexes
H. Striae

For each of the following scenarios, select the sign that you are most likely to find. Each option may be used once, more than once or not at all.

1. A 56-year-old woman presents to her GP with a mass in her neck. She also complains of runs of palpitations. The doctor finds a multinodular goitre on examination.

2. A 24-year-old woman with a long history of inflammatory bowel disease requiring steroids presents to her GP complaining of skin changes on her abdomen. She also has a history of weight gain, low mood and excessive hair growth on her face.

3. A 46-year-old woman with Addison's disease presents with skin changes that affect her palmar creases and buccal mucosa.

4. A 35-year-old woman with Graves' disease develops double vision. On examination, both eyes are protruding.

5. An obese 67-year-old woman with type 2 diabetes develops skin changes on the back of her neck and in her axilla. Her doctor measures her capillary glucose level, which is 17.8 mmol/L.

Theme 7: Features of rheumatoid arthritis

Options

A. Atlantoaxial subluxation
B. Boutonnière deformity
C. Caplan's syndrome
D. Felty's syndrome
E. Palmar erythema
F. Pyoderma gangrenosum
G. Rheumatoid nodules
H. Sjögren's syndrome
I. Spindling
J. Swan-neck deformity
K. Z-deformity

For each of the following scenarios, select the most appropriate feature of rheumatoid arthritis. Each option may be used once, more than once or not at all.

1. You see a 42-year-old woman with rheumatoid arthritis. The fourth digit on her right hand is hyperextended at the proximal interphalangeal joint and flexed at the distal interphalangeal joint.

2. You see a 42-year-old woman with rheumatoid arthritis. She has a 3 cm craggy, hard, painless mass on her left elbow that has grown in size over the last month.

3. You see a 42-year-old woman with rheumatoid arthritis. The second digit on her left hand is flexed at the proximal interphalangeal joint and hyperextended at the distal interphalangeal joint.

4. You see a 42-year-old woman with rheumatoid arthritis. The thumb on her left hand is flexed at the metacarpophalangeal joint and hyperextended at the interphalangeal joint.

5. You see a 42-year-old woman with rheumatoid arthritis. She describes a 'clunking' sound when she flexes her neck and a long history of neck pain.

Theme 8: Management of acute coronary syndromes

Options

A. Aspirin
B. β-Blockers
C. Calcium channel blockers
D. Clopidogrel
E. Cyclizine
F. Emergency coronary artery bypass graft
G. Emergency external pacing
H. Loop diuretics
I. Metoclopramide
J. Past medical history of a haemorrhagic stroke 6 weeks ago
K. Past medical history of ischaemic stroke 2 years ago
L. Past medical history of peptic ulcer disease
M. Percutaneous coronary angioplasty ± stenting
N. Previous thrombolysis with streptokinase
O. Reciprocal ST depression and tall T-waves in lead V2
P. Statins
Q. ST elevation of 2 mm in leads II, III and aVF
R. ST elevation of 2 mm in leads V1–V5
S. Tented T-waves

For each of the following presentations of acute coronary syndrome, select the most appropriate response. Each option may be used once, more than once or not at all.

1. A 62-year-old diabetic man presents to the district general hospital with sudden-onset, central, crushing chest pain that commenced at rest. The junior doctor on call records an ECG, which suggests inferior myocardial ischaemia. Which ECG changes has he seen?

2. A 62-year-old diabetic man presents to a large teaching hospital with sudden-onset, central, crushing chest pain that commenced at rest. An ECG shows significant ST elevation in the inferior leads. Before the attending junior doctor can administer thrombolysis, the cardiology registrar suggests a preferable intervention.

3. A 62-year-old diabetic man presents to the district general hospital with sudden-onset, central, crushing chest pain that commenced at rest. An ECG shows significant ST elevation in the inferior leads, and the attending junior doctor considers thrombolysis. What would be considered as an absolute contraindication to thrombolysis?

4. A 62-year-old diabetic man presents to a large teaching hospital with sudden-onset, central, crushing chest pain that commenced at rest. He is complaining of a variety of symptoms, including pain, breathlessness, nausea and headache. Before considering management, which drug should ideally be avoided in this case?

5. A 62-year-old diabetic man presents to the district general hospital with sudden-onset, central, crushing chest pain that occurred at rest. The attending junior doctor begins management according to an evidence-based hospital protocol, which includes a number of medications. Which class of drug, when given in the acute stage, has been shown to limit the size of an acute myocardial infarction and reduce subsequent mortality?

Theme 9: Pupillary disorders

Options

A. Argyll Robertson pupil
B. Brain-stem death
C. Holmes–Adie pupil
D. Horner's syndrome
E. Marcus Gunn pupil
F. Oculomotor nerve palsy
G. Opiate intoxication

For each of the following scenarios, select the most likely cause of the pupillary abnormality. Each option may be used once, more than once or not at all.

1. A 26-year-old woman presents to the emergency department after falling over in the snow. She says that she hit her head, but now feels well. On examination, one pupil is more dilated than the other. The dilated pupil does not react to light. The accommodation reflex is intact and there is no other neurological deficit.

2. A 64-year-old woman is an inpatient on a surgical ward following a hip replacement. The nursing staff say that she vomited earlier and that she has been unresponsive since her operation 12 hours ago. On examination, you notice that her pupils are small and that she has a respiratory rate of 7/min.

3. A 64-year-old man presents to the GP with a 2-week history of coughing up blood-stained mucus. He has also lost a stone (6 kg) in weight in the last month. He mentions that he cannot fully lift his left eyelid. On examination, the left eyelid is drooping and the associated pupil is smaller than the other. There is no other neurological deficit.

4. A 42-year-old woman presents with a short history of pain and blurring in her left eye. She is known to have multiple sclerosis. On examination, the right pupil appears to react appropriately to light, but shining a torch in the left pupil causes it to dilate.

5. A 62-year-old man is admitted to hospital with difficulty walking and poor coordination. On examination, both of his pupils are small and unreactive to light. The accommodation reflex is present.

Theme 10: Gastrointestinal investigations

Options

A. Abdominal X-ray
B. Anti-endomyseal antibodies
C. Barium swallow and follow-through
D. Colonoscopy
E. CT scan
F. Full blood count
G. Gastrografin swallow
H. *Helicobacter pylori* CLO test
I. *Helicobacter pylori* stool antigen test
J. Non-urgent endoscopy and biopsy
K. Urgent endoscopy

For each of the following scenarios, select the most appropriate investigation. Each option may be used once, more than once or not at all.

1. This investigation should be performed in a 65-year-old man complaining of new-onset dyspepsia and unintentional weight loss.
2. This investigation should be performed in a 28-year-old woman with dyspepsia that has failed to respond to lifestyle adaptations.
3. This investigation should be performed in a patient with suspected Crohn's disease affecting the small bowel.
4. This investigation should be performed in a patient with suspected oesophageal rupture.
5. This investigation should be performed as a first-line investigation in a patient with suspected coeliac disease.

Theme 11: Autoantibodies 1

Options

A. Anti-ACh receptor
B. Anti-adrenal
C. Anti-glomerular basement membrane
D. Anti-Hu
E. Anti-mitochondrial
F. Anti-intrinsic factor/anti-parietal
G. Anti-gliadin
H. Anti-LKM
I. Anti-thyroid peroxidase
J. Antibody to voltage-gated calcium channels
K. Thyroid-stimulating antibody

For each of the following scenarios, select the most specific autoantibody. Each option may be used once, more than once or not at all.

1. A 22-year-old woman has a 3-month history of abdominal discomfort and tiredness associated with passing offensive stools that are difficult to flush. Examination is unremarkable.

2. A 42-year-old woman presents to her GP with a large goitre, which she admits to having had for a long time. More recently, she has been suffering with constipation, lethargy and weight gain.

3. A 44-year-old woman has had multiple faints after standing up from a sitting position. On examination, you notice multiple areas of increased skin pigmentation in the palmar creases and on the elbows.

4. A 37-year-old man who presented with haemoptysis is shown to have 2+ of protein in his urine on dipstick analysis and deteriorating renal function.

5. A 44-year-old woman presents with a 1-month history of jaundice associated with fatigue, itching and dark urine. She has a history of early onset rheumatoid arthritis. On examination, she appears very jaundiced and has multiple xanthelasmas around her eyes.

Theme 12: Investigation of neurological disorders

Options

A. Angiogram
B. CT of the head
C. Copper studies
D. Electroencephalography
E. Lumbar puncture
F. Mini-Mental Test Score
G. MRI of the head
H. Muscle biopsy
I. Nerve conduction study
J. No further investigation required
K. Skull X-ray
L. Tensilon test

For each of the following scenarios, select the most appropriate investigation. Each option may be used once, more than once or not at all.

1. A 20-year-old woman presents with a 10-hour history of severe headache and vomiting. She was previously well. Examination reveals pain on neck flexion. While in the emergency department, she receives appropriate initial management.

2. A 42-year-old woman complains of a weakness in her left hand that has developed over the last few hours. She is otherwise well and has no other symptoms. Last year, she had a similar weakness in her right leg, which lasted for 3 days.

3. A 67-year-old man presents to the emergency department with sudden-onset weakness in his left arm and face. He has no other problems. Examination confirms the weakness, but there is no evidence of sensory deficit.

4. A 38-year-old woman has a 2-week history of intermittent double vision. She also feels generally weaker, particularly after exercise. She demonstrates this by opening and closing her hand repeatedly and showing how the motions get gradually slower. On examination, her eyes appear partially closed. There is no sensory deficit.

5. A 24-year-old man presents to the emergency department with sudden-onset severe headache. He says that it feels as if someone has hit him on the head with the corner of a brick. A CT scan is performed, but shows no abnormality.

Theme 13: Valvular heart disease

Options

A. Aortic regurgitation
B. Aortic stenosis
C. Atrial septal defect
D. Bicuspid aortic valve
E. Coarctation of the aorta
F. Marfan's syndrome
G. Mitral regurgitation
H. Mitral stenosis
I. Prosthetic heart valve
J. Pulmonary stenosis
K. Tetralogy of Fallot
L. Tricuspid regurgitation
M. Tricuspid stenosis

For each of the following scenarios, select the most likely underlying cause. Each option may be used once, more than once or not at all.

1. A 55-year-old man is admitted with tiredness and worsening shortness of breath. On examination, you note gynaecomastia and a midline sternotomy scar. He is subsequently found to have a normocytic anaemia with a number of red cell fragments on the blood film. Coombs' test is negative.

2. A 47-year-old woman has developed aortic stenosis in association with a degree of aortic regurgitation. She is told by her cardiologist that it is likely that she has a congenital abnormality of one of her valves.

3. A 58-year-old man is admitted following an episode of haematemesis. He is a heavy drinker and is already under investigation for heart failure. On examination, he is found to have a murmur that is best heard at the apex and radiates into his axilla.

4. A 35-year-old Indian woman who has known valvular heart disease as a result of rheumatic fever presents to the emergency department with chest pain. An ECG demonstrates bifid P-waves.

5. A 27-year-old woman with known primary pulmonary hypertension is admitted with a long history of abdominal pain. On examination, you find a murmur and peripheral oedema. Her liver is enlarged and tender to palpation.

Theme 14: Substance use

Options

A. Alcohol use
B. Alcohol withdrawal
C. Amphetamine use
D. Amphetamine withdrawal
E. Cannabis use
F. Cannabis withdrawal
G. Cocaine use
H. Cocaine withdrawal
I. Opiate use
J. Opiate withdrawal
K. Sedative use
L. Sedative withdrawal

For each of the following scenarios, select the most likely cause. Each option may be used once, more than once or not at all.

1. A 76-year-old woman is an inpatient on a surgical ward following a hip replacement. The nursing staff say that she vomited earlier and that she has been unresponsive since her operation 12 hours ago. On examination, you notice that her pupils are small and that she has a respiratory rate of 7/min.

2. An 18-year-old man presents to his GP complaining of a dry cough and tiredness. His mother said that he has become very suspicious of those around him. She adds that he has withdrawn himself socially and has not been the same since he met a new group of friends at university.

3. A 34-year-old man presents to the emergency department complaining of a sensation of insects crawling over his skin. He is tachycardic and hypertensive and his pupils are noted to be large.

4. A 74-year-old woman has recently changed GPs and has moved into a nursing home. The doctor is called because she has become unwell: she is sleeping poorly and complaining of nausea and sweating. She subsequently has a seizure.

5. A 63-year-old man is admitted for an elective cholecystectomy. On the second postoperative day, he complains of sweating and tremor. On examination, he is confused, anxious and tachycardic, and appears to be responding to visual hallucinations. He says that he can see thousands of miniature country dancers running around the floor.

Theme 15: Renal manifestations of systemic disease

Options

A. AA amyloidosis
B. AL amyloidosis
C. Diabetic microalbuminuria
D. Diabetic proteinuria
E. Lupus nephritis
F. Multiple myeloma
G. Polyarteritis nodosa
H. Rhabdomyolysis
I. Rhabdomyosarcoma
J. Streptococcal glomerulonephritis
K. Wegener's granulomatosis

For each of the following scenarios, select the most appropriate condition. Each option may be used once, more than once or not at all.

1. A 34-year-old woman with systemic lupus erythematosus presents to her GP complaining of being generally puffy. On examination, there is periorbital oedema and ankle oedema. Her blood pressure is 170/98 mmHg, and a urine dipstick analysis shows 3+ of protein and 2+ of blood.

2. A 56-year-old man with type 1 diabetes is shown to have 150 mg/L of albumin in his urine despite a previous urine dipstick analysis showing no abnormality.

3. A 45-year-old man with Crohn's disease is shown to have deteriorating renal function and proteinuria. A renal biopsy is taken, and the sample stains positively with Congo red.

4. A 78-year-old woman has a long history of bone pain and lethargy. She is found to have deteriorating renal function. On further investigation, there is a monoclonal band on serum electrophoresis and a monoclonal globulin protein in the urine.

5. An 81-year old woman was found collapsed at home following a stroke. She is shown to have a urea of 48 mmol/L, a creatinine of 400 μmol/L and a potassium of 5.8 mmol/L. Her urine is dark red in colour. It has been estimated that she was lying on the floor for at least 36 hours before being found.

Practice Paper 8: Answers

Theme 1: Complications of HIV infection 1

Certain conditions are said to be AIDS-defining (or AIDS indicator) illnesses. These are conditions that are strongly suggestive of AIDS. Examples of AIDS-defining illnesses that are suggestive of AIDS *without* evidence of laboratory HIV infection include *Pneumocystis* pneumonia, Kaposi's sarcoma, cytomegalovirus infection, oesophageal candidiasis, cerebral toxoplasmosis and *Mycobacterium avium intracellulare* infection. Examples of AIDS-defining illnesses that are suggestive of AIDS *with* laboratory evidence of HIV infection include pulmonary tuberculosis, HIV-wasting syndrome, HIV-related dementia, non-Hodgkin's lymphoma and *Cryptosporidium* diarrhoea lasting longer than 1 month.

1. B – *Cryptococcus* infection

This man with HIV presents with features typical of meningitis. In cases of subacute meningitis in immunocompromised patients, one must be wary of *Cryptococcus* infection and tuberculosis. *Cryptococcus neoformans* is an encapsulated fungus found in soil, and infection is by inhalation of contaminated material. *Cryptococcus* is diagnosed by detection of capsular material (e.g. in cerebrospinal fluid or sputum) using India ink stain. Treatment is with intravenous amphotericin B. *Cryptococcus* infection can also result in pulmonary disease.

2. I – *Pneumocystis* infection

Pneumocystis pneumonia (PCP) is the most common AIDS-defining illness, caused by the fungus *Pneumocystis jiroveci* (previously known as *Pneumocystis carinii*). Patients present with a dry cough, fever, shortness of breath, weight loss and night sweats. Oxygen saturations are typically low. If oxygen levels are normal, exercise-induced desaturations will support the diagnosis. Chest X-ray demonstrates widespread infiltrates. The diagnosis is determined by cytological examination of sputum or bronchial washings from bronchoscopy. Treatment is with co-trimoxazole (trimethoprim and sulfamethoxazole). Patients with HIV who have a low CD4 count (<200/μL) receive prophylaxis for *Pneumocystis* (e.g. co-trimoxazole or dapsone).

3. L – Toxoplasmosis

Cerebral toxoplasmosis is the most common central nervous system infection in AIDS, affecting 10% of patients. It is caused by the protozoan *Toxoplasma gondii*, which is mainly found in cats. Features of acute toxoplasmosis in immuno-compromised patients include a flu-like illness, lymphadenopathy and muscle aches. More severe infection can cause eye disease (poor vision and eye pain) and encephalitis. Toxoplasmosis can result in a brain abscess, which shows up on CT as a ring-enhancing lesion. Treatment is with pyrimethamine, often with short-term steroids to help reduce inflammation.

4. A – Candidiasis

This woman with HIV infection, sore mouth, dysphagia and odynophagia has a *Candida* infection affecting her oesophagus. Diagnosis can be confirmed by endoscopy demonstrating white plaques typical of candidiasis. The presence of oesophageal candidiasis in anyone is highly suggestive of immunodeficiency. Treatment is with antifungals, such as fluconazole and amphotericin.

5. K – Stevens–Johnson syndrome

The treatment of HIV infection is with antiretrovirals, which suppress viral replication. Examples of antiretrovirals include nucleoside reverse transcriptase inhibitors (e.g. zidovudine), non-nucleoside reverse transcriptase inhibitors (e.g. nevirapine) and protease inhibitors (e.g. ritonavir). Often, three or more drugs are given simultaneously. This is known as highly active antiretroviral therapy (HAART), and >95% adherence to therapy is required for optimal viral suppression. Side-effects of antiretroviral medications include lipoatrophy, pancreatitis, a fat pad on the dorsum of the neck (buffalo hump) and Stevens–Johnson syndrome (an allergic reaction, with lesions on the skin and mucous membranes).

Theme 2: Scoring systems in medicine

1. E – Glasgow Coma Scale

The Glasgow Coma Scale (GCS) is one of the most widely used scoring systems in medicine, and is used for the initial and continuous assessment of a patient's conscious level. It assesses three main criteria: best eye response, best verbal response and best motor response, and is scored out of 15 (with 3/15 being the lowest score attainable). A GCS of 3/15 implies deep unconsciousness, a score of 3–8/15 implies a significant impairment of consciousness, a score of 9–13/15 implies mild-to-moderate impairment and a score of 14–15/15 is generally regarded as normal. It should be noted that this scoring system has a number of limitations, and must be used in combination with a holistic assessment of the patient's clinical status. For example, patients who are blind, deaf, mute or physically disabled will always score lower than 15 due to an inability to interpret or perform the tasks.

For the full scale, see 'Glasgow Coma Scale' (Paper 4 Answers, Theme 5) .

2. A – Abbreviated Mental Test Score

The Abbreviated Mental Test Score (AMTS) is a quick and easily remembered way of initially and continuously assessing a patient's cognitive function. It involves asking the patient 10 questions that assess several different areas of cognition. It is especially useful in elderly patients suffering from delirium and dementia. A score of less than 7/10 indicates cognitive impairment.

For the full AMTS questionnaire, see 'Dementia 2' (Paper 4 Answers, Theme 10).

3. H – Rockall Score

This scoring system can be used to predict adverse outcome following upper gastrointestinal bleeds by combining a number of independent risk factors (see below). A score >8 indicates a 40% risk of mortality.

	0	*1*	*2*	*3*
Age	<60 years	60–79 years	>80 years	
Shock	BP > 100 mmHg, pulse <100 beats/min	BP > 100 mmHg, pulse >100 beats/min	BP < 100 mmHg	
Comorbidities	None	Ischaemic heart disease, cardiac failure	Renal/liver failure	Metastatic malignancy
Diagnosis	Mallory–Weiss tear	All other except malignancy	Upper gastrointestinal malignancy	
Endoscopy	None		Active bleeding, adherent clot, visible vessels	

Rockall TA, Logan RF, Devlin HB, Northfield TC. Risk assessment after acute upper gastrointestinal haemorrhage. *Gut* 1996; **38**: 316–21.

4. G – Ranson's Criteria

Acute pancreatitis is a condition associated with a high morbidity and mortality in all patients, including those who initially present with relatively mild disease. A number of scoring systems have been developed to identify cases requiring aggressive management. Ranson's Criteria use a combination of patient demographic information and investigation results to calculate a score at the time of presentation and 48 hours later. If the patient scores 7–8 after 48 hours, there is up to a 95–100% risk of mortality. A limitation of Ranson's Criteria is that they cannot be fully determined until 48 hours after presentation. The criteria were developed to allow a more rapid assessment of the patient's prognosis.

Ranson JH, Rifkind KM, Roses DF et al. Prognostic signs and the role of operative management in acute pancreatitis. *Surg Gynecol Obstet* 1974; **139**: 69–81.

5. I – Waterlow Score

The Waterlow Score is an important tool for assessing the risk of pressure sore development. Pressure sores are likely to develop in bedbound patients who have poor mobility, poor nutrition, incontinence and multiple comorbidities. They can cause significant pain and become infected, leading to sepsis and even death. The Waterlow Score is generally used by nurses during the admission of patients, and is especially important in stroke victims, patients with quadriplegia and comatose patients.

Waterlow J. Pressure sores: a risk assessment card. *Nurs Times* 1985; **81**(48): 49–55.

Ranson's Criteria	*Glasgow Criteria*
On admission:	*On admission:*
1 Age >55 years	1. Age >55 years
2 White cell count >16 × 10^9/L	2. $Pa{O_2}$ <8 kPa (60 mmHg)
3 AST >250 IU/L	3. White cell count >15 × 10^9/L
4 LDH >350 IU/L	4. Calcium <2.0 mmol/L
5 Serum glucose >10 mmol/L	5. Urea >16 mmol/L
	6. LDH >600 IU/L
	7. ALT >200 IU/L
	8. Serum albumin <32 mmol/L
At 48 hours:	9. Glucose >10 mmol/L
1. Haematocrit fall >10%	
2. Urea rise of 0.9 mmol/L	
3. Serum calcium <2.0 mmol/L	
4. $Pa{O_2}$ <8 kPa (60 mmHg)	
5. Base deficit >4 mmol/L	
6. Estimated fluid deficit/sequestration >6 L	

Theme 3: Fainting

1. I – Vasovagal attack

'Syncope' is a sudden loss of consciousness. Vasovagal syncope is caused by excessive activation of the parasympathetic nervous system often in response to stimuli such as heat, fear and stress. For details, see 'Causes of collapse' (Paper 1 Answers, Theme 1).

2. H – Stokes–Adams attack

In Stokes–Adams attacks, there is a sudden loss of consciousness with pallor and a death-like appearance. They are due to transient ventricular asystole, which can occur in complete heart block or Mobitz type II second-degree atrioventricular block. Convulsions can occur if there is prolonged asystole due to cerebral ischaemia, but, in contrast to epileptic seizures, recovery is rapid. When the heart starts re-beating, there is a characteristic facial flush. Management of Stokes–Adams attacks is by pacemaker insertion. If untreated, there is a 50% risk of mortality within a year.

William Stokes, Irish physician (1804–77).

Robert Adams, Irish surgeon (1791–1875).

3. J – Vertebrobasilar insufficiency

In vertebrobasilar insufficiency, there is a temporarily reduced flow in the posterior circulation of the brain. It typically affects those aged 60–70 and reflects underlying atherosclerosis. Transient ischaemia in vertebrobasilar insufficiency is precipitated by neck extension, and results in dizziness.

4. G – Postural hypotension

In this scenario, a postural drop in blood pressure after standing from a sitting position resulted in cerebral hypoperfusion and subsequent collapse. For a detailed description of postural hypotension, see 'Symptoms of cardiovascular disease' (Paper 10 Answers, Theme 6).

5. F – Micturition syncope

Micturition syncope describes the uncommon scenario of transient loss of consciousness during or shortly after urination, most commonly affecting middle-aged men. It is thought to be due to increased vagal input, both from the bladder during micturition and from standing up. Micturition syncope is a type of situational syncope. Syncope can also be induced by coughing, burping, defecating and swallowing cold liquids. *Carotid sinus sensitivity* describes hypersensitivity of carotid baroreceptors. It causes recurrent syncope by promoting inappropriate bradycardia and vasodilatation. Triggers of such symptoms include turning the head and wearing garments with tight-fitting collars.

Micturition, from Latin *micturare* = to desire to pass urine.

Urine, from Latin *urina* = sewage.

Theme 4: Management of respiratory disease 2

1. I – Low-molecular-weight heparin

This woman has a new pulmonary embolus. She requires anticoagulation therapy, which begins with low-molecular-weight heparin (LMWH). Warfarin should not be started straight away, as it is prothrombotic in the early stages of treatment. Therefore, heparin (or LMWH) is commenced first, and warfarin is subsequently started under heparin cover.

2. B – Cannula into second intercostal space, mid-clavicular line

This patient has a tension pneumothorax, which is treated immediately with a cannula in the second intercostal space, midclavicular line. A formal chest drain can be inserted after initial decompression.

3. D – Chemotherapy

Small cell lung tumours that cannot be resected are responsive to chemotherapy. Non-small cell lung tumours are given radiotherapy.

4. H – Inhaled β-agonist

This boy has a new diagnosis of asthma and should be started on step 1 of the asthma management ladder (see 'Management of asthma' – Paper 9 Answers, Theme 13). This involves taking an inhaled β-agonist as required, e.g. salbutamol.

5. K – No management required

Pleural plaques are asymptomatic calcified pleural thickenings resembling holly leaves. They are seen on chest X-ray and are associated with previous asbestos exposure. The plaques themselves are asymptomatic and require no treatment.

Theme 5: Non-infective diarrhoea

1. G – Thyrotoxicosis

This patient gives a history that is consistent with hyperthyroidism. Thyrotoxicosis can have significant systemic effects, including weight loss, hair loss, hyperthermia, diarrhoea, oligomenorrhoea, tachycardia and arrhythmia. It is important to test thyroid function when a patient presents with diarrhoea in association with systemic symptoms. In contrast, hypothyroidism usually presents with a history of weight gain, depression, dry skin, lethargy, bradycardia, amenorrhoea and constipation.

2. H – Ulcerative colitis

Ulcerative colitis (UC) is an inflammatory bowel disease in which the colonic mucosa and submucosa become inflamed and ulcerated. During exacerbations, patients suffer from profuse bloody diarrhoea, fever, lethargy, dehydration and hypovolaemic shock. UC may be associated with a number of extraintestinal conditions, including venous thromboembolic disease, pyoderma gangrenosum, erythema nodosum, ankylosing spondylitis, arthritis and episcleritis. The diagnosis of UC is based on the history, the presence of raised inflammatory markers, the exclusion of an infective cause and sigmoidoscopy/colonoscopy findings. During the acute phase, it is also important to take an abdominal X-ray to exclude potentially toxic dilatation (>6 cm) of the colon. Management of UC involves replacing fluid and electrolyte losses and prescribing systemic and local corticosteroids. In acute disease, the 5-ASA (5-aminosalicylic acid) class of drugs (e.g. mesalazine) can increase the speed of remission. Chronic disease usually requires long-term corticosteroid therapy in combination with a 5-ASA and a steroid-sparing agent such as azathioprine. Newer biological treatments such as infliximab are now becoming available. Patients with toxic megacolon, severe disease and frequently relapsing disease should be considered for surgery.

3. C – Laxative abuse

Laxative abuse is often seen in association with eating disorders, and is a relatively common cause of chronic diarrhoea. It may also lead to the development of electrolyte imbalance, protein-losing enteropathy and intestinal paralysis. The abrasions on this patient's knuckles are likely to indicate repeated trauma on the incisors acquired during the induction of vomiting with her fingers. Downy hair (lanugo hair) is a feature of severe disease – it develops to insulate the malnourished patient against heat loss. Other features suggestive of an eating disorder include low mood, weight loss, hair loss, dry skin, pallor, ankle oedema, amenorrhea and signs of iron-deficiency anaemia (e.g. koilonychia, palmar crease pallor, angular stomatitis and tachycardia).

4. B – Irritable bowel syndrome

Irritable bowel syndrome is a functional disease that usually presents with abdominal bloating, abdominal cramps, and alternating constipation and diarrhoea. When considering the diagnosis of irritable bowel syndrome, it is important to exclude organic bowel disease such as coeliac disease and colorectal cancer. If the patient is over 50 years of age and displays any 'red flag' symptoms such as weight loss or rectal bleeding, they should be referred for further investigation. Otherwise, it would be prudent to assess the patient's full blood count, urea and electrolytes, thyroid function, anti-endomyseal antibodies, and do a stool culture to rule out electrolyte imbalance, thyroid disease, coeliac disease and infective causes. If investigation reveals no cause, the patient should be advised to eat a healthy diet with a high fibre content. Antispasmodic medications such as mebeverine hydrochloride or peppermint capsules may provide symptomatic relief. In diarrhoea-prominent disease, loperamide may be used to reduce the frequency of bowel motions (provided that an infective cause has been excluded). In constipation-predominant disease, stool-bulking agents such as methylcellulose may improve symptoms. If no improvement is made with treatment, the patient should be reassessed for an organic cause.

5. E – Overflow diarrhoea

Patients with severe constipation and faecal impaction may suffer from overflow diarrhoea when colonic fluid leaks around the impacted faeces and exits via the anus. Overflow diarrhoea often leads to faecal incontinence, which is embarrassing and negatively affects the patient's quality of life. Affected patients should receive lifestyle advice, including the need to eat a balanced diet, consume plenty of clear fluids and mobilize regularly. Initial medical treatment is with the use of simple laxatives such as senna, sodium docusate and lactulose. If these measures fail, the patient may require suppositories or enemas. In severe and refractory disease, manual faecal evacuation may be indicated.

Theme 6: Signs in endocrinological disease

1. C – Irregularly irregular pulse

It is possible that this woman's palpitations represent atrial fibrillation, which is a known complication of thyrotoxicosis. On examination, patients with atrial fibrillation usually have an irregularly irregular pulse. An ECG would be required to confirm the diagnosis. The risk of developing cardiac complications associated with thyrotoxicosis, such as atrial fibrillation, angina and cardiac failure, increases with age.

2. H – Striae

This woman gives a history of iatrogenic Cushing's syndrome secondary to steroid therapy. The skin changes on her abdomen are likely to be striae, which often have a purple discoloration. Other signs in Cushing's syndrome include central obesity, buffalo hump (accumulation of fat at the back of the neck), thin skin that bruises easily and proximal myopathy.

Striae, from Latin *stria* = scratch or furrow.

3. B – Hyperpigmentation

In Addison's disease, the adrenal cortices are damaged by an autoimmune process. The cortical destruction impairs the synthesis and secretion of mineralocorticoids and glucocorticoids (aldosterone and cortisol). The low circulating levels of cortisol are insufficient to provide negative feedback to the anterior pituitary gland and inhibit the secretion of adrenocorticotropic hormone (ACTH, corticotropin). Thus, patients with Addison's disease synthesize and secrete higher than normal levels of ACTH in a process that produces melanocyte-stimulating hormone (MSH) as a by-product. The excessive production of MSH secondary to ACTH production is responsible for the hyperpigmentation that is characteristic of Addison's disease and other causes of primary adrenal failure. The most common areas to be affected by hyperpigmentation are the palmar creases, buccal mucosa, elbows, knees and old scars. In cases of adrenal failure caused by hypothalamic or pituitary disease, the reduced synthesis/secretion of ACTH means that hyperpigmentation is not a feature.

4. E – Ophthalmoplegia

This patient has thyroid eye disease secondary to Graves' disease. Thyroid eye disease can be bilateral or unilateral, and can present before or after the underlying thyroid disease becomes apparent. Thyroid eye disease is caused by inflammation and lymphocytic infiltration of retro-orbital structures, which pushes the eye forward, causing proptosis, corneal ulceration, conjunctival oedema and optic nerve atrophy. In addition, fibrotic changes in the ocular muscles can cause tethering and eventual ophthalmoplegia, which has happed in this case, as indicated by the presence of reduced eye movements and diplopia. The underlying thyroid disease should be treated, and patients should be advised to stop smoking as this can exacerbate eye disease. Steroids and surgery are occasionally indicated for severe and sight-threatening disease.

5. A – Acanthosis nigricans

Acanthosis nigricans is a dermatological condition associated with insulin resistance, diabetes, Cushing's syndrome, acromegaly and gastrointestinal malignancy. It is a black, velvety papillomatous lesion that is typically seen on the neck, and in the axillary, inguinal and inframammary folds.

Theme 7: Features of rheumatoid arthritis

Rheumatoid arthritis (RA) is the most common inflammatory arthritis, involving the small joints symmetrically. It is three times more common in females and tends to affect the over-40s. There is an increased risk and severity of disease in people expressing HLA-DR4. In RA, there is inflammation of the synovium in the joint, which grows over the adjacent cartilage, forming a pannus. The pannus destroys the articular cartilage and subchondral bone, producing erosions. The typical features are pain, boggy swelling and stiffness in the small hand joints that tends to be worse in the morning.

The diagnosis of RA is made using the American Rheumatism Association criteria, requiring four of the following seven:

1. Morning stiffness for more than 1 hour for more than 6 weeks
2. Arthritis of hand joints (wrist, metacarpophalangeal [MCP] and proximal interphalangeal [PIP]) for more than 6 weeks
3. Arthritis of three or more joint areas for more than 6 weeks
4. Symmetrical arthritis for more than 6 weeks
5. Rheumatoid nodules
6. Characteristic X-ray findings
7. Positive rheumatoid factor.

The four characteristic X-ray findings of RA are soft tissue swelling, narrowed joint space, juxta-articular erosions and subluxation.

Rheumatoid factor is an antibody to the Fc (constant) portion of human immunoglobulin G. Rheumatoid factor is positive in 4% of the normal population, 25% of the elderly population and 70% of those with RA. Everyone who has RA in association with extra-articular features is rheumatoid factor positive.

1. J – Swan-neck deformity

Swan-neck deformities of the fingers are characterized by flexion of the MCP joint, hyperextension of the PIP joint and flexion of the distal interphalangeal (DIP) joint.

2. G – Rheumatoid nodules

Rheumatoid nodules are the most characteristic extra-articular feature of RA, occurring in 30% of cases, and are associated with severe disease. Nodules are made up of a central area of fibrinoid necrosis surrounded by a fibrous capsule. Nodules can occur at any site, but are commonly seen subcutaneously at extensor surfaces and pressure points (e.g. elbows). They can also be found on the fingers and Achilles' tendon externally, and the lung, pleura and pericardium internally. Methotrexate therapy can make rheumatoid nodules worse.

3. B – Boutonnière deformity

The boutonnière deformity is another finger deformity, characterized by fixed flexion of the PIP joint with hyperextension at the DIP joint. This deformity is caused by a central tear in the extensor tendon. The tear in the tendon looks like a buttonhole – hence the name.

Boutonnière, French for 'buttonhole'.

4. K – Z-deformity

The Z-deformity occurs in the thumbs and is characterized by fixed flexion of the MCP joint and hyperextension of the interphalangeal joint.

Other hand deformities seen in RA include spindling of the fingers (MCP and PIP synovitis with DIP sparing). There is ulnar deviation of the MCPs and radial deviation at the wrist. Subluxation at the MCP joints can occur, resulting in prominence of the ulnar styloid ('piano key deformity'). In the foot, the PIP joints can sublux dorsally and the metatarsal heads displace towards the floor. This makes weightbearing uncomfortable – described as 'walking on marbles'. Tenosynovitis of the flexor tendons can result in trigger finger or extensor tendon rupture.

5. A – Atlantoaxial subluxation

In RA, the transverse ligaments between the C1 and C2 vertebrae of the cervical spine can become lax, resulting in atlantoaxial subluxation. This can be seen on X-ray as a gap between the atlas and the odontoid peg greater than 3.5 mm. Atlantoaxial subluxation results in instability of the upper cervical spine, and a sudden impact can cause the odontoid peg (part of the C2 vertebra) to smash into the brain-stem. For this reason, a C-spine X-ray should be taken before general anaesthesia in patients with known RA, so that the anaesthetist can assess and make note of the possible risk during intubation.

Theme 8: Management of acute coronary syndromes

Coronary heart disease is the most common cause of morbidity and mortality in the developed world. It occurs through a process of atherosclerosis. Risk factors for atheromatous disease are stratified as modifiable (e.g. smoking, hypertension, hypercholesterolaemia, diabetes and obesity) or fixed (male sex, family history and increasing age). Coronary heart disease can manifest as stable angina, unstable angina or myocardial infarction. The term 'acute coronary syndrome' (ACS) covers both unstable angina and myocardial infarction.

1. Q – ST elevation of 2 mm in leads II, III and aVF

This man presents with classic features of an ACS. Acute myocardial infarction (MI) should be classified as ST-elevation MI (STEMI) or non-ST-elevation MI (NSTEMI).

STEMI corresponds to a full-thickness MI and NSTEMI to a partial-thickness MI. The ECG changes seen in STEMI are ST-segment elevation, T-wave inversion, pathological Q-wave formation (>2 mm deep and >1 mm wide) and new-onset left bundle-branch block (LBBB). ST elevation in leads II, III and aVF indicates an inferior STEMI, since these leads view the inferior aspect of the myocardium. Similarly, the anterior–septal myocardium is represented by leads V2–V5 and the lateral myocardium by leads V5, V6, I and aVL. Posterior myocardial ischaemia is represented by reciprocal (opposite) changes in V1 and V2. These include a dominant R-wave, ST depression and an upright T-wave.

In cases where the clinical history and serum cardiac enzyme levels suggest MI in the absence of ST elevation, a diagnosis of *NSTEMI* can be made. ECG changes seen in NSTEMI include T-wave flattening/inversion and ST depression. Tented T-waves are seen in hyperkalaemia.

2. M – Percutaneous coronary angioplasty ± stenting

Also known as percutaneous cardiac intervention (PCI), coronary angioplasty with or without coronary artery stenting is widely viewed as the gold standard in reperfusion therapy following STEMI. A number of studies have shown that PCI reduces mortality and significant adverse events following STEMI when compared with thrombolysis. PCI may also be used as a 'rescue' treatment when thrombolysis has failed to reperfuse the myocardium. Complications of PCI include arrhythmia, leg ischaemia, femoral aneurysm formation, allergy to the contrast and sudden death. Significant complications may result in the need for emergency coronary artery bypass grafting. Presently, PCI is available only in a select number of institutions.

3. J – Past medical history of a haemorrhagic stroke 6 weeks ago

Prior to administrating a thrombolytic agent for the first time, the clinician must be familiar with the indications and contraindications of thrombolysis. In the presence of cardiac-sounding chest pain, indications for thrombolysis are:

- ST elevation >2 mm in adjacent chest leads (V1–V6) *or*
- ST elevation >1 mm in adjacent limb leads (I, II, III, aVL, aVR, aVF) *or*
- new-onset LBBB
- true posterior infarct (dominant R-waves, tall T-waves and ST depression in V1 and V2).

Contraindications to thrombolysis can be divided into absolute and relative. Absolute contraindications vary between institutions, but usually include active bleeding from any site, a history of haemorrhagic stroke, ischaemic stroke in the previous 3 months, clotting disturbance and possible dissecting aortic aneurysm. Relative contraindications include a past history of peptic ulcer disease, cerebral neoplasm, liver disease, recent head injury and a systolic blood pressure over 200 mmHg. Thrombolysis should be administered within 20 minutes of presentation and ideally within the first 12 hours of symptoms. Some clinicians make an exception to this rule when the patient is experiencing ongoing chest pain and ST elevation between 12 and 24 hours after the onset of symptoms. Examples of thrombolytic agents include streptokinase and alteplase, and the major risk of such agents is bleeding.

4. E – Cyclizine

Patients experiencing acute MI often feel nauseous secondary to heightened autonomic stimulation and opiate analgesia. Cyclizine is an antihistamine antiemetic drug that has been shown to precipitate tachycardia and increase ventricular filling pressures. This may lead to an increase in myocardial oxygen demand and place additional strain upon the heart. Because of the potential adverse outcomes of using cyclizine in cardiac disease, evidence suggests that it is prudent to prescribe an alternative antiemetic for affected patients.

5. B – β-Blockers

β-Blockers have been shown to reduce infarct size and mortality when given within the first 12 hours following acute MI. They slow the heart rate and reduce myocardial contractibility, thus improving myocardial oxygenation. β-Blockers should not be given to patients with heart rates below 60 beats/min or when the systolic blood pressure is below 100 mmHg. Caution should also be given when considering the use of β-blockers in people with asthma, as they may trigger bronchospasm in sensitive individuals. Angiotensin-converting enzyme inhibitors, regular antiplatelet therapy (aspirin or clopidogrel) and lipid-lowering drugs should be started in the days following infarction, provided that no contraindications exist.

Theme 9: Pupillary disorders

1. C – Holmes–Adie pupil

A Holmes–Adie pupil is a dilated pupil that has impaired accommodation (constriction when the patient focuses on a near object) and reacts slowly (or not at all) to light. Once the pupil constricts, it remains constricted for a long time (tonic pupil). The condition may be unilateral, and is caused by damage to the parasympathetic innervation of the eye. A Holmes–Adie pupil may be associated with absence of the deep tendon reflexes. It occurs most frequently in women, and affected patients can be reassured of its benign nature. The presence of pupils of unequal size is called anisocoria.

William John Adie, British neurologist (1886–1935).

Gordon Morgan Holmes, Irish neurologist (1876–1965).

2. G – Opiate intoxication

Pinpoint pupils are a characteristic feature of opiate use. Other effects of opiates (in addition to analgesia) include euphoria, nausea and vomiting, constipation, anorexia, hypotension, respiratory depression, tremor and erectile dysfunction. Examples of opiates include morphine, heroin, methadone and codeine. For the treatment of opiate overdose, see Case 1 in 'Substance use' (Theme 14 below). The treatment of overdose (after ABC) is with the antidote naloxone. This is ideally given intravenously (but can be given intramuscularly or by inhalation). An infusion of naloxone may be necessary, as its half-life is short. The effects of opiate withdrawal can be very extreme, and include dilated pupils, lacrimation, sweating, diarrhoea, insomnia, tachycardia, abdominal cramp-like pains, nausea and vomiting. Opiate dependence can be managed (once drug use has stopped) by methadone and buprenorphine (a partial agonist).

3. D – Horner's syndrome

Horner's syndrome is caused by an interruption of the sympathetic innervation to the eye. It is characterized by four features: a partial ptosis with ipsilateral anhidrosis (loss of sweating), enophthalmos (the impression that the eye is sunk in) and miosis (constricted pupil). Congenital Horner's syndrome may be associated with heterochromia of the iris – a difference in colour between the two eyes. Causes of non-congenital Horner's syndrome include Pancoast's tumour (a tumour at the lung apex – as in this case), brachial plexus palsies, cervical rib, cluster headache and trauma to the base of the neck.

Johann Friedrich Horner, Swiss ophthalmologist (1831–86).

4. E – Marcus Gunn pupil

A Marcus Gunn pupil is one that reacts poorly to light in comparison with the contralateral pupil. This is elicited on examination using the 'swinging flashlight test': when a pen torch is held towards the good eye, both pupils constrict (as they should), but when it is then held against the affected eye, both pupils appear to dilate. This is because the affected pupil does not perceive the light as well, and so *constricts less* compared with when the light is shone into the normal pupil – hence it appears to dilate. The Marcus Gunn pupil is characteristic of optic nerve lesions (e.g. optic neuritis or compression of the nerve by an aneurysm or tumour).

Robert Marcus Gunn, Scottish ophthalmologist (1850–1909).

5. A – Argyll Robertson pupil

Argyll Robertson pupils are bilateral small pupils that accommodate but do not react to light. They are a feature of neurosyphilis, but can also occur with diabetes mellitus.

Douglas Argyll Robertson, Scottish ophthalmologist (1837–1909).

Theme 10: Gastrointestinal investigations

1. K – Urgent endoscopy

An urgent endoscopy (within 2 weeks) is indicated in a patient of any age presenting with dyspepsia associated with unintentional weight loss, upper gastrointestinal bleeding, dysphagia, persistent vomiting, iron-deficiency anaemia, epigastric mass or a suspicious barium swallow. These findings are usually regarded as 'red flags' due to their association with malignancy, and must be investigated early and appropriately.

2. I – *Helicobacter pylori* stool antigen test

This patient has dyspepsia without any of the 'red flag' features described above. Therefore, she does not require urgent endoscopy. Current guidance advises that such patients be assessed for reversible causes of dyspepsia such as non-steroidal anti-inflammatory drug use, steroid therapy, excess alcohol intake, smoking and poor diet. If a correctable cause exists, appropriate lifestyle advice should be given and any causative drugs stopped. If the symptoms persist despite lifestyle adaptations, the patient should be tested for *Helicobacter pylori* infection. *H. pylori* is a urease-producing, S-shaped, Gram-negative bacterium that is associated with gastritis, peptic ulceration and gastric malignancy. The *H. pylori* stool antigen test and urea breath test are usually the first-line investigations, as they are non-invasive and have high sensitivities and specificities. The CLO test requires a gastric biopsy obtained at endoscopy and is therefore invasive and unpleasant for the patient. If *H. pylori* is detected, the patient should have eradication therapy, which usually involves a 7-day course of two antibiotics and a proton pump inhibitor (e.g. metronidazole, clarithromycin and omeprazole). If the test is negative, the patient should be prescribed a proton pump inhibitor and reassessed after 1 month.

3. C – Barium swallow and follow-through

Crohn's disease is characterized by granulomatous inflammation of the gastrointestinal tract. It can occur anywhere in the gastrointestinal tract from mouth to anus and is most commonly seen in the terminal ileum and proximal colon. Histological characteristics of Crohn's disease include full-thickness inflammation, non-caseating granulomas and skip lesions. The clinical features of Crohn's disease include abdominal pain, abdominal bloating, nausea, vomiting, fever, diarrhoea, lethargy, weight loss, aphthous mouth ulceration, a right iliac fossa mass and pyoderma gangrenosum. The most appropriate imaging technique for the small bowel is a barium swallow and follow-through. This non-invasive test involves the patient swallowing a radio-opaque substance (barium sulphate) and having X-ray images taken of the small bowel after a suitable time interval. The radiological features of small-bowel Crohn's disease include strictures, skip lesions, ulceration and 'cobblestoning' (caused by mucosal ulceration and oedema). Other investigations used in the assessment of Crohn's disease include capsule endoscopy, barium enema, colonoscopy, and the measurement of markers of disease activity such as C-reactive protein, erythrocyte sedimentation rate and white blood cell count.

Comparison between Crohn's disease and ulcerative colitis

	Crohn's disease	*Ulcerative colitis*
Common distribution	Mouth to anus	Distal colon and rectum
Perianal involvement	Yes	No
Inflammation	Transluminal (all three layers)	Mucosa and submucosa
Granulomas	Yes	No
Skip lesions	Yes	No
Smoking	Increases risk	Lowers risk
Risk of malignancy	Low	Higher than in Crohn's disease

4. G – Gastrografin swallow

Oesophageal rupture is a relatively rare but life-threatening condition. Rupture is usually iatrogenic and occurs during instrumentation of the oesophagus (endoscopy). Rarely, it can occur following severe and prolonged bouts of vomiting (Boerhaave's syndrome). The initial investigation of choice in suspected oesophageal rupture is a chest X-ray, which may show pneumomediastinum, plural effusion and subcutaneous emphysema. The next investigation is an oesophageal contrast study to show the size and anatomical location of any perforation. The most commonly used contrast agent in investigating the gastrointestinal tract is barium sulphate. However, barium is contraindicated as a contrast agent in patients with potential perforation, since its leakage outside the tract can result in a severe fibrotic reaction. Gastrografin (diatrizoate meglumine/diatrizoate sodium solution) is an iodine-based water-soluble contrast medium that is used as an alternative when barium is contraindicated. Patients with proven oesophageal rupture often require surgery, as medical management is associated with a poor prognosis.

5. B – Anti-endomyseal antibodies

Coeliac disease causes a gluten-related enteropathy of the small bowel. When the patient consumes gluten-containing foods, a T-cell-mediated autoimmune reaction results in subtotal villous atrophy and crypt hyperplasia of the small-bowel mucosa. The result is malabsorption, leading to malnutrition, anaemia, steatorrhoea, abdominal pain, bloating and fatigue. The initial investigation for coeliac disease is the measurement of serum anti-endomyseal or anti-transglutaminase immunoglobulin A antibodies, which have been shown to have sensitivities and specificities of over 95%. Antibodies to α-gladin and reticulin can also be measured, although they have lower sensitivities and specificities. The gold-standard diagnostic technique is duodenal or jejunal biopsy taken during endoscopy. Since this is an invasive and unpleasant procedure, it is usually performed as a second-line investigation in patients with positive serology. If the biopsy suggests coeliac disease, the patient should be placed on a gluten-free diet and re-biopsied at a later date to assess small-bowel recovery.

Theme 11: Autoantibodies 1

1. G – Anti-gliadin

2. I – Anti-thyroid peroxidase

3. B – Anti-adrenal

4. C – Anti-glomerular basement membrane

5. E – Anti-mitochondrial

The main autoantibodies associated with disease are as follows:

- anti-acetylcholinesterase receptor: myasthenia gravis
- anti-adrenal antibody: Addison's disease
- anti-gliadin and anti-endomyseal: coeliac disease
- anti-glomerular basement membrane: Goodpasture's syndrome
- anti-Hu/anti-Yo/anti-Ri: subacute cerebellar degeneration
- anti-intrinsic factor/anti-parietal: pernicious anaemia
- anti-LKM (liver–kidney–microsomal): autoimmune hepatitis
- anti-mitochondrial: primary biliary cirrhosis
- anti-smooth muscle: autoimmune hepatitis
- anti-thyroid peroxidase: Hashimoto's thyroiditis
- antibody to voltage-gated calcium channels: Lambert–Eaton syndrome
- thyroid-stimulating antibody: Graves' disease.

For the autoantibodies of rheumatological disease specifically, see 'Autoantibodies 2' (Paper 10 Answers, Theme 13).

Subacute cerebellar degeneration is a paraneoplastic syndrome characterized by cerebellar dysfunction (severe ataxia, nystagmus and dysarthria). It is most commonly seen in patients with small cell lung tumours, breast tumours and Hodgkin's lymphoma.

Theme 12: Investigation of neurological disorders

1. B – CT of the head

This woman presents with meningitis. After initial treatment (ABC and antibiotics), a lumbar puncture is required to confirm the diagnosis and help look for the offending cause. Before a lumbar puncture is performed, a CT head scan should be done to rule out raised intracranial pressure. This is because, if lumbar puncture is performed in someone with raised intracranial pressure, the brain-stem can herniate through the foramen magnum ('coning').

2. G – MRI of the head

This woman has had two deficits in anatomically distinct sites consistent with a diagnosis of multiple sclerosis. The best investigation to identify demyelination would be MRI. A lumbar puncture may demonstrate oligoclonal bands of immunoglobulin G, but these are not specific for multiple sclerosis.

3. B – CT of the head

Sudden-onset weakness in a man of this age is suggestive of a stroke (either ischaemic or haemorrhagic). In anyone presenting with suspected stroke, a CT head scan is performed to rule out haemorrhage. If no haemorrhage is seen on the CT scan then aspirin can be administered.

4. L – Tensilon test

This woman has fatigability, the cardinal sign of myasthenia gravis. The diagnosis is confirmed using the Tensilon test, where administration of intravenous edrophonium bromide (a short-acting anticholinesterase) results in transient improvement of symptoms.

5. E – Lumbar puncture

'First-ever, worst-ever' headache is suggestive of subarachnoid haemorrhage (SAH). A CT head scan is negative in up to 15% of cases of SAH. For this reason, anyone with suspected SAH who has a negative CT scan should undergo lumbar puncture after 12 hours to look for xanthochromia (yellow cerebrospinal fluid due to the presence of erythrocyte breakdown products).

Theme 13: Valvular heart disease

1. I – Prosthetic heart valve

The sternotomy scar points to a possible previous valve replacement operation. (The gynaecomastia is a red herring.) There are two main types of replacement heart valve: mechanical and tissue.

Mechanical valves are made from artificial material, whereas tissue valves are made from material retrieved from biological sources, including porcine and human donors. Mechanical valves last longer than tissue valves. However, they are known to cause intravascular haemolysis, which characteristically produces a normocytic anaemia. Coombs' test is negative, as this is not an autoimmune haemolytic anaemia. In addition, mechanical heart valves are thrombogenic and therefore require the recipient to have lifelong anticoagulation therapy (e.g. warfarin, aiming for an international normalized ratio of 3–4).

Tissue valves are not thrombogenic, and therefore patients do not need anticoagulation. They do, however, have a shorter life compared with mechanical valves.

All replacement valves are at risk of bacterial colonization and subsequent bacterial endocarditis. Therefore, patients with replacement valves should receive antibiotic prophylaxis prior to invasive procedures such as catheterization.

2. D – Bicuspid aortic valve

The normal aortic valve has three cusps. In approximately 1–2% of the population, the valve has only two cusps (bicuspid). Bicuspid aortic valves are at increased risk of calcification and subsequent stenosis and/or regurgitation. In addition, due to histological abnormalities of the ascending aorta, people with bicuspid aortic valves are at an increased risk of aortic dissection.

3. G – Mitral regurgitation

Heavy alcohol consumption is linked to dilated cardiomyopathy, in which there is dilatation and impaired contraction of the left ventricle. Apart from alcohol, causes of dilated cardiomyopathy include muscular dystrophy, and the condition can also be inherited in an autosomal dominant manner. Patients present with features of heart failure, arrhythmias and sudden death. The dilated left ventricle prevents the mitral valve cusps from opposing correctly, and thus they cannot produce a seal. This allows regurgitation of blood into the left atrium during ventricular systole.

Other causes of mitral regurgitation include rheumatic fever, myocardial infarction and mitral prolapse. Examination reveals a pansystolic murmur that is heard best at the apex and radiates into the axilla. The apex beat is hyperdynamic (thrusting) and displaced, and an ECG and chest X-ray may demonstrate left ventricular hypertrophy.

Systole, from Greek *systole* = contraction.

4. H – Mitral stenosis

Mitral stenosis is nearly always associated with rheumatic fever. On auscultation, there is a low-pitched (rumbling) mid-diastolic murmur, best heard at the apex with the patient lying on their left-hand side. Other features of mitral stenosis include malar flush (mitral facies), dyspnoea, haemoptysis and right heart failure secondary to increased pressures in the pulmonary vasculature. The classic ECG finding in mitral stenosis is P-mitrale, also referred to as bifid (notched) P-waves. P-mitrale is caused by hypertrophy and dilatation of the left atrium secondary to raised intra-atrial pressure. One of the most common complications of mitral stenosis is atrial fibrillation. Since the ECG tracing of atrial fibrillation shows an irregularly irregular rhythm with no P-waves, it is impossible to have P-mitrale and atrial fibrillation simultaneously

5. L – Tricuspid regurgitation

Pulmonary hypertension can be primary or secondary to cardiac or systemic disease. Increased pressures in the pulmonary vasculature result in a back-pressure that feeds back to the right ventricle. This causes the right ventricle to hypertrophy and dilate, which prevents the tricuspid valve cusps from opposing. Thus, blood is able to regurgitate from the right ventricle into the right atrium during systole. On auscultation, there is a pansystolic murmur that is best heard at the left sternal border in the fifth intercostal space. In severe disease, patients have a raised jugular venous pressure with a prominent v-wave, peripheral oedema and tender, pulsatile hepatomegaly.

Theme 14: Substance use

1. I – Opiate use

This woman is likely to be suffering the effects of opiate use. The effects of opiates (in addition to analgesia) include euphoria, nausea and vomiting, constipation, anorexia, hypotension, respiratory depression, tremor, pinpoint pupils and erectile dysfunction. Examples of opiates include morphine, heroin, methadone and codeine. The treatment of overdose (after ABC) is with the antidote naloxone. This is ideally given intravenously (but can be given intramuscularly or by inhalation). An infusion of naloxone may be necessary, as its half-life is short. The effects of opiate withdrawal can be very extreme, and include dilated pupils, lacrimation, sweating, diarrhoea, insomnia, tachycardia, abdominal cramp-like pains, nausea and vomiting. Opiate dependence can be managed (once drug use has stopped) by methadone and buprenorphine (a partial agonist).

2. E – Cannabis use

Cannabis (Δ^9-tetrahydrocannabinol) has the following effects: dry cough, increased appetite, conjunctival injection and fatigue. Psychological effects include euphoria, relaxation, an altered perception of time, social withdrawal and paranoia.

3. G – Cocaine use

Cocaine intoxication may present with tachycardia, mydriasis, hypertension, nausea and vomiting, euphoria, increased interest in sex and formication (a tactile hallucination described as insects crawling over the skin). Cocaine withdrawal results in a dysphoric mood, cravings, irritability and paranoia. Cocaine use is a risk factor for cardiovascular disease.

4. L – Sedative withdrawal

This woman may be on long-term sedatives (benzodiazepines or barbiturates) that stopped being prescribed when she moved location. Symptoms of sedative withdrawal include nausea and vomiting, autonomic hyperactivity, insomnia, delirium and seizures. Features of sedative use include loss of coordination, slurred speech, decreased attention and memory, disinhibition, aggression, miosis, hypotension and respiratory depression.

Amphetamines are available illegally, but are also prescribed for narcolepsy and hyperkinetic syndromes (e.g. attention deficit hyperactivity disorder) and as appetite suppressants. Features of intoxication include euphoria, insomnia, agitation, hallucinations, hypertension and tachycardia. Symptoms of the withdrawal state include dysphoric mood, fatigue and agitation.

5. B – Alcohol withdrawal

Alcohol withdrawal usually occurs if the blood alcohol concentration falls in someone with alcohol dependence. Symptoms usually start approximately 12 hours after the last intake, and include anxiety, insomnia, sweating, tachycardia and tremor. Seizures may occur after 48 hours. Treatment is supportive with a reducing dose of regular benzodiazepines (e.g. chlordiazepoxide) and vitamin B supplements (intravenous or oral). The mortality rate is approximately 5%.

Delirium tremens may also be a feature of alcohol withdrawal, and occurs after 48 hours, lasting for 5 days. There is tremor, restlessness and increased autonomic activity, fluctuating consciousness with disorientation, a fearful affect and hallucinations. Hallucinations may be auditory, tactile or visual, and delusions may also be present. Lilliputian hallucinations (seeing little people) are characteristic. (Named after the island of Lilliput in Jonathan Swift's novel *Gulliver's Travels*, where the inhabitants were 'not six inches high'.)

Alcohol intoxication presents with mood changes, loss of inhibition, cerebellar signs (dysdiadochokinesis, ataxia, nystagmus, intention tremor, slurred speech, hypotonicity and hyperreflexia) and decreased conscious level.

Alcohol consumption is measured in units; 1 unit = 10 g alcohol (ethanol). Safe levels are 28 units/week for men and 21 units/week for women, with not more than 4 and 3 units/day, respectively. Alcohol-free days are recommended. Excessive drinking can lead to *alcohol dependence syndrome*, which is characterized by the following features:

- increased tolerance (the drug produces less effect per gram ingested)
- repeated withdrawal symptoms
- subjective awareness of compulsion to drink, and cravings if resistance is attempted
- prioritization of alcohol over other aspects of life (e.g. career and family)
- avoidance of withdrawal by continued drinking,
- narrowing of the drinking repertoire (habits develop, including the preference of one particular drink, often as part of a daily routine)
- rapid reinstatement of alcohol if a period of abstinence is successfully achieved.

The *CAGE questionnaire* is a screening tool for alcohol dependence. There are four questions:

- Have you ever felt that you should **C**ut down?
- Have you ever been **A**nnoyed by criticism of your drinking?
- Have you ever felt **G**uilty about your drinking?
- Have you ever had an **E**ye-opener (morning drink)?

Examples of physical morbidity from alcohol use are vomiting, peptic ulcer disease, Mallory–Weiss tears, oesophageal varices, hepatic cirrhosis and liver failure, pancreatitis, repeated trauma, endocrine disturbances and aspiration pneumonias. *Fetal alcohol syndrome* is seen in children whose mothers had drunk excessive amounts of alcohol during pregnancy. Features include microcephaly, small nose, low IQ (mean 70), strabismus and a long philtrum.

Theme 15: Renal manifestations of systemic disease

1. E – Lupus nephritis

Systemic lupus erythematosus (SLE) is a multisystem autoimmune disease characterized by the production of antinuclear antibodies. Up to 50% of patients with SLE have renal involvement. Proteinuria, hypertension, haematuria and peripheral oedema may all be seen. The renal damage is thought to arise from the deposition of immune complexes within the glomeruli that trigger an immunological response, damaging the basement membrane. A renal biopsy is usually required for the diagnosis and staging of the disease. The pattern of glomerulonephritis is mesangial, focal proliferative, diffuse proliferative or membranous. Lupus nephritis is treated by systemic immunosuppression using agents such as prednisolone, ciclosporin and mycophenolate. Some patients require renal replacement therapy and eventual renal transplantation.

2. C – Diabetic microalbuminuria

Microalbuminuria is defined by the presence of 20–300 mg/L of albumin in the urine on two separate occasions or a urine albumin:creatinine ratio >2.5 mg/mmol in males and >3.5 in females. It should be noted that these concentrations of albumin are too low to be identified on urine dipstick and require a specific analysis. Microalbuminuria is an important predictor of renal and cardiovascular disease in diabetes. If it is identified and treated appropriately, the natural progression to persistent albuminuria, diabetic nephropathy and renal failure can be prevented. Treatment involves strict glycaemic and blood pressure control, with the use of angiotensin-converting enzyme inhibitors or angiotensin II receptor antagonists in all patients, including those who are normotensive.

3. A – AA amyloidosis

In amyloidosis, there is deposition of extracellular fibrillar proteins in tissues and organs. The two main types of amyloidosis are AL and AA. *AL amyloidosis*, also incorrectly referred to as primary amyloidosis, is due to the clonal proliferation of plasma cells and particularly affects the cardiovascular system. *AA amyloidosis*, also known as reactive systemic amyloidosis, is due to the production and deposition of amyloid in chronic inflammatory conditions such as Crohn's disease, rheumatoid arthritis and tuberculosis. In AA amyloidosis, amyloid A protein is deposited in the kidneys, liver and spleen, causing renal failure and hepatosplenomegaly. Cardiovascular involvement is rare. The renal complications of amyloidosis include proteinuria, nephrotic syndrome and end-stage renal failure. Amyloidosis is traditionally diagnosed based on a biopsy of the affected tissue. The fibrillar protein shows green birefringence when stained with Congo red and examined beneath a polarised light. AL amyloidosis can be managed with chemotherapy or stem cell transplantation, but is usually fatal within 2 years. AA amyloidosis may respond to treatment of the underlying cause.

Amyloid, from Greek *amylon* = starch.

4. F – Multiple myeloma

Multiple myeloma describes the malignant proliferation of plasma cells that secrete light immunoglobulin chains. It is a multisystem disorder that commonly affects the kidneys, causing renal failure in up to 50% of patients. The pathogenesis of renal failure in multiple myeloma is multifactorial, involving dehydration, hypercalcaemia, hyperuricaemia, ischaemia and light-chain deposition in the nephrons. The treatment of acute renal failure in myeloma requires rehydration with intravenous fluids, renal replacement therapy and treatment of the underlying condition.

5. H – Rhabdomyolysis

Rhabdomyolysis occurs when skeletal tissue breaks down secondary to traumatic, chemical or metabolic injury. Common causes of rhabdomyolysis include crush injury, prolonged immobilization following a fall, prolonged seizure activity, hyperthermia and neuroleptic malignant syndrome. Muscle breakdown results in the rapid release of potassium, phosphate, myoglobin and creatine kinase into the circulation, placing the patient at risk of cardiac arrhythmia and acute renal failure. Diagnosis is based on history, the presence of myoglobin in the urine, hyperkalaemia and raised serum creatine kinase levels (usually >10 000 IU/L). Treatment of rhabdomyolysis is mainly supportive with intravenous fluid hydration, correction of electrolyte imbalance and renal replacement therapy when indicated.

Practice Paper 9: Questions

Theme 1: Symptoms of gastrointestinal disease

Options

A. Coeliac disease
B. Diffuse oesophageal spasm
C. Duodenal ulcer
D. Gastric carcinoma
E. Gastric ulcer
F. Large-bowel obstruction
G. Oesophageal malignancy
H. Pyloric stenosis
I. Rectal carcinoma
J. Small-bowel obstruction

For each of the following descriptions, select the most appropriate diagnosis. Each option may be used once, more than once or not at all.

1. A 68-year-old man attends his GP with a 3-week history of alternating constipation and diarrhoea. He used to open his bowels once daily. On further questioning, he admits to passing fresh blood occasionally per rectum. He occasionally gets the feeling that there is still something left over after he has passed solids.

2. A 25-year-old man presents after three episodes of vomiting that contained altered blood. He has recently started a busy job, which he finds stressful, and he has not had time to eat well. In addition, he complains of a 6-month history of upper abdominal pain, which is exacerbated by eating.

3. A 3-week-old boy presents with a history of projectile vomiting that occurs a few minutes after every feed. There is no bile or blood in the vomit. His mother says that, despite the vomiting, the baby is still hungry for feeds.

4. A 46-year-old woman presents with intermittent severe retrosternal chest pains that occur soon after eating and are accompanied by difficulty swallowing. She complains of no other symptoms. An ECG shows no acute abnormality and cardiac enzymes are normal.

5. A 24-year-old woman presents with a 4-month history of vague abdominal cramps that are worse after eating. This has been accompanied by the passage of foul-smelling stools that float and are difficult to flush away.

Theme 2: Complications of cancer therapy

Options

A. Allergy
B. Alopecia
C. Central venous line infection
D. Chemotherapy-induced emesis
E. Constipation
F. Graft-versus-host disease
G. Infertility
H. Mucositis
I. Neutropenic sepsis
J. Pulmonary fibrosis
K. Tumour lysis syndrome
L. Panhypopituitarism

For each of the following scenarios, select the most likely complication of cancer therapy. Each option may be used once, more than once or not at all.

1. A 65-year-old woman receiving chemotherapy for breast cancer presents to her GP with a painful, inflamed and ulcerated mouth.

2. A 14-year-old girl who received a bone marrow transplant for relapsed acute myeloid leukaemia 6 weeks ago begins to experience significant diarrhoea. On examination, a maculopapular rash is seen on her arms and legs.

3. A 34-year-old man presents to the emergency department with fever and rigors. He reveals that he completed a course of chemotherapy 10 days ago. Blood tests show a haemoglobin of 11 g/dL, a neutrophil count of 0.02×10^9/L and platelets 182×10^9/L.

4. A 72-year-old man is complaining of a dry non-productive cough and shortness of breath after receiving several cycles of palliative radiotherapy for a bronchial carcinoma.

5. A 12-year-old boy who has stage IV Hodgkin's lymphoma develops a temperature of 39.1°C and experiences rigors 30 minutes after having his central venous line accessed for chemotherapy. Blood tests show a haemoglobin of 11 g/dL, a white cell count of 12×10^9/L and a neutrophil count of 9.3×10^9/L.

Theme 3: Pathogens of endocarditis

Options

A. *Candida albicans*
B. Coxsackie B virus
C. *Enterococcus faecalis*
D. *Mycobacterium tuberculosis*
E. *Neisseria meningitidis*
F. *Staphylococcus aureus*
G. *Streptococcus bovis*
H. *Staphylococcus epidermidis*
I. *Streptococcus pyogenes*
J. Viridans streptococcus
K. *Trypanosoma cruzi*

For each of the following scenarios, select the most likely offending pathogen. Each option may be used once, more than once or not at all.

1. A 32-year-old male intravenous drug user presents with a 4-week history of fever, lethargy and weight loss. On examination, you find that he has swollen ankles and a raised jugular venous pressure. On auscultation, you notice a pansystolic murmur that is best heard over the left sternal border.
2. A 45-year-old woman presents with a 3-week history of night sweats, weight loss and palpitations approximately 1 month after having a dental abscess removed. On auscultation, you notice a pansystolic murmur that is best heard at the apex. She had rheumatic fever as a child.
3. A 64-year-old man presents to the emergency department with fever. The observations include temperature 40.2°C, blood pressure 100/48 mmHg and heart rate 114 beats/min. Examination reveals a thoracotomy scar from a metallic aortic valve replacement 1 month previously. Transoesophageal echocardiography shows a number of vegetations that are visualized at the insertion point of the metallic ring.
4. A 72-year-old man with known benign prostatic hypertrophy and a past history of rheumatic fever presents to the emergency department. He was last admitted 3 weeks ago with acute urinary retention, for which he was catheterized and then taught intermittent self-catheterization. He is lethargic, feverish and has lost a stone (6 kg) in weight since his discharge. On examination, you notice a diastolic murmur and signs of left ventricular failure that were not documented on his previous admission.
5. A 65-year-old woman, who was diagnosed with sigmoid carcinoma 5 years previously, presents with a 5-week history of malaise, fever, palpitations and weight loss. On examination, you notice a number of splinter haemorrhages under her fingernails. Auscultation reveals a diastolic murmur that is best heard over the second intercostal space on the left-hand side while in expiration. The murmur was not present at her last colonoscopy 2 years ago.

Theme 4: Sexually transmitted infections 2

Options

A. Bacterial vaginosis
B. Cervical cancer
C. Chancroid
D. Chlamydia infection
E. Epstein–Barr virus
F. Genital candidiasis
G. Genital herpes
H. Genital warts
I. Gonorrhoea
J. Granuloma inguinale (donovanosis)
K. HIV
L. Lymphogranuloma venereum
M. Molluscum contagiosum
N. Phthiriasis
O. Reiter's syndrome
P. Scabies
Q. Syphilis
R. Trichomoniasis

For each of the following scenarios, select the most likely diagnosis. Each option may be used once, more than once or not at all.

1. A 30-year-old man presents with a 2-day history of left knee pain and a burning sensation on passing urine. On examination, his temperature is 37.2°C and you notice that his eyes are red.

2. A 42-year-old woman presents with multiple lesions on her face. The lesions are raised and shiny, non-tender, non-erythematous, and around 3 mm in diameter. They have an umbilicated centre. The patient is known to be HIV positive.

3. A 29-year-old woman presents with pain on passing urine and increased frequency. She is started on a course of trimethoprim and a urine sample is sent to the laboratory. She returns 4 days later complaining of 'extreme itching down there' and pain when having sexual intercourse. On speculum examination, there is redness of the vulva and a thick white discharge is seen within the vagina.

4. A 27-year-old man presents with a single ulcer on his penis, which he says developed from a spot. He denies any pain in the area. On examination, lymphadenopathy is palpable in the left groin, with evidence of a discharging sinus. A culture of the discharge reveals *Chlamydia trachomatis*.

5. A 54-year-old woman attends the GP with a persistent headache. She denies any other symptoms. She recently completed a 10-year round-the-world expedition. On examination, you notice that her pupils are small and unequal in size. The light reflex is absent.

Theme 5: Airway management

Options

A. Cricothyroidotomy
B. Endotracheal tube
C. Head tilt and chin lift
D. Laryngeal mask airway
E. Nasopharyngeal airway
F. Oropharyngeal airway
G. Suction
H. Tracheostomy

For each of the following scenarios, select the most appropriate adjunct to airway management. Each option may be used once, more than once or not at all.

1. An 18-year-old man is post-ictal following an epileptic seizure. He is making snoring noises when breathing. His Glasgow Coma Scale score is 6.

2. An 18-year-old man is post-ictal following an epileptic seizure. He is making snoring noises when breathing. His Glasgow Coma Scale score is 12.

3. A 65-year-old man collapsed unconscious in a restaurant toilet after complaining of chest pain. An ambulance has been called, but has yet to arrive.

4. A 30-year-old woman has significant facial and upper airway burns. An attempt at bag-and-mask ventilation and intubation has failed due to laryngeal oedema.

5. A 67-year-old woman is in ventricular fibrillation. An anaesthetist has yet to arrive.

Theme 6: Pathogens in pneumonia

Options

A. *Chlamydophila pneumoniae*
B. *Chlamydophila psittaci*
C. *Haemophilus influenzae*
D. *Klebsiella pneumoniae*
E. *Legionella pneumophila*
F. *Mycobacterium tuberculosis*
G. *Mycoplasma pneumoniae*
H. *Pneumocystis jiroveci*
I. *Pseudomonas aeruginosa*
J. *Staphylococcus aureus*
K. *Streptococcus pneumoniae*

For each of the following scenarios, select the most likely causative pathogen. Each option may be used once, more than once or not at all.

1. A 26-year-old man has a 2-day history of malaise, fever and shortness of breath associated with pain over the right side of his chest. He has developed a cough and is expectorating rusty sputum. A chest X-ray confirms consolidation of the right lower lobe.

2. A 67-year-old woman presents with a 5-day history of malaise and a cough productive of yellow sputum. Examination is unremarkable. A chest X-ray shows two cavities with air–fluid levels.

3. A 42-year-old woman has a 2-month history of worsening shortness of breath and a dry cough. She also complains of night sweats. On examination, her oxygen saturations are 89%. She has no other symptoms and no history of respiratory disease, but is known to have HIV infection.

4. A 53-year-old man is brought to the emergency department after a fit. His wife says that he has been complaining of malaise, muscle aches and a dry cough for the last 7 days since they returned from holiday. Blood tests reveal a sodium of 124 mmol/L and a potassium of 4.2 mmol/L.

5. A 62-year-old man presents with a 2-week history of shortness of breath associated with a dry cough and widespread joint ache. He has felt somewhat feverish and unwell over this time. Examination reveals an enlarged liver and spleen. A chest X-ray demonstrates patchy consolidation of both lower lobes.

Theme 7: Gastrointestinal malignancy

Options

A. Carcinoid tumour
B. Colorectal carcinoma
C. Gallbladder carcinoma
D. Gastric carcinoma
E. Insulinoma
F. Oesophageal adenocarcinoma
G. Pancreatic carcinoma
H. Small-bowel carcinoma
I. Zollinger–Ellison syndrome

For each of the following scenarios, select the most appropriate diagnosis. Each option may be used once, more than once or not at all.

1. A 67-year-old man presents to his GP with a 2-month history of difficulty swallowing and significant weight loss. He has had no other symptoms and examination is unremarkable.

2. A 68-year-old woman with a long history of dyspepsia, anorexia and weight loss presents to her GP after developing epigastric pain. On examination, she appears cachexic. In addition, the skin on her neck and axillae is dark and velvety.

3. A 58-year-old man presents to the emergency department complaining of sudden-onset severe abdominal pain, abdominal distension and constipation. He denies vomiting. On further questioning, he admits to a recent history of weight loss.

4. A 57-year-old man presents to the emergency department with severe upper abdominal pain and haematemesis. An emergency endoscopy is organized, and showed multiple peptic ulcers in his stomach, duodenum and jejunum.

5. A 46-year-old woman presents to her GP complaining of episodes of flushing and shortness of breath. On further questioning, she admits to occasional episodes of explosive diarrhoea.

Theme 8: Visual defects 2

Options

A. Amaurosis fugax
B. Bitemporal hemianopia
C. Cataract
D. Central scotoma
E. Cortical blindness
F. Fortification spectra
G. Homonymous hemianopia
H. Hypermetropia
I. Myopia
J. Presbycusis
K. Tunnel vision

For each of the following scenarios, select the most appropriate visual defect. Each option may be used once, more than once or not at all.

1. A 67-year-old man complains of a 12-month history of worsening vision. He says that his vision is becoming more blurry and that he is finding it especially difficult focusing when reading the newspaper. Fundoscopy is unremarkable.

2. A 71-year-old woman presents with her second episode of visual loss. She describes two occasions in the last month where she briefly lost vision in her right eye. Both episodes resolved spontaneously. Fundoscopy is unremarkable.

3. A 74-year-old man is brought by his wife to the emergency department with dizziness that started suddenly earlier in the day. He has had a stroke in the past that presented with similar symptoms. On examination, he is clearly unable to see out of either eye, although he denies that he is blind. Fundoscopy is unremarkable.

4. A 59-year-old woman complains of worsening of vision. Her sight has deteriorated over the last 2 years, and now she finds it difficult to drive at night, especially with the glare of headlamps in the other lanes. Fundoscopy demonstrates a reduced red reflex bilaterally.

5. A 38-year-old woman presents with a visual problem. She complains that she has a dark patch of visual loss within her field of vision in the right eye. Despite this, the rest of her vision is fine.

Theme 9: Endocrine investigations

Options

A. 24-hour catecholamine collection
B. Aldosterone levels
C. Clotting screen
D. Glucose tolerance test
E. High-dose dexamethasone suppression test
F. Low-dose dexamethasone suppression test
G. Random cortisol level
H. Random glucose
I. Short Synacthen test
J. Thyroid function tests
K. Water deprivation test

For each of the following scenarios, select the most appropriate investigation. Each option may be used once, more than once or not at all.

1. A 3-year-old boy is noticed to be drinking excessively and passing large amounts of dilute urine on a daily basis. His capillary blood glucose level is 5 mmol/L.

2. A 29-year-old man presents to the GP with a 2-month history of malaise. On examination, he has hyperpigmentation in his mouth and on his palms. Blood tests show a sodium of 124 mmol/L and a potassium of 5.7 mmol/L.

3. A 48-year-old woman presents to the GP with weight gain and increased hair on her abdomen and face. On examination, she has thin skin and multiple bruises.

4. A 14-year-old boy is brought to the GP complaining of intermittent headaches and anxiety. These episodes are accompanied by facial flushing and sweating. An abdominal mass is felt on examination.

5. A 56-year-old man with hypertension, hyperglycaemia and facial changes is referred to the general medicine clinic for investigation.

Theme 10: Diagnosis of neurological disease

Options

A. Acoustic neuromas
B. Arnold–Chiari malformation
C. Ataxia telangiectasia
D. Brown-Séquard syndrome
E. Friedreich's ataxia
F. Neurofibromatosis type 1
G. Neurofibromatosis type 2
H. Shy–Drager syndrome
I. Subacute sclerosing panencephalitis
J. Syringomyelia
K. Von Hippel–Lindau disease

For each of the following scenarios, select the most likely diagnosis. Each option may be used once, more than once or not at all.

1. A 22-year-old woman attends the dermatology outpatient clinic with multiple skin lesions on her body. On examination, she has eight light-brown macules on her arms and trunk, and four firm rubbery lesions.

2. A 42-year-old woman has a 2-month history of shoulder pain associated with sensory loss in her arms. On examination, you note that she is insensate to pain and temperature in both hands, although her joint position sense is intact. There is no other motor or sensory loss.

3. A 34-year-old man is referred to the general medical clinic by his GP for uncontrollable hypertension. He is presently on ramipril and bendroflumethazide. On further questioning, he admits to having paroxysms of anxiety, sweating and palpitations that are brought on by stress, which he describes as 'panic attacks'. He has a past medical history of kidney cancer and 'tumours in his eyes'.

4. An 8-year-old boy is brought to the GP with a 6-month history of difficulty walking and increasing clumsiness. He was previously developing normally. On examination, he appears to have some thin, red, spidery lesions on his cheeks.

5. A 47-year-old woman complains of a tremor in her hands that is worse at rest, and she is finding it increasingly difficult to play the piano. She also complains of dizziness when standing up and of intermittent incontinence.

Theme 11: Overdose and antidotes

Options

A. Atropine
B. Desferrioxamine
C. Digibind
D. *N*-Acetylcysteine
E. Ethanol
F. Flumazenil
G. Glucagon
H. Naloxone
I. Sodium bicarbonate infusion
J. Vitamin K

For each of the following scenarios, select the most appropriate antidote. Each option may be used once, more than once or not at all.

1. A 35-year-old man took 60 paracetamol tablets 6 hours ago in an attempt to end his life. He has now changed his mind regarding suicide and wishes to receive treatment.

2. A 3-year-old boy is admitted to the emergency department having consumed a large quantity of his mother's iron tablets. He is complaining of severe abdominal pain and passes some blood per rectum.

3. A 21-year-old woman took a significant overdose of propranolol that she was prescribed for anxiety. On admission, she has a heart rate of 50 beats/min and a blood pressure of 86/42 mmHg.

4. In an attempt to sedate a 76-year-old delirious woman, the nursing staff at her care home gave her an accidental overdose of diazepam. She is now unresponsive and her airway appears compromised.

5. A 45-year-old man presents to the emergency department having reportedly taken an overdose of morphine sulphate tablets that were originally prescribed for his mother, who has chronic back pain. He is unresponsive, has small pupils and has a respiratory rate of 5/min.

Theme 12: Extra-articular manifestations of rheumatoid arthritis

Options

A. Amyloidosis
B. Anaemia of chronic disease
C. Atlantoaxial subluxation
D. Caplan's syndrome
E. Episcleritis
F. Felty's syndrome
G. Mononeuritis multiplex
H. Palmar erythema
I. Pyoderma gangrenosum
J. Rheumatoid nodules
K. Scleritis
L. Scleromalacia perforans
M. Sjögren's syndrome

For each of the following scenarios, select the most appropriate condition. Each option may be used once, more than once or not at all.

1. A 52-year-old woman with rheumatoid arthritis has noticed that she can no longer lift her right foot at the ankle. Last week, she had problems using the first three digits of her right hand.

2. A 37-year-old man with rheumatoid arthritis is complaining of dry, itchy eyes. He has had two recent bouts of conjunctivitis, and wants treatment.

3. A 58-year-old woman with rheumatoid arthritis is admitted with a chest infection. Routine blood tests show haemoglobin 9.4 g/dL, white cell count 6.2×10^9/L and platelet count 128×10^9/L. Examination reveals a large abdominal mass in the left upper quadrant.

4. A 46-year-old woman with rheumatoid arthritis presents with painless reddening in her eyes. Examination reveals dilated vessels in both eyes.

5. A 61-year-old man with rheumatoid arthritis has a 3-month history of worsening shortness of breath and a cough productive of grey sputum. Examination reveals widespread crackles bilaterally.

Theme 13: Management of asthma

Options

A. Inhaled high-dose steroids
B. Inhaled low-dose steroids
C. Inhaled short-acting β_2-agonist
D. Intravenous magnesium sulphate
E. Nebulized short-acting β_2-agonist
F. No further management required
G. No treatment required
H. Oral leukotriene receptor antagonist
I. Oral steroids
J. Oxygen via facemask and inhaled short-acting β_2-agonist
K. Oxygen via facemask, inhaled short-acting β_2-agonist and steroids
L. Oxygen via facemask and nebulized short-acting β_2-agonist
M. Oxygen via facemask, nebulized short-acting β_2-agonist and steroids

For each of the following scenarios, select the most appropriate management. Each option may be used once, more than once or not at all.

1. An 8-year-old boy presents to his GP with a 6-month history of night cough and intermittent wheeze. He has previously been well. On examination, he is small for his age and has mild eczema on his upper limbs.

2. A 16-year-old boy attends the GP with poorly controlled chronic asthma. He is currently being managed with an inhaled long-acting β_2-agonist and high-dose inhaled steroids. His parents want to know if there is anything else that he can be given.

3. A 14-year-old girl attends the GP with poorly controlled chronic asthma. She is currently being managed with an inhaled long-acting β_2-agonist and high-dose inhaled steroids and monteleukast. Her parents want to know if there is anything else that can be done to help.

4. A 23-year-old man with known asthma is brought to the emergency department with shortness of breath. He has widespread wheeze, is too breathless to talk, and has a heart rate of 115 beats/min and a respiratory rate of 36/min.

5. A 21-year-old women with known asthma is brought to the emergency department with shortness of breath. She can barely talk, has a silent chest and has a respiratory rate of 36/min. Although there appears to be some improvement with oxygen, nebulized salbutamol and steroids, her peak flows are still 30% of her best.

Theme 14: Investigation of cardiovascular disease

Options

A. 24-hour ECG tape
B. Ambulatory blood-pressure monitoring
C. Chest X-ray
D. CT pulmonary angiogram
E. Doppler ultrasound scan
F. Exercise (stress) ECG
G. Myocardial biopsy
H. Myocardial perfusion scan
I. Resting ECG
J. Serum brain-type natriuretic peptide (BNP)
K. Serum D-dimer levels
L. Serum lactate dehydrogenase
M. Serum myoglobin
N. Serum troponin
O. Thrombophilia screen
P. Transoesophageal echocardiography
Q. Transthoracic echocardiography

For each of the following scenarios, select the most appropriate investigation. Each option may be used once, more than once or not at all.

1. A 63-year-old man presents to his GP following several episodes of central chest pain that occurred while gardening. On each occasion, the pain was relieved by rest. The admission ECG, full blood count and thyroid function tests reveal no abnormality.

2. A 67-year-old woman presents to the emergency department with a 12-hour history of central chest pain that commenced at rest and radiated to both arms. She is nauseated and appears pale and sweaty. The resting ECG shows an ST depression of 1 mm in leads II, III and aVF, associated with non-specific T-wave changes. A chest X-ray is normal.

3. A 40-year-old female inpatient develops a red, tender swelling of her left leg 10 days after a hysterectomy. The affected leg is painful and hard to touch, and the peripheral veins appear engorged. A full blood count is unremarkable and her observations are stable.

4. A 50-year-old man with a past history of rheumatic fever becomes acutely unwell 5 days after an elective tooth extraction. On examination, he has a temperature of 38.3°C and has a pansystolic murmur that was not documented on his previous admission. Blood cultures have been sent, but the results are not yet available.

5. A 56-year-old man with hypertension and ischaemic heart disease presents to his GP following several episodes of palpitations. Each episode lasts approximately 1 hour and terminates spontaneously. A resting ECG performed in the practice shows no abnormalities. Routine blood tests taken a week previously were within normal limits.

Theme 15: Gait disturbance 1

Options

A. Antalgic gait
B. Cerebellar ataxia
C. Extrapyramidal gait
D. Gait apraxia
E. High-stepping gait
F. Marche à petit pas
G. Pyramidal gait
H. Sensory ataxia
I. Spastic gait
J. Trendelenburg gait
K. Waddling gait

For each of the following scenarios, select the most appropriate gait disturbance. Each option may be used once, more than once or not at all.

1. A 59-year-old woman is having difficulty walking and has had multiple falls recently. On gait examination, you notice that she is walking very slowly and is carefully watching and placing her feet. On examination, there is no weakness or sensory deficit.

2. A 62-year old woman is having extreme difficulty walking up stairs. She also finds it difficult to stand up, and says that her legs feel weak. She has a history of severe chronic obstructive pulmonary disease, for which she has taken frequent courses of prednisolone.

3. A 65-year-old woman attends the orthopaedic follow-up clinic. She had a left hip replacement 2 weeks ago. As she enters the room, you notice that she is walking with a limp on one side. On examination, there is no evidence of sensory or motor impairment.

4. A 27-year-old woman presents with a 48-hour history of leg weakness, which started in her feet. She is unable to walk properly and she keeps tripping over her feet. On examination, there is marked weakness of ankle plantarflexion and dorsiflexion, as well as loss of tendon reflexes and some sensory deficit.

5. A 12-year-old boy is brought to the emergency department with abdominal pains. When he walks into the room, you notice that he has a characteristic posture. His knees are slightly flexed, his hips are adducted and his ankles are plantarflexed bilaterally. This results in his legs crossing each other when he walks.

Practice Paper 9: Answers

Theme 1: Symptoms of gastrointestinal disease

1. I – Rectal carcinoma

Tenesmus is an uncomfortable sensation of incomplete evacuation of the rectum that results in a strong desire to defecate. It is usually caused by a mass within the rectum, such as a rectal carcinoma or polyp, but may be found in association with functional bowel disease, such as irritable bowel syndrome, and prostatic disease, such as prostatitis.

Tenesmus, from Latin *tenesmos* = to strain or stretch.

2. E – Gastric ulcer

Gastric ulcers are usually found in the lesser curvature of the stomach and account for approximately 20% of peptic ulcers (the remaining 80% are duodenal). They are associated with epigastric pain that is exacerbated by eating and relived by vomiting. Weight loss is often a feature, due to a fear of food and its association with pain. In contrast, the pain associated with duodenal ulcers is classically exacerbated by hunger and relieved by eating – so that weight gain is often a feature. Investigation of suspected gastric ulceration is important because of the risk of malignancy. The patient should have a barium meal or endoscopy to identify any lesion. If there is radiological or endoscopic evidence of gastric ulceration, biopsies should be taken and investigated for malignant change. Duodenal ulcers are rarely malignant and do not require compulsory biopsy.

3. H – Pyloric stenosis

Non-bile-stained projectile vomiting soon after feeds in a hungry baby is indicative of pyloric stenosis. Pyloric stenosis is hypertrophy of the circular muscle of the pylorus, causing gastric outflow obstruction. It presents in the first few weeks of life and most commonly affects first-born males. Apart from projectile vomiting, affected babies may be constipated and lose weight. A characteristic hypochloraemic, hypokalaemic, metabolic alkalosis results from vomiting stomach acid. Pyloric stenosis is diagnosed by giving the baby a 'test feed': when the baby is given milk, visible gastric peristalsis may be seen over the epigastrium, and the pylorus is felt as an olive-shaped mass in the upper abdomen. If the diagnosis is in doubt, an ultrasound can be performed. After initial rehydration, management is by Ramstedt's pyloromyotomy (in which the muscle of the pylorus is cut longitudinally down to the mucosa). The baby can tolerate milk feeds a few hours after the operation.

Pyloric stenosis can also occur in adults, in whom it is usually due to gastric ulceration and the formation of fibrotic tissue that contracts and distorts the stomach architecture. Adults tend not to experience projectile vomiting, but do vomit undigested food many hours after it was consumed.

4. B – Diffuse oesophageal spasm

Diffuse oesophageal spasm (DOS), also known as 'nutcracker oesophagus', is an idiopathic condition characterized by intermittent, uncontrolled spasm of the distal half of the oesophagus without any structural stenosis. Patients present with severe retrosternal chest pain lasting 30 minutes, with or without dysphagia. Symptom frequency can vary from every few days to every time that the patient eats. A barium swallow in active disease will show diffuse spasm known as the 'corkscrew oesophagus'; however, as symptoms are intermittent, barium studies are often normal. Manometry will show prolonged, powerful, oesophageal contractions induced by swallowing. The condition may respond to medical therapies such as nitrates or calcium channel blockers, but severe or refractory disease indicates the need for more invasive treatments such as botulinum toxin injection and surgery (oesophagomyotomy or oesophagectomy).

5. A – Coeliac disease

Dietary fats are broken down by lipases and are emulsified by bile salts before being absorbed in the small intestine. Conditions that cause reduced bile or lipase secretion (e.g. chronic pancreatitis) or damage to the small-intestinal mucosa (e.g. coeliac disease) can result in malabsorption of fats, which then enter the stool in excessive amounts. This is referred to as steatorrhoea and describes the passage of loose, pale and foul-smelling stools that do not flush away. The investigation of steatorrhoea involves the assessment of faecal fat content and the search for a cause of malabsorption.

Theme 2: Complications of cancer therapy

1. H – Mucositis

Chemotherapy generally works by inducing apoptosis and inhibiting mitosis, thus preventing the division and proliferation of malignant cells. The chemotherapeutic agents currently used do not specifically target malignant cells, and therefore also exert their cytotoxic actions on healthy cells. The most commonly affected cells are those with a high turnover, i.e. those of the gastrointestinal mucosa, hair follicles, bone marrow and reproductive system. The damage that chemotherapy exerts on these cell lines can result in mucositis, alopecia, pancytopenia and infertility. In this case, the patient is suffering from mucositis – inflammation and ulceration of the gastrointestinal mucosa secondary to chemotherapy. In addition to causing mouth pain, vomiting and diarrhoea, mucositis places the patient at an increased risk of infection and sepsis secondary to the breakdown of the protective gastrointestinal epithelium. Treatment of mucositis is supportive (mouth care and analgesia). Broad-spectrum antibiotics should be prescribed if infection is suspected.

2. F – Graft-versus-host disease

Graft-versus-host disease (GVHD) is usually seen following allogeneic bone marrow transplantation, but may occur following any form of allogeneic transplantation. It is caused by T cells within the graft bone marrow cross-reacting with the host's tissues and organs. GVHD commonly affects the skin, gastrointestinal tract and liver. Patients have severe diarrhoea and abdominal pain associated with a maculopapular rash and desquamation of the skin. Treatment involves high-dose corticosteroids, antithymocyte globulin and ciclosporin.

3. I – Neutropenic sepsis

Neutropenic sepsis is one of the most common emergencies in oncology. Neutropenia in malignancy is usually secondary to bone marrow infiltration by tumour cells or chemotherapy-/radiotherapy-induced marrow suppression. Neutropenic sepsis must be suspected in any patient with malignancy presenting with a temperature >38°C on two separate occasions or a single reading >38.5°C. Neutropenia is generally recognized as a neutrophil count $<1 \times 10^9$/L. Severe neutropenia is defined as a count $<0.5 \times 10^9$/L. If neutropenic sepsis is suspected, the patient should be assessed for a potential source of infection. The most common causes of sepsis are urinary tract infection, respiratory tract infection and central line infections. Treatment with intravenous broad-spectrum antibiotics should begin immediately.

4. J – Pulmonary fibrosis

Radiotherapy uses ionizing radiation to induce DNA damage and apoptosis in malignant cells via the production of oxygen free radicals. It is used in both the curative and the palliative treatment of malignancy. Side-effects of radiotherapy can be divided into short-term and long-term effects. Examples of short-term side-effects include lethargy, nausea, vomiting, skin damage, mucositis and oedema. Long-term side-effects include tissue fibrosis, infertility, chronic skin disease and secondary malignancy. The side-effect profile of radiotherapy is largely dependent on the area exposed to radiation. For example, radiotherapy to the bladder may result in fibrosis of the bladder, causing dysuria and frequency, radiotherapy to the bowel can cause diarrhoea, and radiotherapy to the head can cause xerostoma (reduced saliva production) and panhypopituitarism. The patient in this case has developed pulmonary fibrosis secondary to irradiation of the thorax. Pulmonary fibrosis typically presents with exertional dyspnoea and dry cough after a patient has received thoracic radiotherapy. Management is with high-dose corticosteroids.

5. C – Central venous line infection

Patients receiving chemotherapy often have central venous lines inserted to improve the delivery of chemotherapy and improve their quality of life. Despite the benefits of central venous lines, they represent a permanent indwelling foreign body that is prone to bacterial colonization and infection. A central venous line infection presents with fever and rigors soon after the line is accessed. Common pathogens include *Staphylococcus epidermidis* and *S. aureus*. Treatment is with broad-spectrum intravenous antibiotics, e.g. vancomycin with a third-generation cephalosporin.

Theme 3: Pathogens of endocarditis

1. F – *Staphylococcus aureus*

Intravenous drug users are at risk of developing bacterial endocarditis secondary to *S. aureus* bacteraemia introduced during non-sterile venepuncture. The valves that are affected tend to be (previously) normal and are often right-sided. In this case, the tricuspid valve is affected, causing significant regurgitation and right heart failure. The antibiotics of choice in acute *S. aureus* endocarditis are intravenous flucloxacillin and gentamicin. If resistant bacteria, such as meticillin-resistant *S. aureus* (MRSA), are suspected or proven, intravenous vancomycin plus gentamicin should be initiated.

Staphylococcus, from Greek *staphyle* = bunch of grapes + *coccus* = berry (or round). Staphylococci are round organisms that arrange themselves into clusters resembling bunches of grapes.

Aureus, from Latin *aureus* = gold. Also gives rise to Au, the chemical symbol for gold.

2. J – Viridans streptococcus

Viridans streptococci are a large group of bacterial organisms that are usually commensals in the oral cavity. They are the most common cause of bacterial endocarditis, being responsible for approximately 60% of cases. Individuals with pre-existing valvular disease are at risk of viridans streptococcal endocarditis following invasive dental procedures such as tooth extraction. Antibiotic treatment is usually with intravenous benzylpenicillin, with the addition of gentamicin if resistant bacteria are present. Patients with known valvular heart disease should always receive prophylactic antibiotics prior to any invasive procedure.

Streptococcus, from Greek *strepto* = twist. The round organisms of streptococci assemble into long chains.

Viridans, from Latin *viridis* = green. Colonies of viridans streptococci appear green on agar culture.

3. H – *Staphylococcus epidermidis*

This organism is a skin commensal. It commonly infects prosthetic valves and other indwelling foreign bodies such as peritoneal dialysis lines and venous lines. This is due to the bacterium's ability to adhere to, and grow on, prosthetic surfaces. *S. epidermidis* should therefore be suspected in all patients with prosthetic valves who present with the signs and symptoms of bacterial endocarditis. Antibiotic therapy is with benzylpenicillin and gentamicin. If infection occurs within the initial weeks following valve replacement, an urgent surgical opinion should be sought.

Epidermis, from Greek *epi* = upon + *dermis* = skin.

4. C – *Enterococcus faecalis*

This organism originates from the gastrointestinal tract and causes approximately 10% of cases of bacterial endocarditis. It tends to occur in patients with pre-existing valvular disease following instrumentation of the genitourinary or gastrointestinal tract – catheterization, cystoscopy, colonoscopy, etc. – which causes an enterococcus bacteraemia. In order to prevent bacteraemia and valve colonization during instrumentation, patients with a history of valvular damage or prosthetic valves should be given antibiotic prophylaxis.

5. G – *Streptococcus bovis*

S. bovis belongs to the viridans streptococci – so if you checked option J as your answer, give yourself the mark! It is a rare cause of bacterial endocarditis that has been shown to have links with bowel malignancy. In the case described here, it is improbable that instrumentation was involved in producing a bacteraemia, since the patient's last colonoscopy was 2 years ago and the symptoms have been present for only 5 weeks. *S. bovis* bacteraemia is associated with bowel cancer in 25% of cases. Therefore, if it is grown in the blood culture of any patient, with or without suspected bacterial endocarditis, further investigation is warranted to rule out underlying gastrointestinal tract malignancy.

Theme 4: Sexually transmitted infections 2

1. O – Reiter's syndrome

Reiter's syndrome, or reactive arthritis, is a triad of urethritis, seronegative (i.e. rheumatoid factor-negative) arthritis and conjunctivitis resulting from a pathological immune response to an infectious agent ('can't see, can't pee, can't climb a tree!'). Two other associated features of Reiter's syndrome are circinate balanitis (erythematous lesions on the penis) and keratoderma blenorrhagicum (hard nodules on the soles of the feet that are clinically and histologically indistinguishable from plantar psoriasis). There are two main causes of Reiter's syndrome: genitourinary infection (*Chlamydia* or *Neisseria gonorrhoeae*) or gastrointestinal infection (*Salmonella, Shigella, Yersinia* or *Campylobacter*). Reiter's syndrome is much more common in males (25:1). Diagnosis is normally clinical, although the erythrocyte sedimentation rate is raised and HLA-B27 is often present.

Hans Conrad Reiter, German military physician (1881–1969). Reiter was convicted of war crimes for his medical experiments on concentration camp detainees. Because of this association, the term 'reactive arthritis' is now becoming preferred.

2. M – Molluscum contagiosum

Molluscum contagiosum is caused by a DNA-containing poxvirus. Spread is by sexual contact, personal contact and fomites (an inanimate object that is contaminated with disease-causing microorganisms, e.g. a used towel). Hemispherical papules of 2–5 mm diameter that are pearly, raised and firm develop on the face, abdomen, buttocks and genitals. There is a latent period of 15–50 days. Spontaneous regression generally occurs, but lesions can be present for several months. The lesions can be extensive and persistent in immunocompromised patients, including those with HIV.

3. F – Genital candidiasis

Candidiasis (thrush) is caused by yeasts, particularly *Candida albicans* and *C. glabrata*, and produces vulval pruritis, burning, swelling and dyspareunia. White discharge and plaques are seen in the vagina, with redness of the vulva and labia minora. Candidiasis is seen more commonly with pregnancy, tissue maceration, diabetes mellitus, HIV infection, and use of antimicrobial agents and immunosuppressive drugs. Diagnosis is confirmed by culture, and treatment is with antifungals, e.g. topical imidazoles (Canesten) or oral fluconazole.

Candida, from Latin *candidus* = clear and white.

4. L – Lymphogranuloma venereum

Lymphogranuloma venereum (LGV) is a sexually transmitted infection caused by serovars L1, L2 and L3 of *Chlamydia trachomatis*. It is mainly found in the tropics. In one-third of people infected, a small painless papule appears between 3 and 21 days after infection; this ulcerates and heals after a few days. Lymphadenopathy then develops; it is unilateral in two-thirds of cases. Inguinal abscesses (buboes) may form, and a sinus may develop. Acute ulcerative proctitis may develop when infection takes place via the rectal mucosa. Treatment is with appropriate antibiotics.

Bubo, from Greek *boubon* = groin or swollen groin. Also gives rise to the 'bubonic plague' and, allegedly, the American colloquial 'boo boo', used to describe little cuts and scrapes.

Venereal, from Latin *venereus* = desire (derived from Venus, the goddess of love).

5. Q – Syphilis (specifically neurosyphilis)

Syphilis is caused by the bacterium *Treponema pallidum* and is spread by sexual contact (it can also be acquired congenitally). There are many stages of syphilis infection:

- *Primary syphilis*: this occurs 10–90 days post-infection. A dull, red papule develops on the external genitalia and forms a single, well-demarcated, painless ulcer associated with bilateral inguinal lymph node enlargement. This lesion heals within 8 weeks.
- *Secondary syphilis*: this develops 7–10 weeks after primary infection, and involves malaise, mild fever, headache, a pruritic skin rash, hoarseness, swollen lymph nodes, patchy or diffuse hair loss, bone pain and arthralgia.
- *Latent syphilis*: there is no clinical evidence of disease, but it is still detectable by serological testing.
- *Tertiary syphilis*: this comprises cardiovascular, gummatous and neurological syphilis.
- *Cardiovascular syphilis*: this is characterized by aortitis and aortic aneurysms.

- *Gummatous syphilis*: this is a late stage of infection, when the host resistance to the infection begins to fail. Areas of syphilitic granulation tissue develop on the scalp, upper aspect of the leg or sternoclavicular region. These so-called 'gummatous' lesions are copper coloured. Granulation can also occur internally, e.g. on heart valves and bone. At this stage, there is still a good response to treatment.
- *Neurosyphilis*: this is where disease is detectable in the cerebrospinal fluid. Patients complain of headache, cranial nerve palsies, 'general paralysis of the insane' (psychosis with muscular reflex abnormality, dementia and seizures), tabes dorsalis (degeneration of the dorsal column of the spinal cord, resulting in poor coordination), trophic ulcers, Charcot's joints (a peripheral neuropathy resulting in excessive trauma to distal joints, with subsequent bony destruction) and Argyll Robertson pupils (bilateral small, irregular pupils that *do* accommodate but *do not* react to light).

Initial diagnosis of syphilis is by dark-ground microscopy (which shows the bluish coiled treponema organisms against the dark-brown background) and the Venereal Disease Research Laboratory (VDRL) test, which detects the presence of anticardiolipin, an antibody produced by people with syphilis. False positives to the VDRL test can occur with infectious mononucleosis, antiphospholipid syndrome and leprosy. Treatment of syphilis is with benzylpenicillin (or doxycycline if there is a penicillin allergy).

Congenital syphilis occurs in babies born to mothers with secondary or tertiary syphilis. Manifestations of congenital syphilis include Hutchinson's triad (deafness, notched upper incisors and keratitis of the cornea), frontal bossing, saddle nose deformity, rhagades (linear scars at the angles of the mouth and nose) and sabre shins (bowing of the legs).

Trichomoniasis is a sexually transmitted infection caused by the flagellated protozoan *Trichomonas vaginalis,* which invades superficial epithelial cells of the vagina, urethra, glans penis, prostate and seminal vesicles. Affected women present with an offensive greeny-grey discharge, vulval soreness, dyspareunia, dysuria, vaginitis and vulvitis. On examination, the cervix may have a punctate erythematous appearance ('strawberry cervix'). Men are mostly asymptomatic. Treatment is with metronidazole.

Granuloma inguinale (donovanosis) is caused by the bacterium *Klebsiella granulomatis.* A flat-topped papule develops on the genitalia (days to months post-infection), and then degenerates into a painless ulcer. The ulcer spreads along skin-folds, and heals with scarring.

Gonorrhoea is caused by the Gram-negative diplococcus *Neisseria gonorrhoeae.* The majority of infected women are asymptomatic, but some complain of vaginal discharge and urethritis. Complications include Bartholin's abscess and gonococcal salpingitis with irreversible tube damage. Infected men present with dysuria, frequency and/or a mucopurulent discharge after 3–5 days, coupled with urethritis and meatal oedema. Disseminated gonococcal infection occurs in <1% cases and causes pyrexia, a vasculitic rash and polyarthritis. Gonorrhoeal infection is confirmed by culture (Gram-negative diplococci), and treatment is with appropriate antibiotics (e.g. ciprofloxacin).

Phthiriasis ('crabs') is caused by the crab-louse *Phthirus pubis,* which lives mainly in the thick hairs of the pubic and perianal areas. Most cases are due to sexual transmission, but any close contact with an infected person can transmit the lice. Clinically, there is itching in the affected areas. The lice feed on blood, and can leave spots on the skin (pediculosis pubis).

Phthirus, from Greek *phtheir* = louse.

Theme 5: Airway management

1. F – Oropharyngeal airway

Snoring noises in any patient suggest partial upper airway obstruction. In order to maintain airway patency, an oropharyngeal airway can be used to prevent the tongue and soft tissues from collapsing and obstructing the airway. The correct size of airway is determined by measuring the distance from the angle of the jaw to the level of the incisors. In adults, the oropharyngeal airway is introduced with the curvature away from the hard pallet. Once the airway has passed the tongue, it is rotated 180°and left in situ. Since this type of airway can initiate a cough-and-gag reflex, it can be used only in patients with a reduced Glasgow Coma Scale score.

2. E – Nasopharyngeal airway

This patient has upper airway obstruction in association with a Glasgow Coma Scale score of 12/15. He is therefore unlikely to tolerate an oropharyngeal airway, for the reasons described above. A nasopharyngeal airway is a flexible plastic tube that is inserted into the nostril and passed into the pharynx, where it maintains the patency of the airway. It is usually inserted into the right nostril with the aid of a lubricating jelly. The phalange at the nostril end is fitted with a safety-pin to prevent the airway from being inhaled. Nasopharyngeal airways are also indicated in patients with significant maxillofacial injuries and other conditions that prevent adequate mouth opening. They are often better tolerated than oropharyngeal airways, but are contraindicated when a basal skull fracture is suspected, because of the theoretical possibility of the airway passing through the fracture into the brain.

3. C – Head tilt and chin lift

The head tilt and chin lift is the airway manoeuvre of choice when cervical spine trauma is not suspected. To achieve this, the patient is placed on the back, and the rescuer simultaneously lifts the patient's chin while extending the patient's head. This simple manoeuvre lifts the collapsed soft tissues and restores airway patency. Once the manoeuvre has been completed, the rescuer can reassess the airway by looking for chest movement and feeling for breath on their cheek. If the airway is patent and the patient is breathing spontaneously, they can be placed in the recovery position. If the patient is not breathing, basic life support should commence.

4. A – Cricothyroidotomy

A needle cricothyroidotomy involves inserting a cannula directly into the trachea through the cricothyroid membrane, which is located between the cricoid and thyroid cartilage. The needle is removed from the cannula, which is then used as a port for ventilation. This is a temporary invasive airway that is used when there is massive facial trauma or when laryngeal obstruction is preventing ventilation. It is imperative that the larynx remain at least partially patent, as exhalation must occur through the upper airway (since the cannula is too narrow to allow adequate exhalation). If the upper airway is completely obstructed, the intrathoracic pressure will increase to a level that can impede venous return to the heart and compromise cardiac output. If there is a complete laryngeal obstruction, a surgical cricothyroidotomy can be performed. This involves making vertical and horizontal incisions in the cricothyroid membrane to form a cross through which a cuffed endotracheal tube is inserted. The wide bore of this endotracheal tube will allow exhalation.

5. D – Laryngeal mask airway

Laryngeal mask airways are inserted into the mouth and form a cuff around the laryngeal opening. They require little training in their use and are technically easy to insert. Laryngeal mask airways allow more efficient ventilation compared with bag-and-mask ventilation techniques. They are also less likely to cause gastric distension and reflux, as lower pressures are generated. It should be noted that laryngeal masks lie above the glottis and therefore do not protect the airway against reflux of gastric contents.

Theme 6: Pathogens in pneumonia

1. K – *Streptococcus pneumoniae*

S. pneumoniae is the most common cause of community-acquired pneumonia. It often affects young and middle-aged people, and presents as a rapid-onset illness with high fevers, rigors and pleuritic chest pain. The production of rusty-coloured sputum (blood stained) is characteristic. Chest X-ray often shows lobar consolidation.

Chlamydophila pneumoniae (previously known as *Chlamydia pneumoniae*) causes a mild pneumonia in younger people, and may be associated with sinusitis, pharyngitis and laryngitis. Chest X-ray shows small segmental infiltrates. *Mycoplasma pneumoniae* affects adolescents and young adults, and tends to cause epidemics in 3-year cycles. Patients often present with few chest signs, but can develop erythema nodosum, pericarditis and haemolytic anaemia. Chest X-ray shows patchy or lobar consolidation and hilar lymphadenopathy.

In 40% of community-acquired pneumonias, no causative organism is found.

2. J – *Staphylococcus aureus*

S. aureus often complicates an underlying viral pneumonia. Infection can arise from other foci, such as osteomyelitis. The characteristic feature is the X-ray finding of abscesses, seen as cavities with air–fluid levels.

3. H – *Pneumocystis jiroveci*

Pneumocystis pneumonia (PCP) is the most common AIDS-defining illness, caused by the fungus *Pneumocystis jiroveci* (previously known as *Pneumocystis carinii*). Patients present with a dry cough, fever, shortness of breath, weight loss and night sweats. Oxygen saturations are typically low. If oxygen levels are normal, exercise-induced desaturations will support the diagnosis. Chest X-ray demonstrates widespread infiltrates. The diagnosis is determined by cytological examination of sputum or bronchial washings from bronchoscopy. Treatment is with co-trimoxazole (trimethoprim and sulfamethoxazole). Patients with HIV who have a low CD4 count (<200/μL) receive prophylaxis for *Pneumocystis* (e.g. co-trimoxazole or dapsone).

4. E – *Legionella pneumophila*

Legionella pneumophila pneumonia (Legionnaire's disease) tends to occur in localized epidemics. Patients present with a dry cough, myalgia, malaise and gastrointestinal symptoms. Confusion and hepatitis can also occur. Blood tests characteristically show a low sodium and low albumin.

Legionnaire's disease is so called as it was first recognized as causing an outbreak of pneumonia is a group of elderly men attending an American Legion (war veterans') conference in Philadelphia.

5. B – *Chlamydophila psittaci*

Psittacosis is caused by the bacterium *Chlamydophila psittaci* (previously known as *Chlamydia psittaci*), which is contracted from parrots, pigeons, seagulls and other birds. The bacteria are shed through faeces and nasal discharges, which can remain infectious for many months. Patients present with fever, arthralgia, diarrhoea, conjunctivitis and headache. Hepatosplenomegaly is a recognized finding. Chest X-ray shows patchy lower lobe consolidation.

Klebsiella pneumoniae causes a marked systemic disturbance and is a recognized cause of hospital-acquired infections and aspiration pneumonia. Patients are very unwell with a cough productive of purulent dark sputum. Chest X-ray can show widespread consolidation, often in the upper lobes.

Theme 7: Gastrointestinal malignancy

1. F – Oesophageal adenocarcinoma

A history of rapidly progressive dysphagia with weight loss in a patient of this age (60–80 years) suggests a diagnosis of oesophageal carcinoma. Oesophageal carcinomas are mostly of the squamous cell type, and risk factors for their development include male sex, smoking, achalasia, alcohol use, coeliac disease and a Chinese origin. Squamous cell carcinomas of the oesophagus occur most frequently in the mid-oesophagus, and spread of tumours is to local structures, such as the trachea and recurrent laryngeal nerve (blood metastases occur late). Diagnosis of oesophageal carcinoma is by endoscopy and biopsy, with a CT scan performed later to stage the disease. A barium swallow will show an irregular filling defect. Treatment is by oesophagecomy, with re-anastomosis of the stomach to the upper oesophagus. Unresectable tumours may be given palliative stenting or radiotherapy to improve dysphagia. Oesophageal tumours have a poor prognosis.

Oesophageal adenocarcinoma can occur against a background of Barrett's oesophagus. Barrett's oesophagus refers to metaplasia of the distal oesophageal mucosa in which the usual squamous cells are replaced by intestinal columnar cells. It is caused by chronic gastro-oesophageal reflux disease (GORD) and has the potential to undergo malignant change to oesophageal adenocarcinoma. Some patients with Barrett's oesophagus are completely asymptomatic, whereas others suffer from debilitating GORD, dyspepsia, weight loss and haematemesis. Diagnosis is by direct visualization of the mucosa and by biopsy during endoscopy. If dysplastic (premalignant) or malignant changes are identified on biopsy, the patient may require oesophageal resection. Other treatment options, such as mucosal ablation therapy, may be used in patients who are not suitable candidates for invasive surgery. Surveillance schemes involving regular endoscopy for patients with Barrett's oesophagus have been shown not to affect survival.

Normal Rupert Barrett, British surgeon (1903–79).

2. D – Gastric carcinoma

Gastric carcinoma is one of the most common malignancies in the UK. Common clinical features include new dyspepsia, weight loss, vomiting, haematemesis and iron-deficiency anaemia. Rarer non-gastric features include the presence of Virchow's node (a palpable left supraclavicular lymph node caused by tumour spread), acanthosis nigricans (a black velvety rash usually seen on the neck and in the axillary and submammary folds) and Sister Joseph's nodule (a metastatic deposit found in the umbilicus). Patients with features suggestive of gastric malignancy should undergo urgent endoscopy within 2 weeks of referral. CT/MRI is usually indicated for the staging of disease and to help plan surgery. Curative treatment requires partial or complete gastrectomy. Chemotherapy and radiotherapy are largely ineffective, but may have a role in palliation.

3. B – Colorectal carcinoma

This patient has presented with abdominal pain, abdominal distension and constipation, which is highly suggestive of bowel obstruction. This presentation in association with the history of weight loss suggests the presence of a colorectal malignancy that has acutely obstructed the bowel. Colorectal carcinoma can present in a number of ways, depending upon the site of the lesion, but should always be considered in patients presenting with a change in bowel habit, rectal bleeding, iron-deficiency anaemia and unintentional weight loss.

4. I – Zollinger–Ellison syndrome

Zollinger–Ellison syndrome describes peptic ulceration secondary to a gastrin-secreting adenoma (gastrinoma). The adenoma is usually located in the pancreas, but can be found in the stomach or small bowel. Approximately 60% of gastrinomas are malignant and have the potential to metastasize to local lymph nodes and the liver. The unregulated secretion of gastrin simulates the parietal cells in the gastric antrum to produce excessive amounts of hydrochloric acid. This disrupts the gastric and duodenal mucosa, causing peptic ulceration. The acid can also denature pancreatic enzymes, such as lipase, resulting in malabsorption and chronic diarrhoea. Diagnosis is often based upon endoscopic identification of multiple peptic ulcers in association with a raised fasting serum gastrin level. Treatment involves high-dose protein pump inhibitors and surgical resection of the adenoma. Patients with Zollinger–Ellison syndrome associated with multiple endocrine neoplasia (MEN) type 1 often have multiple adenomas that are not suitable for resection. In this situation, the patient can usually be managed using a somatostatin analogue (e.g. octreotide), which decreases gastrin secretion. Metastatic disease necessitates systemic chemotherapy.

Robert Milton Zollinger, American surgeon (1903–92).

Edwin Homer Ellison, American surgeon (1918–70).

5. A – Carcinoid tumour

Carcinoid tumours are serotonin-secreting neoplasms derived from the enterochromaffin cells of the gastrointestinal tract. They are usually found in the terminal ileum, appendix or rectum, but can occur in extraintestinal sites such as the bronchi, testes and ovary. If the tumour is limited to the gastrointestinal tract, the serotonin that is secreted enters the portal vein and is metabolized by the liver. If there are liver metastases, or if the primary tumour is extra-intestinal, the secreted serotonin escapes hepatic metabolism and enters the systemic circulation, causing flushing, tachycardia, wheeze, diarrhoea, heart valve fibrosis and right heart failure. This is known as carcinoid syndrome. Diagnosis is based on the history and elevated levels of 5-hydroxyindole acetic acid (5-HIAA), a serotonin metabolite, in the urine. Management is by resection or, in widespread disease, symptomatic treatment with octreotide. Carcinoid tumours are slow growing so, even if disseminated disease is present, patients can live for many years.

Theme 8: Visual defects 2

1. H – Hypermetropia

Hypermetropia is 'long-sightedness' – inability of the lens to focus on nearby objects. This causes the eye to focus the image on a point behind the retina. When long-sightedness occurs as a result of the ageing process, it is known as *presbyopia*. Presbyopia is thought to occur secondary to a loss of lens elasticity. *Presbycusis* is age-related hearing loss. *Myopia* is 'short-sightedness' – an inability to focus faraway objects.

Presby-, from Greek *presbyos* = older person.

Myopia, from Greek *myein* = to close + *opia* = vision

2. A – Amaurosis fugax

Amaurosis fugax describes a transient, sudden vision loss in one eye. It is often described in the literature as a 'curtain coming down vertically', although this classic description is infrequently reported by patients, who instead may complain of transient blindness, dimming or blurring of vision. The underlying cause of this symptom can be embolic (passage of an embolus through the retinal or ophthalmic artery), vascular (giant cell arteritis and other vasculitides), ocular (e.g. acute glaucoma) or neurological (e.g. optic neuritis).

Amaurosis fugax, from Greek *amaurosde* = darkness + Latin *fugere* = fleeting.

3. E – Cortical blindness

Cortical blindness describes the loss of vision in a normal eye caused by bilateral damage to the visual cortex in the occipital lobe. The patient in this scenario has had bilateral posterior circulation strokes, which have caused his symptoms. Affected people have no vision, but can suffer with visual hallucinations and a vehement denial of visual loss (Anton's syndrome).

Gabriel Anton, Austrian neurologist (1858–1953).

4. C – Cataract

A cataract is an opacification of the lens. It is the most common cause of blindness in the world. Risk factors include older age, diabetes, trauma, smoking and steroid eye drops. Some cases are congenital. Cataracts result in painless blurring or loss of vision, glare and a change in the refractive error (focusing ability of the eye). Examination reveals a reduced visual acuity – especially in bright rooms, due to glare. The cataract appears black against the red light reflex on fundoscopy. Cataracts can be treated by removing the affected lens and replacing it with a plastic lens implant under local anaesthetic.

Cataract, from Latin *cataracta* = waterfall (it was previously thought that the cataract was caused by humour from the eye flowing in front of the lens).

5. D – Central scotoma

A scotoma describes an area of visual field loss within a field of normal vision. The blind spot is an example of a scotoma that is present in every human. Pathological scotomata can be caused by problems of the retina or optic nerve, e.g. multiple sclerosis, optic nerve glioma, glaucoma and vascular lesions. A *scintillating scotoma* describes an area of flashing lights within the field of vision, often seen in migraine. This can take the form of zigzag lines, in which case it is known as a *fortification spectrum.*

Scotoma, from Greek *skotos* = darkness, gloom.

Tunnel vision describes loss of the peripheral visual field with preservation of central vision. Causes of tunnel vision include chronic glaucoma and retinitis pigmentosa. *Retinitis pigmentosa* is a genetic condition characterized by night blindness, tunnel vision and eventual blindness. Patients pathognomonically have dark spicule pigmentation of the retina. The combination of retinitis pigmentosa with progressive deafness is called *Usher's syndrome.*

For descriptions of bitemporal hemianopia and homonymous hemianopia, see 'Visual defects 1 (Paper 7 Answers, Theme 8)'.

Theme 9: Endocrine investigations

1. K – Water deprivation test

Antidiuretic hormone (ADH, also known as arginine vasopressin) is secreted from the posterior pituitary gland in response to a high plasma osmolality, hypovolaemia or stress. Its main function is to stimulate the reabsorption of water from the collecting ducts of the nephron into the circulation. This results in a reduction in plasma osmolality and urine output and an increase in urine osmolality and blood pressure. Diabetes insipidus (DI) is a condition caused by either an absolute lack of ADH secretion (cranial DI) or renal insensitivity to its actions (nephrogenic DI). DI usually presents with massive polyuria, as water cannot be reabsorbed from the collecting ducts. As a result, patients with DI are often dehydrated, and consume massive amounts of water in order to maintain their fluid balance. Other conditions that may present in a similar manner include diabetes mellitus, hypercalcaemia and psychogenic polydipsia. DI is usually diagnosed using the water deprivation test. This involves measuring the patient's urine volume, concentration and plasma osmolality while depriving the patient of water. A positive result is recorded when water deprivation fails to concentrate urine due to a lack of ADH or insensitivity to its actions. If the initial test is positive, the patient is given a dose of desmopressin – a synthetic ADH analogue. If the patient concentrates their urine in response to desmopressin, the defect must be central and a diagnosis of cranial DI can be made. If, however, the urine is not concentrated following desmopressin administration, there is end-organ resistance to ADH, i.e. nephrogenic DI.

Diabetes insipidus, from Greek *diabainein* = to siphon + Latin *in* = not + *sapere* = to taste – in other words, to pass tasteless urine.

2. I – Short Synacthen test

Hyponatraemia, hyperkalaemia and hyperpigmentation in a patient presenting with non-specific symptoms indicate a possible diagnosis of primary adrenal insufficiency (Addison's disease). To diagnose adrenal insufficiency, the short Synacthen test is used. Synacthen, a synthetic analogue of adrenocorticotrophic hormone (ACTH, corticotrophin), is given to the patient and the cortisol response is noted. In normal individuals, Synacthen will stimulate the adrenal cortex to secrete cortisol. In patients with adrenal insufficiency, the cortex is unable to respond, and the cortisol levels remain low. A cortisol level >550 nmol/L 30 minutes after Synacthen administration excludes adrenal insufficiency. If the result is positive or equivocal, the patient should have a long Synacthen test. In this investigation, cortisol is measured at 1, 4, 8 and 24 hours after Synacthen administration. In primary adrenal insufficiency (Addison's disease), the cortisol will never exceed 550 nmol/L. If the insufficiency is caused by corticotrophin-releasing hormone (CRH) or ACTH deficiency, it is termed secondary adrenal deficiency. In secondary adrenal insufficiency, the cortisol level is likely to exceed 550 nmol/L, but the response is delayed.

3. F – Low-dose dexamethasone suppression test

This patient could have glucocorticoid excess (Cushing's syndrome), which can be diagnosed using the dexamethasone suppression test. This involves measuring a baseline serum cortisol level at 09:00 before giving 0.5 mg of dexamethasone (a synthetic glucocorticoid) four times daily for 48 hours. At 48 hours, the serum cortisol level is repeated. In healthy individuals, the dexamethasone suppresses cortisol secretion by negatively feeding back to the anterior pituitary gland and inhibiting ACTH release. In Cushing's syndrome, the cortisol levels remain elevated and the test is positive. If the low-dose dexamethasone suppression test is positive a *high-dose dexamethasone suppression test* can be performed to differentiate between Cushing's syndrome caused by pituitary disease (Cushing's disease) and Cushing's syndrome caused by the ectopic secretion of ACTH from a non-pituitary tumour (e.g. small cell lung carcinoma). This test involves measuring a baseline serum cortisol level at 09:00 before giving 2 mg of dexamethasone four times daily for 48 hours and then measuring a repeat serum cortisol level. If the 48-hour cortisol level is significantly lower than the pre-test sample, it is likely that pituitary disease is responsible, since it is partially sensitive to negative feedback. If the cortisol is not suppressed at 48 hours, it is likely that ectopic ACTH secretion is occurring, since it is completely unresponsive to negative feedback.

4. A – 24-hour catecholamine collection

It is possible that this patient has a phaeochromocytoma – a catecholamine-secreting tumour of the adrenal medulla that presents with paroxysms of sweating, headache, palpitations, anxiety and hypertension. The first-line investigation for this condition is a 24-hour urine collection for catecholamines (specifically vanillylmandelic acid, VMA). If the first collection is negative, a second should be performed. MRI or CT will help localize the tumour.

5. D – Glucose tolerance test

It is possible that this patient has acromegaly. Growth hormone (GH) opposes the action of insulin, resulting in high plasma glucose levels. Features of acromegaly include swelling of the hands and feet, lower jaw protrusion, macroglossia (large tongue), bitemporal hemianopia, carpal tunnel syndrome, hypertension, hyperglycaemia and cardiomegaly. In health, high plasma glucose levels feed back to suppress GH secretion. In acromegaly, there is autonomous secretion of GH, usually from a pituitary adenoma, that escapes the control of negative feedback. The glucose tolerance test can be used to help diagnose acromegaly. Failure to suppress GH levels to below 1 μg/L 2 hours after a 75 g oral glucose bolus is considered a positive result. Other investigations used in the diagnosis of acromegaly include insulin-like growth factor 1 levels and cranial MRI.

Theme 10: Diagnosis of neurological disease

1. F – Neurofibromatosis type 1

Neurofibromatosis is an autosomal dominant disorder characterized by the development of multiple neurofibromas from the neurilemmal sheaths of central and peripheral nerves. There are two types: in type 1 (NF1, also known as von Recklinghausen's disease), the mutation is on chromosome 17; in type 2 (NF2), the mutation is on chromosome 22. NF1 is the 'peripheral form', accounting for 70% of cases. Features include multiple cutaneous neurofibromas, café-au-lait patches (at least six), axillary freckling and fibromas on the iris (Lisch nodules). Affected patients are also at risk of developing scoliosis and neural tumours (e.g. phaeochromocytoma, acoustic neuromas). NF2 is the 'central form' and has few or no cutaneous lesion. Instead, patients develop bilateral neural tumours (acoustic neuromas, optic nerve gliomas and meningiomas).

Acoustic neuromas are benign tumours of the Schwann cells of cranial nerve VIII. They can occur in conjunction with neurofibromatosis or as isolated tumours. Because of their close relationship to cranial nerves VII and VIII, acoustic neuromas can result in hearing loss, motor symptoms of the face and vertigo. The investigation of choice is MRI and treatment is by surgical removal (although permanent unilateral deafness and facial weakness often result).

Friedrich Daniel von Recklinghausen, German pathologist (1833–1910).

2. J – Syringomyelia

Syringomyelia describes the presence of a fluid-filled cavity within the spinal cord, usually in the cervical segments. The expanding cavity disrupts spinothalamic neurons, resulting in sensory loss (pain and temperature) in the affected distribution. Syringomyelia may be associated with congenital herniation of the cerebellar tonsils (*Arnold–Chiari malformation*). The best investigation is MRI. Management is by surgical decompression of the syrinx.

Syringomyelia, from Greek *syrinx* = tube + *myelos* = marrow (pertaining to the spinal cord).

3. K – Von Hippel–Lindau disease

This man presents with a phaeochromocytoma and has a history of other tumours. Von Hippel–Lindau disease is caused by an autosomal dominant defect on chromosome 3. The syndrome is characterized by retinal and intracranial haemangiomas and haemangioblastomas, renal cysts, renal cell adenocarcinoma, pancreatic tumours and phaeochromocytoma.

Eugen von Hippel, German ophthalmologist (1867–1939).

Arvid Lindau, Swedish pathologist (1892–1958).

4. C – Ataxia telangiectasia

Ataxia telangiectasia is an example of a hereditary ataxia. It is autosomal recessive and presents in childhood with progressive ataxia and athetosis (slow writhing movements). It is associated with the presence of telangiectasias on the conjunctiva, cheeks and ears. Patients also have immunodeficiency and are significantly predisposed to lymphoma and leukaemia.

Friedreich's ataxia is an autosomal recessive condition that presents in adolescence with ataxia and muscle weakness, hearing loss, dysarthria and optic atrophy. It is also associated with diabetes mellitus and cardiomyopathy. Examination may reveal areflexia, scoliosis and pes cavus (high-arched feet). Affected people are often wheelchair bound by 20 years.

Nikolaus Friedreich, German neurologist (1825–82).

5. H – Shy–Drager syndrome

Shy–Drager syndrome is a degenerative disease of the autonomic nervous system. It presents with parkinsonian symptoms (tremor, bradykinesia and rigidity) and features of autosomal failure (e.g. incontinence, postural hypotension, gastroparesis and erectile dysfunction).

Glenn Albert Shy, American physician (1917–67).

George Milton Drager, American neurologist (1919–67).

Theme 11: Overdose and antidotes

1. D – *N*-Acetylcysteine

Paracetamol is widely available, cheap and extremely toxic in overdose. It is one of the most common drugs implicated in intentional overdose, and is usually taken in combination with alcohol and other substances. There are usually no initial symptoms of paracetamol overdose, which often leads to the patient believing that they have caused no harm. Late features of overdose include vomiting, abdominal pain, bruising, jaundice and encephalopathy. If a patient presents with paracetamol overdose, a serum paracetamol level should be tested 4 hours after the overdose was taken, in addition to a full blood count, liver function tests, glucose and a coagulation screen. When a therapeutic dose of paracetamol is taken, the hepatotoxic metabolites are conjugated with glutathione, which neutralizes their toxicity. In paracetamol overdose, the endogenous glutathione pathways become saturated, allowing the hepatotoxic metabolites to build up and cause hepatic necrosis. *N*-Acetylcysteine is the first-line antidote in paracetamol overdose, and works by restoring the levels of glutathione. It should ideally be started within 8 hours of the patient taking the overdose, but can be given up to 24 hours after the overdose. If a patient presents more than 24 hours after overdose, a specialist liver unit should be contacted for advice.

The decision to treat with *N*-acetylcysteine is usually based upon the serum paracetamol level taken at least 4 hours after the overdose. The paracetamol level is applied to a normogram that plots the time since overdose against the serum paracetamol level. On the normogram, there is a low-risk treatment line and a high-risk treatment line. If the patient's paracetamol level is plotted above the treatment line, they will require *N*-acetylcysteine. If the patient is taking enzyme-inducing drugs or has pre-existing liver disease, the 'high-risk' treatment line should be used (which in practice means that this group are treated in the presence of lower serum paracetamol levels compared with patients who are not considered to be high risk). In cases of delayed presentation, extreme overdose, staggered overdose or unconsciousness, it is often appropriate to treat prior to taking a 4-hour paracetamol level. If the patient has had a prior allergic reaction to *N*-acetylcysteine, the alternative antidote is methionine.

2. B – Desferrioxamine

This patient has had a significant iron overdose requiring treatment. Although the exact number of tablets taken is not known it can be deduced that it was large, based upon the symptoms of severe abdominal pain and gastrointestinal bleeding caused by necrosis of the gastrointestinal mucosa. In severe disease, the patient can become encephalopathic and develop fulminant liver failure within days. Desferrioxamine is a chelating agent that binds free iron in the bloodstream and is used to treat significant iron overdose. It can be given as an intramuscular or intravenous preparation, with 100 mg binding approximately 8 mg of iron. Some patients will eventually require haemofiltration or haemodialysis.

3. A – Atropine

β-Blockers antagonize β-adrenergic receptors and, if taken in overdose, can result in bradycardia, hypotension, syncope and eventual heart failure. If a patient is haemodynamically unstable following a β-blocker overdose, they should be attached to a cardiac monitor, be given a 3 mg dose of intravenous atropine and receive intravenous fluid resuscitation. Atropine inhibits the parasympathetic vagal stimulation of the heart by competitively blocking muscarinic receptors. In the absence of vagal stimulation, the sinoatrial node depolarizes at a faster rate, which counteracts the actions of β-blockers, improving the heart rate and haemodynamic stability. If the atropine fails to reverse the bradycardia and haemodynamic stability, the patient can be given a dose of glucagon. Glucagon has been shown to improve heart rate, myocardial contraction and conduction in β-blocker overdose.

4. F – Flumazenil

This patient has had an overdose of a benzodiazepine. Benzodiazepine overdose can present with mild symptoms (e.g. blurred vision, lethargy and dizziness) or more significant symptoms (confusion, coma and cardiorespiratory arrest). The specific antidote for benzodiazepine overdose is flumazenil, which works by competitively inhibiting the benzodiazepine binding sites (γ-aminobutyric acid type A receptors: $GABA_A$). This drug has a number of contraindications and potentially life-threatening complications, and therefore should be used only in a life-threatening overdose when it can be confirmed that only a benzodiazepine has been taken. If prescribed to patients dependent on benzodiazepines, flumazenil can cause a rapid withdrawal, which can induce seizures. Flumazenil should never be given to patients who have a mixed overdose involving benzodiazepines and tricyclic antidepressants, since tricyclic antidepressants are known to lower the seizure threshold. In this situation, the antiepileptic properties of the benzodiazepine may be all that is preventing a life-threatening tricyclic-induced seizure. If flumazenil is administered, the antiepileptic benefit is lost.

5. H – Naloxone

This patient is suffering from a morphine overdose and is exhibiting the classic features of reduced responsiveness, pinpoint pupils and respiratory depression. This is a significant and potentially life-threatening overdose that will require treatment with naloxone. Naloxone competes with opiates for the μ receptors. It should be noted that naloxone has a very strong affinity for μ receptors and can therefore rapidly induce opiate withdrawal and trigger seizures. It has been known for intravenous drug users to be extremely annoyed at medical staff for ruining their 'high' with naloxone. Naloxone also has a shorter half-life compared with opiates, so repeated doses or an infusion may be required to maintain its beneficial effect.

Examples of antidotes for other substances used in overdose

- Antimuscarinic overdose: physostigmine
- Aspirin overdose: sodium bicarbonate
- Carbon monoxide poisoning: oxygen
- Digoxin overdose: Digibind (an anti-digoxin antibody fragment)
- Heparin overdose: protamine
- Methanol overdose: ethanol
- Warfarin overdose: vitamin K.

Theme 12: Extra-articular manifestations of rheumatoid arthritis

1. G – Mononeuritis multiplex

Mononeuritis multiplex is a form of peripheral neuropathy where there is damage to at least two anatomically distinct peripheral or spinal nerves. Apart from rheumatoid arthritis (RA), other causes include diabetes mellitus, polyarteritis nodosa and systemic lupus erythematosus.

2. M – Sjögren's syndrome

Sjögren's syndrome is characterized by dry eyes and a dry mouth. It can occur in isolation, but is associated with RA. For more information, see 'Connective tissue disease' (Paper 4 Answers, Theme 13).

3. F – Felty's syndrome

Anaemia in RA has four main underlying causes. There can be an anaemia of chronic disease, which tends to cause a normochromic normocytic anaemia (although 25% of cases are associated with a hypochromic microcytic picture). There may be an autoimmune haemolysis associated with the disease process. Some drug treatments of RA can result in anaemia, especially non-steroidal anti-inflammatory drugs and gold. The final reason is Felty's syndrome.

Felty's syndrome is a triad of RA, splenomegaly and hypersplenism (which results in pancytopenia). Sequelae of pancytopenia include anaemia and recurrent infections. Felty's syndrome is also associated with leg ulcers and lymphadenopathy. In some cases, splenectomy can improve symptoms.

Augustus Roi Felty, American physician (1895–1964).

4. E – Episcleritis

Episcleritis describes inflammation of the episclera, a thin membrane that covers the sclera. It presents with painless reddening of the eye. Episcleritis is common with autoimmune conditions, such as RA (as in this scenario). On examination, dilated blood vessels will be seen only in the superficial layer of the sclera. When a cotton bud is placed against the eye, these vessels can be moved over the sclera. Steroid eye drops provide symptomatic relief and aid recovery.

Scleritis is inflammation of the sclera, which is less common but more serious than episcleritis. Patients present with redness of the sclera (i.e. if you try moving the dilated vessels with a cotton bud, they will not budge), severe ocular pain and photophobia. Repeated episodes of scleritis can result in thinning of this membrane over time – *scleromalacia* – which is seen as a blue-tinged area in the sclera. This area is prone to perforation (*scleromalacia perforans*). All of these changes can occur with RA.

5. D – Caplan's syndrome

Caplan's syndrome (rheumatoid pneumoconiosis) is a combination of RA with large fibrous nodules in the peripheries of the lung seen in coal workers. It is very rare.

Other extra-articular manifestations of RA include amyloidosis, vasculitis and cardiopulmonary disease (e.g. pleural effusion and pericarditis).

Theme 13: Management of asthma

Asthma is the most common chronic respiratory disorder affecting children. The British Thoracic Society guidelines for the management of asthma are the gold standard in the UK. These can be found at www.brit-thoracic.org.uk.

1. C – Inhaled short-acting β_2-agonist

This boy has a new diagnosis of asthma and should be started on step 1 of the management ladder. He should be reassessed later and, if this has not been effective, inhaled steroids should be added.

For reference, the management of asthma follows a stepwise approach, summarized as follows:

Step 1: short-acting β_2-agonist (salbutamol, terbutaline)
Step 2: step 1 + low-dose inhaled steroids (budesonide, fluticasone)
Step 3: step 2 + high-dose inhaled steroids or long-acting β_2-agonist (salmeterol)

Step 4: high-dose inhaled steroids + long-acting β_2-agonist + other drugs: e.g. theophyllines, anticholinergics (ipratropium), leukotriene antagonists (montelukast), mast cell stabilizers (sodium cromoglicate)

Step 5: step 4 + oral steroids (prednisolone).

2. H – Oral leukotriene receptor antagonist

This boy is on step 3 of the stepwise approach to managing asthma. He needs escalation to step 4, with the addition of another drug. Examples of available medications include theophyllines (e.g. Uniphyllin Continus), anticholinergics (e.g. inhaled ipratropium bromide), leukotriene receptor antagonists (e.g. montelukast) and mast cell stabilizers (e.g. sodium cromoglicate). The aim of treatment in early asthma is to abolish or minimize symptoms, permit unrestrictive exercise and prevent exacerbations. In more severe disease, such as this, the aim is to achieve the best possible stable peak expiratory flow rate (PEFR) and improve symptoms with the fewest side-effects.

3. I – Oral steroids

This girl is being treated on step 4 unsuccessfully. Step 5 involves the addition of oral steroids (prednisolone) in the lowest dose that controls symptoms. This patient should be referred to a respiratory paediatrician if she is not already being seen by one. She should also have her inhaler technique reviewed and compliance checked.

4. M – Oxygen via facemask, nebulized short-acting β_2-agonist and steroids

This is a severe exacerbation of asthma. Features of severe asthma are:

- the patient is too breathless to finish sentences
- respiration rate ≥25/min
- pulse ≥100 beats/min
- peak flow ≤50% predicted or best.

Acute exacerbations of asthma should be treated immediately with 60% oxygen (via a mask), back-to-back nebulizers and systemic steroids (either oral prednisolone or intravenous hydrocortisone). Patients should have their oxygen saturations measured continuously, and have regular PEFR readings (e.g. every 15–30 minutes) and serial arterial blood gases.

5. D – Intravenous magnesium sulphate

This is a life-threatening exacerbation of asthma. Features of life-threatening asthma are:

- fatigue or exhaustion
- central cyanosis
- decreasing consciousness
- bradycardia
- silent chest or poor respiratory effort
- peak flow ≤33% predicted or best.

Additional treatment is required in this case, as the patient is not responding well. This can be provided with intravenous magnesium sulphate. If the patient deteriorates, she may require intubation and ventilation.

Theme 14: Investigation of cardiovascular disease

1. F – Exercise (stress) ECG

The resting ECG in patients with suspected ischaemic heart disease (IHD) is often normal and of limited diagnostic value. The exercise ECG was developed to aid in the diagnosis of IHD. The patient is placed on a treadmill and exercised according to a predetermined protocol while their blood pressure, heart rate and ECG are monitored. The most widely used programme is the Bruce protocol, where the speed and incline of the treadmill are increased every 3 minutes through a maximum of seven stages. A positive test is indicated by the development of ischaemic symptoms, ST elevation/depression, arrhythmia and a failure of the blood pressure to rise in response to exercise. The test should be stopped when there is ST elevation >2 mm in any lead, worsening ST depression, chest pain, shortness of breath or arrhythmia. Resuscitation equipment and glyceryl trinitrate spray should always be available when carrying out this investigation.

Robert A Bruce, American cardiologist (1916–2004).

2. N – Serum troponin

The most likely diagnosis in this scenario is a non-ST-elevation myocardial infarction (NSTEMI). Since the ECG in this condition is often non-specific, the diagnosis is based on the triad of history, examination and the presence of serum markers of myocardial necrosis (i.e. cardiac enzymes). Troponin is the most sensitive and cardiospecific marker currently available, and should be used in preference to the more traditional markers such as creatine kinase, lactate dehydrogenase and aspartate transaminase. Following myocardial infarction, troponin is released into the circulation from necrotic myocytes.

Serum troponin levels peak at 12 hours post-infarct and remain elevated for up to 10 days. The sensitivity of troponin in the diagnosis of myocardial infarction has been shown to be as high as 100% when measured 12 hours after the onset of symptoms. This compares with sensitivities as low as 21% when measured within the first 6 hours of symptoms. Therefore, serum troponin levels should be measured no less than 12 hours after the onset of symptoms. A negative serum troponin measured 12 hours after the onset of symptoms means that infarction is unlikely, but not impossible. Therefore, in this situation, a second troponin sample should be taken after a further 12 hours if the diagnosis remains uncertain. Troponin may also be elevated in other conditions, such as myocarditis, arrhythmia and pulmonary infarction, but to a lesser extent than with myocardial infarction.

3. E – Doppler ultrasound scan

This patient has a deep vein thrombosis (DVT). DVT usually presents with a red, swollen and painful leg with engorged superficial veins. Other conditions with similar presentations include cellulitis, ruptured Baker's cyst and peripheral oedema. The diagnosis of DVT is based upon the history, risk factor profile, examination findings and investigation. Risk factors include immobilization (e.g. after surgery), use of the oral contraceptive pill and hormone replacement therapy, smoking, malignancy, and thrombophilic conditions such as factor V Leiden mutation, antithrombin III deficiency and protein C or S deficiency.

The investigation of DVT usually consists of measuring serum D-dimer levels, followed by Doppler ultrasonography. D-dimers are fibrin degradation products that increase in the presence of thrombosis. However, they are a non-specific marker and also rise in a number of other conditions, such as infection, trauma, disseminated intravascular coagulation, and postoperatively. Despite being non-specific, D-dimers are rarely normal in patients with DVT/pulmonary embolism (PE). Therefore, patients with normal levels are very unlikely to have a DVT. Patients with plausible history and raised D-dimer levels require Doppler ultrasonography, which can identify a thrombosis and accurately locate its anatomical position. The management of DVT should begin immediately so as to reduce the risk of complications such as PE and post-thrombotic phlebitis. Treatment is with warfarin anticoagulation, aiming for an international normalized ratio (INR) between 2 and 3. During the first few days of treatment, when the INR is subtherapeutic, a low-molecular-weight heparin must also be prescribed. Warfarin therapy is usually continued for 6 months unless a clearly defined risk factor is identified and corrected, in which case, a 3-month period of treatment is usually sufficient.

Christian Doppler, Austrian physicist (1803–53). Described the Doppler effect – the apparent change in frequency and wavelength of a wave that is perceived by an observer moving relative to the source of the waves.

4. P – Transoesophageal echocardiography

This is a case of subacute bacterial endocarditis. Transoesophageal echocardiography (TOE) is the most accurate way to image the heart valves and view vegetations that may be present. TOE is a semi-invasive investigation in which an ultrasound probe is passed down the oesophagus to gain a better view of the heart. It is usually employed to look for cardiac sources of emboli, investigate valvular heart disease and review prosthetic valves. TOE also has a role in the investigation of aortic dissection, and is sometimes used to aid cardiothoracic surgery. Transthoracic echocardiography (TTE) is simpler and quicker to perform, especially in the emergency setting, but the views are not as accurate.

5. A – 24-hour ECG tape

This patient is experiencing episodic palpitations. The paroxysmal nature of his symptoms means that accurate diagnosis is difficult, as the resting ECG is often normal. An ambulatory ECG (Holter monitor) allows an ECG tracing to be taken continuously over 24 hours. The patient can go about their daily activities while being monitored. The longer period of monitoring increases the likelihood of gaining ECG evidence of an arrhythmia if indeed one exists.

Norman J Holter, American biophysicist (1914–83).

Theme 15: Gait disturbance 1

1. H – Sensory ataxia

Sensory ataxia occurs with a loss of joint position sense. Affected patients literally have to watch their feet, and they tend to place the foot on the ground with greater emphasis, especially in conditions of poor lighting. This can lead to stamping of the feet with walking ('stomping gait'). Sensory ataxia occurs with disorders affecting the dorsal column of the spinal cord (which controls joint position sense and vibration). Causes include tabes dorsalis of neurosyphilis and vitamin B_{12} deficiency (pernicious anaemia).

2. K – Waddling gait

Difficulty standing from a sitting position and trouble walking up stairs is indicative of proximal muscle weakness (i.e. hip girdles). This is a known side-effect of steroid use. If the muscles that stabilize the hip joint (the gluteus medius and minimus) are weak, the hips will not be fixed when the contralateral leg is lifted off the ground. This results in exaggerated trunk movements bilaterally, described as a waddling gait.

3. A – Antalgic gait

This woman has recently had a hip operation, and it is likely that there is some residual pain in the joint. When the manner of walking is adjusted to avoid acute pain, it is known as an antalgic gait.

Antalgic, from Greek *an* = without + *algos* = pain.

4. E – High-stepping gait

In the normal gait cycle, the toe strike follows the heel strike. If there is weakness of ankle dorsiflexion, there is poor control of foot descent and it becomes easy to catch the toes on the floor. In order to avoid this, the foot has to be lifted higher off the ground to allow space for the inadequately dorsiflexed foot to swing through. This is known as a high-stepping gait, and is caused by any condition that results in distal lower limb muscle weakness, including Guillain–Barré syndrome (this case), multiple sclerosis, Friedreich's ataxia and peroneal nerve injury.

5. I – Spastic gait

This child has cerebral palsy. The described deformity is characteristic of spasticity (hips adducted and internally rotated, knees flexed and ankles plantarflexed). In these circumstances, both lower limbs are moved slowly and dragged along the ground, with crossing of the legs due to adduction at the hip. Movement in the patient with bilateral spasticity is known as a scissoring gait.

Gait apraxia describes the case where there is normal power and sensation in the lower limbs and no evidence of cerebellar dysfunction, but the patient cannot formulate the motor action of walking. This represents a higher cerebral dysfunction where the patient 'forgets' how to walk. Gait apraxia occurs in bilateral hemisphere disease, e.g. normal-pressure hydrocephalus.

Practice Paper 10: Questions

Theme 1: Classification of stroke

Options

A. Lacunar stroke
B. Partial anterior circulation stroke
C. Posterior circulation stroke
D. Total anterior circulation stroke
E. Transient ischaemic attack

For each of the following scenarios, select the most appropriate type of cerebral infarction. Each option may be used once, more than once or not at all.

1. A 74-year-old man attends the emergency department after experiencing sudden-onset dizziness earlier in the day. He also has problems articulating his words and swallowing food.

2. A 68-year-old man presents with weakness in his left arm and leg. He also appears confused, and his wife says that this is new. On examination, there is no evidence of visual field deficit.

3. A 62-year-old man woke up one morning and noticed in the mirror that the right side of his face was drooping. He had no other problems. By the time he called his GP later that afternoon, the defect had resolved.

4. A 79-year-old woman suffers sudden-onset weakness in her left arm and leg. She denies any other problems. Examination reveals no cognitive or sensory impairment, or any visual field defect.

5. An 81-year-old woman is unable to get out of bed one morning because she is weak in her right arm and leg. You notice that she has trouble understanding what you ask her, although she can speak comprehensively. On examination, she is blind in the lateral half of the visual field of the right eye.

Theme 2: Psychiatric signs of physical illness

Options

A. Cushing's syndrome
B. Delirium
C. Hyperthyroidism
D. Hypothyroidism
E. Multiple sclerosis
F. Neurosyphilis
G. Pellagra
H. Punch-drunk syndrome
I. Space-occupying lesion
J. Systemic lupus erythematosus

For each of the following scenarios, select the most likely underlying physical cause. Each option may be used once, more than once or not at all.

1. A 58-year-old woman presents to the emergency department hearing voices. Her partner has noticed increased irritability, restlessness, change in behaviour and loss of libido over the past 2 months. On examination, she has a fine tremor, is underweight and has an irregular pulse.

2. A 45-year-old woman presents with low mood and tearfulness. She is upset about severe pains in her knees and hands and an embarrassing red rash over her face. She also complains of worsening shortness of breath.

3. A 42-year-old man presents with memory loss, and his wife says that he has been pointing at things in the room that are not there. For over a month, he has also had a headache that is worse in the mornings.

4. A 77-year-old woman is found by her carers confused and disorientated. She is usually lucid. The carers notice that she has been incontinent of urine.

5. A 34-year-old woman presents to her GP complaining of feeling sad all the time, difficulty sleeping, and weight gain. She has a history of Crohn's disease and is taking medication regularly for frequent exacerbations.

Theme 3: Respiratory diseases of childhood

Options

A. Aspiration of vomit
B. Asthma
C. Bronchiolitis
D. Croup
E. Cystic fibrosis
F. Epiglottitis
G. Infectious mononucleosis
H. Inhalation of foreign body
I. Pertussis

For each of the following scenarios, select the most appropriate diagnosis. Each option may be used once, more than once or not at all.

1. A 5-year-old unimmunized boy presents to the GP with a chronic cough. His mother reports that he has had this cough for 3 months. It started with a normal 'cold and cough', but he has not managed to shake it off. For the first 4 weeks, the cough would occur in bursts and he would get very distressed, occasionally going blue and vomiting.

2. A 2-year-old boy presents with a non-productive cough that started suddenly yesterday afternoon. He is otherwise well and has a temperature of 36.5°C. On examination, there are reduced breath sounds on the right side.

3. An 18-month-old girl presents with a non-productive cough and stridor. The cough is described as 'barking' in nature. She has a temperature of 38°C and is restless. She does not appear systemically unwell and is not cyanotic, but there is a moderate stridor on exertion.

4. A 7-year-old boy presents to the emergency department. His mother says that he has become very unwell very quickly. It started with a high fever and a sore throat. He is now very quiet, and is drooling while sitting upright on the edge of the bed. You examine him briefly, and he appears shocked and tachypnoeic and has a very faint stridor. He has a past medical history of asthma and has never been immunized.

5. A 6-month-old baby presents with a cough. The illness began 4 days ago with a runny nose and a mild fever. Over the last 24 hours, he has developed a high-pitched cough associated with a wheeze. On examination, crepitations are heard throughout the lung fields.

Theme 4: Haematemesis

Options

A. Arteriovenous malformation
B. Boerhaave's syndrome
C. Duodenal ulcer
D. Mallory–Weiss tear
E. Gastric ulcer
F. Gastric malignancy
G. Oesophageal varices
H. Oesophagitis
I. Peutz–Jeghers syndrome
J. Reactive gastritis

For each of the following scenarios, select the most likely diagnosis. Each option may be used once, more than once or not at all.

1. A 26-year-old man stumbles into the emergency department following an episode of blood-stained vomiting that occurred after a prolonged bout of retching. He is otherwise well.

2. A 45-year-old woman presents to the emergency department after vomiting blood. She suffers from chronic back pain, for which she takes regular analgesia. There is no other significant past history.

3. A 59-year-old man presents to the emergency department vomiting large amounts of blood. He has a history of alcoholic liver disease. On examination, he is tachycardic and hypotensive.

4. A 35-year-old man presents to the emergency department with severe upper abdominal pain and blood-stained vomit. On questioning, he admits to a long history of dyspepsia that is worse when he is hungry and at night.

5. A 69-year-old man presents to the emergency department after vomiting blood. On questioning he admits to a 4-month history of severe dyspepsia and has lost two stone (12 kg) in weight over this period.

Theme 5: Managing symptoms in palliative care

Options

A. Cyclizine
B. Diclofenac
C. Do nothing
D. Hyoscine butylbromide
E. Metoclopramide
F. Midazolam
G. Naloxone
H. Morphine, as oral solution, 5 mg as required
I. Morphine, as oral solution, 10 mg as required
J. Morphine, as oral solution, 15 mg as required
K. Patient-controlled analgesia system
L. Propofol infusion
M. Urgent chemotherapy
N. Urgent radiotherapy

For each of the following scenarios, select the most appropriate management option. Each option may be used once, more than once or not at all.

1. A 37-year-old man who is receiving palliative care for metastatic melanoma is complaining of nausea, and is vomiting several times a day. There are no signs of raised intracranial pressure. He is not taking any medication that may trigger nausea and has no neurological symptoms.

2. A 78-year-old woman with metastatic breast cancer who is receiving end-stage palliative care is noticed to be producing a gurgling sound on breathing. She does not appear to be distressed, but her family are concerned and worried that she is uncomfortable.

3. A 57-year-old man who is being managed in a hospice for metastatic lung cancer is complaining of pain that occurs towards the end of the day before he takes his night-time pain killers. He currently takes paracetamol 1 g four times daily, diclofenac 50 mg three times daily and modified-release morphine sulphate tablets 30 mg twice daily.

4. A 65-year-old man who is being palliatively managed for end-stage metastatic disease of unknown origin is restless and anxious during what is thought to be the last few hours of his life. The nurses believe that he is at significant risk of injury to himself.

5. A 68-year-old woman with pancreatic carcinoma and liver metastases is complaining of right upper quadrant abdominal pain that is preventing her from eating and interacting with her family.

Theme 6: Symptoms of cardiovascular disease

Options

A. Acute angina
B. Acute mesenteric infarction
C. Acute myocardial infarction
D. Acute pulmonary oedema
E. Chronic left ventricular failure (NYHA class I)
F. Chronic left ventricular failure (NYHA class III)
G. Drug side-effect
H. Epilepsy
I. Hypertrophic cardiomyopathy
J. Infective endocarditis
K. Mesenteric ischaemia
L. Postural hypotension
M. Rheumatic fever
N. Stokes–Adams collapse
O. Vasovagal syncope

For each of the following scenarios, select the most appropriate diagnosis. Each option may be used once, more than once or not at all.

1. A 75-year-old man wakes from sleep feeling extremely breathless and anxious. His breathlessness resolves after a few minutes of walking around the bedroom. He also mentions that he becomes very breathless during day-to-day activities such as climbing the stairs.

2. A 65-year-old man presents with a 6-hour history of shortness of breath and palpitations, and is coughing up pink frothy sputum. He refuses to be laid flat.

3. A 70-year-old man with known angina, hypertension and hyper-cholesterolemia is experiencing severe episodic abdominal pains. These occur approximately 30 minutes after eating. A gastroscopy and colonoscopy show no abnormalities.

4. A 12-year-old girl is complaining of lethargy, fever and shortness of breath. These symptoms were initially associated with painful and swollen knee joints, which have now resolved to be replaced by a swollen elbow joint. Apart from a recent sore throat, she is otherwise fit and well.

5. A 45-year-old woman with known Addison's disease collapsed while getting out of bed in the morning. She denies any chest pain or palpitations. She was unresponsive for 40 seconds, during which her 'legs twitched a little'. She recovered fully after 2 minutes. This has happened on several previous occasions when standing up from a lying or sitting position.

Theme 7: Statistics

Options

A. 15%
B. 25%
C. 50%
D. 67%
E. 50%
F. 87.5%
G. 1.5
H. 2.5
I. 3.0
J. 4.0
K. 6.0

A new blood test is being developed to help detect the presence of tuberculosis lung infection. In a trial, 1000 patients have been tested. The trial produces 200 positive results and 800 negative results. Of the 200 positive results, 100 are false positives. Of the 800 negative results, 100 are false negatives.

What is the:

1. Sensitivity
2. Specificity
3. Positive predictive value
4. Negative predictive value
5. Likelihood ratio.

Theme 8: Scoring the severity of pneumonia

Options

A. CURB 0 pneumonia
B. CURB 1 pneumonia
C. CURB 2 pneumonia
D. CURB 3 pneumonia
E. CURB 4 pneumonia
F. CURB 5 pneumonia
G. Not a pneumonia

For each of the following scenarios, select the most appropriate degree of severity of the pneumonia. Each option may be used once, more than once or not at all.

1. A 55-year-old man presents with a cough productive of purulent sputum. A chest X-ray shows left basal consolidation. Other investigations show a blood pressure of 118/78 mmHg, respiratory rate 18/min and urea 5.4 mmol/L. He scores 10/10 on the Abbreviated Mental Test Score (AMTS).

2. A 69-year-old man presents with a cough productive of purulent sputum. A chest X-ray shows left basal consolidation. Other investigations show a blood pressure of 86/62 mmHg, respiratory rate 34/min and urea 9.6 mmol/L. He scores 6/10 on the AMTS.

3. A 71-year-old man presents with a cough productive of purulent sputum. A chest X-ray shows no evidence of consolidation. Other investigations show a blood pressure of 96/68 mmHg, respiratory rate 28/min and urea 6.6 mmol/L. He scores 9/10 on the AMTS.

4. A 71-year-old man presents with a cough productive of purulent sputum. A chest X-ray shows left basal consolidation. Other investigations show a blood pressure of 96/68 mmHg, respiratory rate 32/min and urea 8.3 mmol/L. He scores 9/10 on the AMTS.

5. A 42-year-old man presents with a cough productive of purulent sputum. A chest X-ray shows left basal consolidation. Other investigations show a blood pressure of 106/78 mmHg, respiratory rate 24/min and urea 7.3 mmol/L. He scores 10/10 on the AMTS.

Theme 9: Complications of HIV infection 2

Options

A. Candidiasis
B. Cryptococcus infection
C. Cryptosporidiosis
D. Cytomegalovirus infection
E. HIV dementia
F. HIV-wasting syndrome
G. Kaposi's sarcoma
H. Lichen planus
I. *Mycobacterium avium* complex
J. Pneumocystis infection
K. Seroconversion
L. Stevens–Johnson syndrome
M. Toxoplasmosis

For each of the following people with HIV infection, select the most likely complication. Each option may be used once, more than once or not at all.

1. A 37-year-old man presents to the GP with lumps in his neck. He says that he had the flu last month and the lumps appeared only since then. He is otherwise well. On examination, cervical lymphadenopathy is palpable. A subsequent HIV test returns positive.

2. A 25-year-old man presents to the GP with abdominal pain and watery diarrhoea. He has had these symptoms for 6 weeks and there is no sign of improvement. The patient has lost a stone (6 kg) in weight over the last month. On examination, he is significantly dehydrated. He is known to be HIV positive.

3. A 31-year-old woman presents to the emergency department with severe bilateral eye pain and blurring of vision. This was preceded by 3 days of flu-like symptoms. On examination, there are palpable cervical lymph nodes and there is some vague abdominal tenderness. She is known to be HIV positive.

4. A 45-year-old man presents to the GP with a skin rash. He has two purple lesions on his left upper arm that developed over the last week. The lesions are both 2 cm in size. There is no pain or itching. The man is known to have HIV infection.

5. A 52-year-old woman presents to the GP with a 3-week history of worsening shortness of breath and cough productive of sputum. She has also developed fevers and night sweats. Auscultation of the lungs reveals crackles in the upper zones on both sides. She is known to have HIV infection.

Theme 10: Management of cardiovascular disease

Options

A. Adenosine
B. Atenolol
C. Digoxin
D. Non-steroidal anti-inflammatory drugs
E. Paracetamol
F. Streptokinase
G. Sublingual glyceryl trinitrate
H. Synchronized DC cardioversion
I. Tenecteplase alone
J. Tenecteplase followed by intravenous heparin infusion
K. Unsynchronized DC cardioversion
L. Verapamil
M. Warfarin

For each of the following presentations, select the most appropriate management plan. Each option may be used once, more than once or not at all.

1. A 67-year-old man presents to the emergency department with palpitations. He has known ischaemic heart disease and hypertension. On examination, he is pale and appears confused, and his hands are cool and clammy. His pulse is 160 beats/min and irregularly irregular, his blood pressure is 70/40 mmHg and his capillary refill time is 6 s.

2. A 45-year-old woman presents to her GP with a 2-day history of central chest pain. The pain does not radiate and there is no associated shortness of breath. She only gains relief by sitting forward in bed at night. Examination is unremarkable, and an ECG performed in the practice shows ST elevation in V1, V4 and aVL. She has a past history of rheumatoid arthritis.

3. A 25-year-old asthmatic man presents to the emergency department with palpitations. Examination reveals a regular heart rate of 168 beats/min. The ECG shows a regular narrow complex tachycardia with no obvious P-waves. The Valsalva manoeuvre and carotid sinus massage have failed to slow the heart rate.

4. A 69-year-old man presents with central chest pain radiating to his left arm that came on suddenly at rest 1 hour ago. He is nauseous, sweaty and short of breath. He describes the pain as similar to that when he had a heart attack 4 years previously, during which he received a 'clot-busting' drug that he was instructed never to have again. The ECG shows ST elevation of 4 mm in V2, V3 and V4. On questioning, he has no contraindications to thrombolysis. Aspirin, clopidogrel, morphine and metoclopramide have been given so far.

5. A 57-year-old man with known end-stage renal failure awaiting renal transplantation collapses at home with chest pain. He is brought to the emergency department attached to a cardiac monitor. The monitor shows a regular broad complex tachycardia with a rate of 230 beats/min. On examination, the carotid pulse is not palpable.

Theme 11: Gait disturbance 2

Options

A. Antalgic gait
B. Cerebellar ataxia
C. Extrapyramidal gait
D. Gait apraxia
E. High-stepping gait
F. Marche à petit pas
G. Pyramidal gait
H. Sensory ataxia
I. Spastic gait
J. Trendelenburg gait
K. Waddling gait

For each of the following scenarios, select the most appropriate gait disturbance. Each option may be used once, more than once or not at all.

1. A 66-year-old man presents with recurrent falls. He denies any other problems. On examination, he has multiple spider naevi on his face and gynaecomastia. There is no neurological weakness, but he does display past-pointing. You notice that he places his feet wide apart when he walks.

2. A 66-year-old man presents with recurrent falls. He says that he has difficulty starting to walk and that, once he has started, he speeds up uncontrollably. On examination, he has a tremor in his arms.

3. A 66-year-old man presents with recurrent falls. Since an operation for a left hip replacement last year, he has been finding it difficult to walk. He cannot manage to stabilize his body when he lifts his right leg. There is no pain in his lower limbs.

4. A 66-year-old man presents with recurrent falls. He was admitted to hospital only last month with weakness in his right arm and leg. On examination, his right arm is flexed at the elbow and his right leg is extended at the hip. When he walks, he swings his right leg out to stop it from dragging.

5. A 66-year-old man presents with recurrent falls. On examination, he walks with small, slow steps, but there is no inconsistency in his speed. He has a history of ischaemic heart disease and is currently under follow-up for dementia.

Theme 12: Treatment of gastrointestinal disease

Options

A. Colectomy
B. Infliximab
C. Intravenous antibiotics
D. Intravenous fluids
E. Lifestyle advice
F. Oesophageal stenting
G. Oesophagectomy
H. Oral antibiotics
I. Oral rehydration therapy
J. Phosphate enema
K. Prednisolone enema
L. Sulfasalazine

For each of the following scenarios, select the most appropriate management. Each option may be used once, more than once or not at all.

1. A 16-year-old boy presents with a 4-day history of diarrhoea and vomiting. On examination, his mucous membranes are slightly dry, but his skin turgor is good. There is vague generalized abdominal tenderness. Prior to this illness, he was well.

2. A 54-year-old man presents with severe abdominal pain and bloody diarrhoea. He is already taking regular oral prednisolone and sulfasalazine for ulcerative colitis. Examination reveals diffuse abdominal tenderness. An abdominal X-ray is unremarkable.

3. A 67-year-old man is having increasing difficulty swallowing, and this is adversely affecting his eating habits and making him miserable. He has recently been diagnosed with metastatic oesophageal adenocarcinoma.

4. A 45-year-old woman has a long history of constipation. This is the first time that she is telling a doctor about it, and she wants to know what can be done. She is otherwise well and physical examination is unremarkable.

5. A 24-year-old woman has Crohn's disease of the small bowel. She is on steroid therapy and mesalazine, but is still having frequent severe symptoms.

Theme 13: Autoantibodies 2

Options

A. Anti-centromere
B. Anti-dsDNA
C. Anti-Jo-1
D. Anti-Ro
E. Anti-topoisomerase II
F. Anti-U1-RNP
G. Anticardiolipin
H. cANCA
I. pANCA
J. Rheumatoid factor

For each of the following scenarios, select the autoantibody that is most specific. Each option may be used once, more than once or not at all.

1. A 47-year-old woman complains that the skin of her fingers is becoming tight and it is becoming difficult for her to type. She is also having some problems swallowing. On examination, you notice that she has tight skin on both arms distal to the elbow and a furrowed mouth.

2. A 56-year-old woman has a 2-month history of progressive weakness in her hips. She finds it especially difficult to walk up the stairs at home. On examination, both hips are tender. She also has a purple rash over her eyelids.

3. A 28-year-old man presents with a 2-month history of pain in the small joints of his hand. He has also developed a rash on his cheeks and nose, which he feels gets worse in the sun.

4. A 41-year-old man has had frequent nosebleeds over the last month. He has never had one before this. In addition, he has recently started coughing up blood. Examination is unremarkable.

5. A 26-year-old woman presents with sudden left-sided weakness, and a stroke is diagnosed. She has a past history of a left-sided deep vein thrombosis and a pulmonary embolus. Routine blood tests show a haemoglobin of 12.5 g/dL, a white cell count of 8×10^9/L and a platelet count of 68×10^9/L.

Theme 14: Diagnosis of endocrine disorders

Options

A. Acromegaly
B. Addison's disease
C. Carcinoid tumour
D. Congenital adrenal hyperplasia
E. Conn's syndrome
F. Cushing's syndrome
G. Hyperparathyroidism
H. Hypoparathyroidism
I. Multiple endocrine neoplasia type 1
J. Multiple endocrine neoplasia type 2A
K. Multiple endocrine neoplasia type 2B
L. Nelson's syndrome
M. Phaeochromocytoma

For each of the following scenarios, select the most appropriate diagnosis. Each option may be used once, more than once or not at all.

1. A 54-year-old man presents to the clinic complaining of paraesthesiae in both of his hands and a headache. He has also noticed a slight change in his appearance, mentioning that his nose looks bigger. He has a past medical history of hypertension and diabetes. On examination, you find abnormal sensation in the lateral three-and-a-half digits of the hands.

2. A 52-year-old woman presents with increased skin pigmentation. She denies using sunbeds or sunbathing. You note that she has been treated for Cushing's disease in the past.

3. A 34-year-old man presents to the emergency department with epigastric pain. He admits having had brain surgery in the past for a tumour that caused him to produce milk. While you are taking a history, the patient suffers a large haematemesis, and an urgent endoscopy is arranged. The endoscopist notes multiple large ulcers throughout the stomach, duodenum and jejunum.

4. A 48-year-old woman presents with frequency of urine and excessive thirst. She also complains of occasional muscle cramps. She has history of hypertension, but is not on any regular medication. Her capillary glucose is 4.2 mmol/L, and routine blood tests show a sodium of 148 mmol/L and a potassium of 3.2 mmol/L.

5. A 24-year-old man presents to his GP with a lump in his neck that has been growing slowly over a few weeks. On examination, you note that he is tall and has long digits. He tells you that his father died of adrenal cancer.

Theme 15: Dermatomes 2

Options

A. C1
B. C2
C. C4
D. C5
E. C7
F. C8
G. T4
H. T6
I. T10
J. L1
K. L3
L. L5
M. S1
N. S3
O. S5
P. Trigeminal nerve

For each of the following descriptions, select the most appropriate dermatome. Each option may be used once, more than once or not at all.

1. This dermatome supplies the dorsum of the foot.

2. This dermatome supplies the middle finger.

3. This dermatome supplies the cheek.

4. This dermatome supplies the skin over the inguinal ligament.

5. This dermatome supplies the little finger.

Practice Paper 10: Answers

Theme 1: Classification of stroke

1. C – Posterior circulation stroke

2. B – Partial anterior circulation stroke

3. E – Transient ischaemic attack

4. A – Lacunar stroke

5. D – Total anterior circulation stroke

An *acute focal stroke* is characterized by a sudden focal deficit, usually vascular in origin. The majority are ischaemic in origin (85%) and the remainder haemorrhagic (15%). A *transient ischaemic attack* (TIA) is a focal deficit that resolves within 24 hours. This deficit may include focal weakness (e.g. facial drooping) or amaurosis fugax (transient sudden vision loss in one eye due to passage of embolus through the retinal artery). A *complete stroke* is one with a persisting deficit that is not worsening. An *evolving stroke* is one where the deficit continues to worsen 6 hours after the onset (due to progressive artery occlusion).

The classification of acute stroke was first described by Bamford and the Oxfordshire Community Stroke Project in the 1990s as follows. A *total anterior circulation stroke (TACS)* results in a triad of hemiplegia, hemianopia and higher cortical dysfunction (e.g. aphasia and visuospatial problems). A *partial anterior circulation stroke (PACS)* displays two of the above three features. A *posterior circulation stroke (POCS)* affects the brain stem, resulting in vertigo, dysphagia, dysarthria and facial weakness. A *lacunar stroke (LACS)* is a pure motor stroke (hemiparesis), a pure sensory stroke or a combination of the two. The deficit in an LACS must involve two of the face, leg and hand. Furthermore, there must be no visual field defect, no higher cortical dysfunction, no brain stem disturbance and no drowsiness in an LACS.

John Bamford, British neurologist.

Theme 2: Psychiatric signs of physical illness

1. C – Hyperthyroidism

Thyroid disease is one of the most common endocrine disorders. Thyroid dysfunction results in systemic symptoms. Psychological symptoms of hyperthyroidism include irritability, behavioural changes, restlessness, loss of libido, weight loss despite an increased appetite and, in extreme cases, psychosis (mania). Psychological symptoms of hypothyroidism include depression, tiredness, reduced libido, cognitive impairment, and occasionally psychosis or coma. The accompanying physical symptoms of tremor, weight loss and atrial fibrillation in this case confirm hyperthyroidism. Investigations should proceed with measurement of thyroid hormones, expecting to find a raised thyroxine with low levels of thyroid-stimulating hormone.

2. J – Systemic lupus erythematosus

Systemic lupus erythematosus (SLE) is an autoimmune connective tissue disease. There is a very broad range of physical signs and symptoms. It can also cause depression, seizures and psychosis. A few of the possible physical manifestations mentioned in this case are malar (butterfly) rash, arthralgia, and shortness of breath, which could be caused by lung fibrosis or several other pulmonary conditions.

3. I – Space-occupying lesion

Cerebral tumours should be considered as a differential diagnosis of psychiatric illness. Such space-occupying lesions present with headache that is worse in the mornings and exacerbated by bending, straining and coughing. Possible psychological and psychiatric manifestations include impaired consciousness, irritability, apathy, hallucinations, seizures, neuroses and psychosis.

4. B – Delirium

This woman has a urinary tract infection causing delirium. Delirium is characterized by fluctuating impairment of consciousness, mood changes and abnormal perceptions. It affects 10–25% of people aged over 65 years on medical wards. The patient may be obviously confused, with disruptive behaviour and expressing bizarre ideas, but it is important to recognize that it can also cause a decreased level of activity and speech. It develops over a short period of time and is caused by an underlying physical condition. Common causes are infection, hypoxia, electrolyte disturbances, constipation, drugs and central nervous system disease. The main principle of management is to investigate and treat the cause, but also to concurrently help relieve distress to the patient by optimizing their ability to orientate themselves. There should be a calm environment with adequate lighting, even at night. Patients should be wearing their glasses and hearing aids (if applicable), have continuity of staff contact where possible, and ideally have family members or familiar belongings around them. In some circumstances, oral or intramuscular haloperidol or benzodiazepines can be used to relieve severe agitation, but they should be avoided where possible. The average duration of delirium is 7 days. Around 40% of patients with delirium die of the underlying condition and 5% go on to develop dementia.

5. A – Cushing's syndrome

The features of Cushing's syndrome are due to raised levels of glucocorticoids from any sources. Causes include steroid use, ectopic adrenocorticotrophic hormone secretion and a pituitary tumour (Cushing's disease). In addition to the physical features (hirsutism, striae, acne, plethora, bruising, thin skin and cataracts), psychological features include depression, insomnia, reduced libido and occasionally psychosis.

Punch-drunk syndrome (also known as post-traumatic dementia or boxing encephalopathy) occurs after repeated blows to the head. Brain atrophy is a feature. Clinical features are cognitive impairment and personality deterioration with cerebellar, extrapyramidal and pyramidal signs. Occasionally, pathological jealousy and rage reactions are associated. *Pellagra* is a disorder caused by niacin (vitamin B_3) deficiency. It is most common in South America, where maize forms the staple diet. The main physical features are weakness, dermatitis and diarrhoea. There can also be personality changes, progressing to dementia. Treatment is with niacin. Death can occur within a few years if the condition is untreated.

Theme 3: Respiratory diseases of childhood

1. I – Pertussis

Whooping cough is caused by the bacterium *Bordetella pertussis*. The illness usually begins with coryza, and a dry cough develops a few days later. This cough becomes more pronounced and occurs in paroxysms. Repeated episodes of coughing classically then end with an inspiratory 'whoop'. Another name for pertussis is the '100-day cough', as the symptoms often continue for that duration. There is no treatment that will change the course of the illness, although erythromycin is said to reduce the period of infectivity. Complications are uncommon, but include pneumonia and bronchiectasis. Immunization does not give total protection, and protection is not necessarily lifelong.

Pertussis, from Latin *per* = throughout + *tussus* = cough ('intensive coughing').

2. H – Inhalation of foreign body

Foreign-body inhalation is most common in toddlers, as they are prone to putting objects in their mouths. The most common offenders are small toys and peanuts. Most foreign bodies present immediately. However, some may be delayed by weeks to months before symptoms develop. At the time of swallowing, the child has sudden-onset cough, wheeze or breathlessness. If the object is stuck in the larynx, it causes a croupy cough and stridor. If the object becomes stuck in the bronchus, there may initially be no symptoms until an infection develops several days later. Inhaled foreign bodies may be diagnosed radiologically, but rigid bronchoscopy will confirm the diagnosis and remove the offending object.

3. D – Croup

Croup (laryngotracheobronchitis) typically follows a viral upper respiratory tract infection, and accounts for 95% of laryngeotracheal infections in children. The main causative pathogen is parainfluenza virus. Croup commonly affects children under the age of 2 years, and can be very distressing for parents. These children often have a barking cough, harsh stridor and a low-grade fever (compared with the high-grade fever in epiglottitis). Various croup scores have been devised to assess for the degree of stridor, cyanosis, respiratory distress, air entry and consciousness. Management options include humidified air and steroids (nebulized or oral) to relieve the inflammation. In severe cases, the airway compromise can be significant enough to require adrenaline. Antibiotics are of no use.

4. F – Epiglottitis

Acute epiglottitis is a life-threatening emergency caused by *Haemophilus influenzae* type b. A toxic-looking child with stridor, drooling and fever strongly suggests acute epiglottitis. The child sits upright and immobile to optimize the airway. *Do not* be reassured by a quiet stridor or a quiet wheeze. This is often a sign that the airway is almost closed and very little air can be moved. Examination of the throat should only be performed by an ENT surgeon in an intensive care unit with facilities to intubate and protect the airway. *Do not* attempt to examine the throat yourself or make the child lie down, as this may precipitate airway obstruction. Treatment is with intravenous antibiotics (e.g. a cephalosporin), with rifampicin prophylaxis being given to all contacts.

5. C – Bronchiolitis

Bronchiolitis is very common, and can be life threatening, especially to at-risk groups (premature babies, heart disease, etc.). Bronchiolitis is caused by viruses, most commonly respiratory syncytial virus (RSV). Respiratory distress (intercostal recession, head bobbing and nasal flaring) and wheezing are caused by obstruction of the small airways. Auscultation may reveal fine inspiratory crepitations. Bronchiolitis can be confirmed by taking swabs of nasopharyngeal secretions. Most infants do not require admission, although some may need support for hydration and oxygenation. Antibiotics, steroids and bronchodilators are not effective.

Infectious mononucleosis (glandular fever) is caused by the Epstein–Barr virus (EBV). Symptoms are varied, and include fever, malaise, pharyngitis, tonsillitis and lympadenopathy. Other features are petechiae on the soft palate, jaundice, splenomegaly and hepatomegaly Symptoms may persist for as long as 3 months. Infectious mononucleosis is diagnosed by finding atypical lymphocytes on the blood film or by demonstrating the presence of heterophile antibodies (i.e. antibodies that agglutinate sheep or horse erythrocytes but that are not absorbed by guinea-pig kidney extracts). This is known as the monospot test or the Paul Bunnell test. Treatment is symptomatic.

Theme 4: Haematemesis

1. D – Mallory–Weiss tear

A Mallory–Weiss tear is a superficial tearing of the oesophageal mucosa at the gastro-oesophageal junction secondary to prolonged and forceful vomiting, such as that associated with alcohol intoxication and bulimia nervosa. It usually presents with a history of vomiting followed by haematemesis. The majority of patients recover with supportive treatment. A minority will require endoscopic or surgical repair of the defect.

George Kenneth Mallory, American pathologist (1900–86).

Soma Weiss, Hungarian physician (1898–1942).

2. J – Reactive gastritis

The most likely diagnosis in this case is reactive gastritis with gastric erosions secondary to non-steroidal anti-inflammatory drug (NSAID) use. NSAIDs cause gastritis by inhibiting the synthesis of gastroprotective prostaglandins. Patients with NSAID-related gastritis may be asymptomatic or experience dyspepsia, haematemesis and melaena. If gastritis or peptic ulceration is suspected in patients taking NSAIDs, the drug should be stopped immediately and the patient should be prescribed a proton pump inhibitor. If the drug is necessary for the management of an underlying condition, it may be reintroduced with caution in combination with a proton pump inhibitor once the acute phase has resolved, but should be reviewed regularly. Other medications associated with gastritis and peptic ulceration include corticosteroids, calcium channel blockers, nitrites and theophylline.

3. G – Oesophageal varices

Patients with cirrhosis of the liver and portal hypertension are at risk of developing oesophageal varices due to portosystemic shunting. The distended and tortuous varices are usually found at the gastro-oesophageal junction and are prone to acute and torrential bleeding, causing haematemesis and melaena. The initial management of severe upper gastrointestinal bleeding involves securing the patient's airway and assessing breathing before establishing good venous access and initiating fluid resuscitation with a crystalloid or a colloid until matched blood products are available. If blood products are required urgently, unmatched O-negative blood can be given until cross-matched products are available for administration. Patients with liver disease may also have deranged coagulation due to impaired production of clotting factors. If clotting derangement is suspected, fresh frozen plasma or cryoprecipitate can be given to correct clotting factor deficiency. Definitive management requires therapeutic endoscopy, during which the bleeding varices are sclerosed or banded. If endoscopy cannot be achieved quickly, or if the patient suffers a torrential re-bleed, a Sengstaken–Blakemore tube can be inserted into the oesophagus to provide temporary balloon tamponade of the bleeding vessels.

4. C – Duodenal ulcer

Duodenal ulcers account for 80% of peptic ulcers, and usually present with a history of cyclic dyspepsia that is exacerbated by hunger and relieved by eating. The major risk factors for developing duodenal ulceration are *Helicobacter pylori* infection and NSAID use. Patients with proven uncomplicated duodenal ulceration should be offered lifestyle advice (healthy diet, smoking cessation and reduced alcohol intake) and should be started on a proton pump inhibitor. If *H. pylori* infection is confirmed, eradication therapy should be started (e.g. a 7-day course of metronidazole, clarithromycin and omeprazole). Patients who present with acute haematemesis secondary to a suspected bleeding ulcer should be stabilized and undergo urgent endoscopy, during which the operator can attempt to establish haemostasis by injecting adrenaline (epinephrine) or initiating coagulation. An intravenous proton pump inhibitor should be started in the acute setting, especially if there are endoscopic signs of active bleeding or a significant risk of re-bleeding. If haemostasis cannot be achieved, or there is evidence of duodenal perforation, surgical repair may be required. Once stabilization has been achieved, long-term management is as for uncomplicated duodenal ulcers.

5. F – Gastric malignancy

Haematemesis that is preceded by a history of new dyspepsia, significant weight loss and prolonged vomiting should raise the suspicion of gastric malignancy. Acute haematemesis secondary to gastric malignancy usually occurs when the lesion erodes through a vessel, although it is more common for chronic bleeding to occur, resulting in iron-deficiency anaemia and melaena. The acute management of haematemesis is the same as for any other cause of upper gastrointestinal bleeding. During endoscopy, multiple biopsies should be taken from suspicious lesions, including gastric ulcers. Once stable, the patient should be examined and investigated for other features of gastrointestinal malignancy such as iron-deficiency anaemia, Virchow's node, hepatomegaly, acanthosis nigricans and Sister Joseph's nodule.

Theme 5: Managing symptoms in palliative care

1. A – Cyclizine

Vomiting is a common symptom in patients with cancer. It can be secondary to metabolic disturbance, raised intracranial pressure, chemotherapy and mechanical obstruction of the gastrointestinal tract. Nausea and vomiting are distressing, and can have a severe impact on a patient's quality of life. Regular antiemetics are the mainstay of treatment. In cases where the mechanical effects of the tumour are to blame, other methods such as radiotherapy and surgery may be indicated. Cyclizine is an antihistamine antiemetic that acts centrally to inhibit the histamine-dependent stimulation of the vomiting centre via the chemoreceptor trigger zone. It is particularly useful in vomiting due to metabolic disturbance and chemotherapy. Prokinetic antiemetics such as metoclopramide, which are useful in vomiting due to gastric stasis, should be avoided if bowel obstruction is suspected. If vomiting is not improved by a single agent, a second agent should be added. The 5-HT_3 (serotonin receptor) antagonists such as ondansetron are very effective, but are also very expensive. Other antiemetics available include dexamethasone, haloperidol and domperidone.

2. D – Hyoscine butylbromide

The presence of uncleared respiratory secretions in dying people can produce unpleasant sounds when the patient breathes ('death rattle'), which can cause distress to the patient's family and loved ones. Hyoscine butylbromide is an antimuscarinic drug that reduces the production of secretions. It is fast acting and can be given via the oral, subcutaneous or intravenous route. Dyspnoea is also a common symptom at the end of life, and can be secondary to position, respiratory tract obstruction and anxiety. Opiate medication can help relax the patient and reduce the sensation of dyspnoea. Radiotherapy may be used to reduce the size of tumours obstructing the respiratory tract.

3. I – Morphine, as oral solution, 10 mg as required

Pain is one of the most feared symptoms in patients diagnosed with cancer. The management of pain in palliative care should involve the analgesic ladder, starting off with drugs such as paracetamol and stepping up the ladder if pain is not controlled until opiate medication is required. The key to good pain management is prevention rather than cure, i.e. regular analgesia should be prescribed rather than 'as required' analgesia. Morphine is available as modified-release ('slow-release') oral preparations of morphine sulphate given in one or two regular doses each day (e.g. MST Continus tablets or MXL capsules, respectively). The patient in this case is taking such a preparation, but is still suffering from breakthrough pain. Breakthrough pain can be initially controlled using a single dose of a short-acting opiate, such as an oral solution of morphine (Oramorph) or standard ('immediate-release') tablets. The dose of short-acting opiate should be one-sixth of the total daily dose of regular opiates. In this case, the patient is taking a total of 60 mg of morphine sulphate daily, and will therefore require 10 mg of morphine in oral solution for breakthrough pain. If the patient is consistently requiring additional opiates, they should have their regular analgesia increased or changed. Alternative routes of delivery of analgesia should also be considered, such as continuous delivery via a syringe driver or using a patient-controlled analgesia system (PCA).

4. F – Midazolam

Terminal restlessness is a common feature in dying patients. It is a multi-aetiological condition that can involve anxiety, metabolic disturbance, infection and the presence of brain pathology. It is often distressing to relatives and may place the patient at risk of injury and harm. Once other causes of confusion have been eliminated and environmental conditions optimized (familiar faces and items, a well-lit room, a clock, etc.) it is often necessary to sedate the patient. Midazolam, a benzodiazepine, is commonly used in the management of terminal restlessness. If there are significant psychotic features then haloperidol, a neuroleptic drug, may be used. These medications can be given subcutaneously and intramuscularly, either as a one-off dose or as a continuous infusion using a syringe driver.

5. B – Diclofenac

This patient is suffering from liver capsule pain secondary to the presence of liver metastases. This kind of pain may reduce a patient's quality of life and suppress their appetite. Non-steroidal anti-inflammatory drugs, such as diclofenac, are particularly effective at treating liver capsule pain.

Theme 6: Symptoms of cardiovascular disease

1. F – Chronic left ventricular failure (NYHA class III)

This patient is experiencing paroxysmal nocturnal dyspnoea (PND), a symptom of significant left ventricular failure, where the patient suddenly wakes from sleep with severe breathlessness. To relieve this symptom, the patient usually sits upright, and often opens a window in an attempt to improve breathing. PND is caused by pulmonary oedema. During the night, the reabsorption of dependent oedema into the circulation causes the pulmonary venous pressure to gradually increase and force fluid into the alveolar spaces. Since the patient is asleep and has a lower level of consciousness, the pulmonary oedema is able to build up to significant levels before the patient becomes aware. In addition to PND, this patient is complaining of a severe limitation of activities of daily living, which places him in class III according to the New York Heart Association (NYHA) classification of heart failure.

NYHA classification of heart failure

Class	*Symptoms and activities of daily living (ADL)*
I	No symptoms, with ordinary physical activity and no limitation of ADL
II	Mild symptoms, with ordinary activity and slight limitation of ADL. Asymptomatic at rest
III	Symptoms occur at less than normal activity and there is significant limitation of ADL. Asymptomatic at rest
IV	Severe limitation of ADL. Symptoms present at rest

2. D – Acute pulmonary oedema

Acute pulmonary oedema can be caused by a number of conditions, including myocardial infarction, endocarditis, cardiac tamponade, acute renal failure, acute respiratory distress syndrome and inhalation of toxins. In this condition, there is a build-up of fluid in the alveolar spaces, causing the patient to become acutely short of breath and have a cough that is productive of pink, frothy sputum. On examination, the patient is usually peripherally shut down, hypotensive, tachypnoeic, tachycardic and oxygenating poorly. On auscultation, there are usually widespread fine crackles throughout the lung fields. There may also be a gallop rhythm caused by the presence of third and fourth heart sounds on auscultation of the heart.

The treatment of acute pulmonary oedema aims to reduce the amount of fluid in the lung, improve myocardial oxygenation and maintain vital organ perfusion until the underlying condition can be corrected, e.g. thrombolysis in myocardial infarction. The treatment usually includes oxygen, furosemide, nitrates and opiates. Furosemide causes systemic vasodilatation, which reduces cardiac preload and improves cardiac output. Nitrates are prescribed if the systolic blood pressure is above 90 mmHg; they work by initiating systemic vasodilatation and reducing preload. Intravenous opiates, i.e. morphine or diamorphine, reduce anxiety and improve the sensation of dyspnoea. In addition, opiates cause vasodilatation of the coronary arteries and therefore improve myocardial oxygenation. If the patient fails to respond to standard therapies, inotropic agents such as dobutamine should be considered with senior input.

3. K – Mesenteric ischaemia

Mesenteric ischaemia is caused by atherosclerotic disease of the coeliac trunk and mesenteric arteries. Stenosis of the mesenteric arteries leads to inadequate perfusion of the bowel at times of increased oxygen demand, such as when digesting food. The condition usually presents with severe, griping abdominal pain 15–45 minutes after eating. Patients often fear to eat, because of the anticipation of pain, and can lose significant amounts of weight as a result. Mesenteric ischaemia must be differentiated from acute mesenteric infarction, which occurs when a local atherosclerotic plaque ruptures or when the artery becomes occluded by an embolus from a distant source, e.g. the left atrium in atrial fibrillation. Mesenteric infarction is extremely painful and typically lacks clinical signs. If it is suspected, an urgent surgical opinion is warranted.

Mesentery, from Greek *mesos* = middle + *enteron* = intestine.

4. M – Rheumatic fever

Rheumatic fever is predominantly a disease of the developing world, and is usually seen in children between 5 and 15 years of age. The condition develops 2–4 weeks after a group A β-haemolytic streptococcal pharyngitis. In susceptible individuals, the antibodies formed against the bacterial carbohydrate cell wall cross-react with antigens in the heart, joints and skin in a process known as molecular mimicry. The immune response in the heart causes myocarditis, pericarditis and endocarditis, resulting in valve destruction, conduction defects, arrhythmia and congestive cardiac failure.

The diagnosis of rheumatic fever is made using the modified Duckett Jones criteria, requiring either two major criteria *or* one major and two minor criteria *PLUS* evidence of streptococcal infection (e.g. anti-streptolysin-O titres).

Modified Duckett Jones criteria

Major:

- Pancarditis
- Polyarthritis
- Sydenham's chorea (St Vitus' dance)
- Erythema marginatum
- Subcutaneous nodules.

Minor:

- Fever
- Arthralgia
- High erythrocyte sedimentation rate or white cell count
- Heart block.

Pancarditis can present with murmurs, including mitral regurgitation, aortic regurgitation (in 50%) and the Carey Coombs' murmur (a soft mid-diastolic murmur that is due to nodule development on mitral valve leaflets). Sydenham's chorea includes choreiform movements, emotional lability and explosive speech. The polyarthritis is often fleeting, affects the large joints and is characteristically responsive to aspirin. Subcutaneous nodules are small, firm and painless, and are best felt over the tendons or bones.

Treatment of rheumatic fever requires antibiotics (usually penicillin), analgesia, non-steroidal anti-inflammatory drugs and bed rest. Steroids are sometimes indicated in severe cases. Following the acute phase, patients require prophylactic antibiotics prior to invasive procedures such as tooth extraction in order to protect against bacteraemia and subsequent bacterial endocarditis.

Chorea, from Latin *chorea* = dance.

Saint Vitus' dance (*chorea sancti viti* in Latin) was a mediaeval festival that celebrated St Vitus, the patron saint of dancers, actors and comedians.

Carey Franklin Coombs, English cardiologist (1879–1932).

Thomas Sydenham, English physician (1624–89).

T Duckett Jones, American physician (1899–1954).

5. L – Postural hypotension

In this scenario, a postural drop in blood pressure after standing from a lying position resulted in cerebral hypoperfusion and subsequent collapse. The history of Addison's disease, which is known to cause postural hypotension secondary to hypovolaemia, is likely to be an important factor in this case. Other causes of postural hypotension include age-related degeneration of autonomic reflexes, medication side-effects (e.g. vasodilatation caused by nitrates), hypovolaemia and multisystem atrophy. Postural hypotension is usually defined as a 20 mmHg drop in systolic blood pressure after standing from a lying position. In this case, the patient is noted to have been 'shaken' while unconscious. Although this feature, usually in combination with urinary incontinence and tongue biting, is commonly attributed to seizure activity, it is important to note that all of these can occur in vasovagal and postural hypotensive collapse. Prior to the diagnosis of idiopathic postural hypotension, other reversible causes of collapse must be ruled out, such as cardiac disease, neurological disease, pharmacological side-effects and metabolic conditions. Postural hypotension is usually managed with lifestyle advice and treatment of any underlying condition, such as hydrocortisone and fludrocortisone in Addison's disease. Regular review of medications in elderly people help to reduce polypharmacy and collapse secondary to drugs.

Theme 7: Statistics

1. E – 50%

The *sensitivity* of an investigation is its ability to detect a true-positive result. It is calculated as follows:

$$\text{sensitivity} = \frac{\text{number of true positives}}{\text{number of true positives} + \text{number of false negatives}} \times 100\%$$

So, here:

$$\text{sensitivity} = \frac{100}{100 + 100} \times 100\% = 50\%$$

2. F – 87.5%

The *specificity* is the ability of an investigation to detect a true-negative test result:

$$\text{specificity} = \frac{\text{number of true negatives}}{\text{number of true negatives} + \text{number of false positives}} \times 100\%$$

So, here:

$$\text{specificity} = \frac{700}{700 + 100} \times 100\% = \frac{7}{8} = 100\% = 87.5\%$$

3. E – 50%

The *positive predictive value (PPV)* describes the probability that a condition can be confirmed given a positive test result:

$$\text{PPV} = \frac{\text{number of true positives}}{\text{total number of positive results}} \times 100\%$$

So, here:

$$\text{PPV} = \frac{100}{200} \times 100\% = 50\%$$

4. F – 87.5%

The *negative predictive value (NPV)* describes the probability that a condition can be ruled out given a negative test result:

$$\text{NPV} = \frac{\text{number of true negatives}}{\text{total number of negative results}} \times 100\%$$

So, here:

$$\text{NPV} = \frac{700}{800} \times 100\% = \frac{7}{8} \times 100\% = 87.5\%$$

5. J – 4.0

The *likelihood ratio* is the likelihood that a given test result will be positive in a patient with a certain disorder compared with the likelihood that the same positive result would be expected in a patient without that disorder:

$$\text{likelihood ratio} = \frac{\text{sensitivity}}{1 - \text{specificity}}$$

So, here:

$$\text{likelihood ratio} = \frac{0.50}{1 - 7/8} = 4.0$$

Theme 8: Scoring the severity of pneumonia

1. A – CURB 0 pneumonia

2. F – CURB 5 pneumonia

3. G – Not a pneumonia

4. D – CURB 3 pneumonia

5. B – CURB 1 pneumonia

The CURB-65 score is a simple clinical prediction tool that has been validated for predicting mortality in community-acquired pneumonia. It is recommended by the British Thoracic Society for use in the assessment of severity of pneumonias.

The CURB-65 score is as follows (1 point for each):

- **C**onfusion: Abbreviated Mental Test Score <8
- **U**rea: urea >7 mmol/L
- **R**espiratory rate: respiratory rate ≥30/min
- **B**lood pressure: systolic <90 mmHg or diastolic ≤60 mmHg
- **65**: age ≥65 years.

The risk of death increases as the score increases, and the CURB score can be used to help guide treatment. A CURB score of 0 or 1 is associated with a low mortality rate (1.5%), and such patients are likely to be suitable for home treatment with oral antibiotics. A CURB score of 2 indicates an intermediate mortality rate (9%), and these patients should be considered for hospital admission. A CURB score of 3 or more is associated with a 22% mortality rate (50% if the CURB score is 5). These patients should be managed in hospital as cases of severe pneumonia, with appropriate intravenous antibiotics. Other indications for intravenous antibiotics are malabsorption, impaired consciousness and impaired swallowing.

The patient in Case 3 does not have evidence of consolidation on his chest X-ray – this is a required feature for the diagnosis of pneumonia. The patient's diagnosis is rather that of a lower respiratory tract infection.

Theme 9: Complications of HIV infection 2

The human immunodeficiency virus (HIV) is a retrovirus, i.e. a virus that possesses an RNA genome but whose replication involves a DNA intermediate (the viral RNA is 'reverse transcribed' into DNA, which is then integrated into the genome of an infected cell). HIV is transmitted via bodily fluids (sexually, via blood products and from mother to baby, especially during breastfeeding). Around 40% of HIV infections are in women, and heterosexual contact is the most common form of spread. Risk factors for HIV infection include multiple partners, the presence of other sexually transmitted infections and intravenous drug use, and not using contraception. HIV directly targets T-helper cells (CD4+ cells), which play an active role in cellular immunity.

1. K – Seroconversion

There are four stages in the natural course of HIV infection. The first is seroconversion – the development of specific anti-HIV antibodies in the serum. This is often accompanied by a flu-like illness, and is often identified only retrospectively after a diagnosis of HIV. It is only after seroconversion that an HIV test will detect specific antibodies, so someone newly infected with HIV who has not undergone seroconversion will have a negative test result. After seroconversion, patients enter the asymptomatic phase. During this phase, there is often generalized lymphadenopathy, defined as lymph nodes of 1 cm or more in diameter in two or more non-contiguous extrainguinal sites that cannot be explained by any other infection or condition. The most common sites of lymphadenopathy are the axillary and cervical regions. In most patients who do not receive therapy, HIV-associated illnesses develop within 10 years. These include fever, night sweats, weight loss and minor opportunistic infections (e.g. oral candidiasis and oral hairy leukoplakia).

When the CD4+ cell count ('CD4 count') falls to <200/μL (normal range 700–1200/μL), AIDS-defining illnesses ensue, e.g. Kaposi's sarcoma, oesophageal candidiasis, cerebral toxoplasmosis and *Pneumocystis* pneumonia (PCP). HIV is monitored using the CD4 count and viral load. Antiretroviral therapy is given when the CD4 count is <350/μL, and prophylaxis for PCP is provided when the CD4 count is <250/μL. When the CD4 count drops to <50/μL, infection with low-pathogenicity infections (cytomegalovirus and *Mycobacterium avium*) occurs. The viral load (number of viral copies per millilitre of blood) can be used to measure treatment efficacy, with a load of <50 copies/mL being the aim of therapy.

2. C – Cryptosporidiosis

Cryptosporidium is a single-celled protozoan that is transmitted by the faeco-oral route (by ingesting pathogen oocysts). Cryptosporidiosis causes gastroenteritis, with nausea, abdominal pain and profuse, watery, foul-smelling diarrhoea. Normally, symptoms can persist for days, and even a couple of weeks. Symptomatic cryptosporidiosis lasting longer than a month is strongly indicative of underlying immunocompromise. Treatment is with paramomycin.

3. D – Cytomegalovirus infection

Cytomegalovirus (CMV) is a human herpesvirus (HHV-5), which is usually transmitted by saliva, genital secretions or blood products. In normal hosts, CMV infection causes a mild or subclinical infection. In fact, half of adults in the developed world show evidence of previous CMV infection. In immunocompromised patients, CMV can cause more severe disease, with fever, diarrhoea, pneumonitis, retinitis, hepatitis and encephalitis. The inflammation of the retina leads to a so-called 'pizza pie' appearance on fundoscopy (haemorrhages and yellowish retinal infiltrates). CMV is determined microscopically by demonstrating intranuclear inclusion bodies. These are known as 'owl's eye' bodies. Treatment of CMV infection is with the antiviral drug ganciclovir.

4. G – Kaposi's sarcoma

Kaposi's sarcoma is a malignant tumour of vascular endothelium. It gives rise to painless, non-itchy purple–brown plaques and nodules on the skin and mucous membranes. Pulmonary or gastrointestinal involvement can result in breathlessness and intestinal haemorrhage. Kaposi's sarcoma is associated with underlying infection with human herpesvirus 8 (HHV-8; also known as Kaposi's sarcoma-associated herpesvirus, KSHV) in people who are immunosuppressed (e.g. HIV infection or patients on immunosuppressant drugs following organ transplantation). Before the advent of AIDS, Kaposi's sarcoma was a rare sporadic tumour that occurred in Italian males and Ashkenazi Jews. Biopsy of the lesions is required to confirm diagnosis, and symptomatic treatment is with radiotherapy and antiretroviral drugs. *Lichen planus* also results in purple lesions, but these are intensely itchy.

Moriz Kohn Kaposi, Hungarian dermatologist (1837–1902).

5. I – *Mycobacterium avium* complex

Mycobacterium avium complex (MAC) is a group of related airborne bacteria that includes *Mycobacterium avium–intracellulare*. Because of the low pathogenicity of these bacteria, clinical symptoms are usually found only in immunocompromised patients. Features are similar to those of tuberculosis: productive cough, shortness of breath, fever, lethargy, night sweats, weight loss, diarrhoea and abdominal pain. A chest X-ray may demonstrate the pulmonary MAC lesions. Sputum stain and culture can also help establish diagnosis. Treatment is with antituberculous drugs, including rifampicin, ethambutol and amikacin.

Theme 10: Management of cardiovascular disease

1. H – Synchronized DC cardioversion

This patient with palpitations is in fast atrial fibrillation causing haemodynamic compromise. This is an emergency, and requires prompt action. Once the airway and breathing have been assessed and secured, the patient requires emergency DC cardioversion. DC cardioversion can be either synchronized (performed at a specific point of the cardiac cycle) or unsynchronized (done at any point, regardless of the cardiac cycle). In acute, unstable atrial fibrillation, shocks are synchronized with an R-wave on the ECG in order to reduce the chance of ventricular fibrillation. The patient needs to be adequately anticoagulated with intravenous heparin before the procedure, as cardioversion may precipitate systemic embolization from an intracardiac thrombus. An initial synchronized shock of 50–100 J is delivered to the sedated patient while they are attached to a cardiac monitor. If the initial attempts at cardioversion are unsuccessful, the voltage can be increased to 200 J then 300 J.

2. D – Non-steroidal anti-inflammatory drugs

This is a classic history of acute pericarditis. The pain is typically sharp and central, and is usually relieved by sitting forward. The examination in patients with pericarditis is usually unremarkable, although some patients may be mildly pyrexial or have a pericardial rub (high-pitched scratching noise) on auscultation. Investigation may reveal elevated markers of inflammation or clues to the underlying diagnosis. The ECG is usually normal, although some cases show saddle-shaped ST elevation (in no particular distribution) that can be confused with the ST elevation seen in myocardial infarction. Pericarditis is usually secondary to a viral infection (e.g. Coxsackie), but is also seen in connective tissue disease, metabolic disease and renal failure. All forms of pericarditis can result in a pericardial effusion. Treatment involves correcting the underlying cause and symptomatic management with non-steroidal anti-inflammatory drugs (NSAIDs). NSAIDs should be avoided in people with asthma, as they can precipitate bronchospasm in sensitive individuals. They should also be prescribed with caution in elderly patients, patients with renal disease and those with a history of peptic ulcer disease or gastritis.

3. L – Verapamil

This patient is experiencing a supraventricular tachycardia that is most likely to be an atrioventricular nodal re-entrant tachycardia (AVNRT) or atrioventricular re-entrant tachycardia (AVRT). The typical ECG findings are of a regular narrow complex tachycardia with no obvious P-waves. Provided that the patient is haemodynamically stable, the initial treatment is with vagal manoeuvres such as the Valsalva manoeuvre, and carotid sinus massage. The Valsalva manoeuvre, where the patient forcefully exhales against a closed epiglottis by blowing hard on a syringe, is the most commonly employed and safest vagal manoeuvre available.

If such methods fail to slow the heart rate, or if the patient is haemodynamically compromised, they will require cardioversion. The first-line method in AVNRT and AVRT is chemical cardioversion with adenosine. Adenosine is given as an intravenous bolus of 6 mg, increasing to 12 mg if cardioversion does not occur. Before administrating adenosine, the patient should be placed on a cardiac monitor and warned that they will experience significant chest tightness and dyspnoea. It must be noted that adenosine is contraindicated in asthmatic patients, as it may precipitate bronchospasm. In such patients, chemical cardioversion should be with verapamil, which should be administered as a 2.5–5 mg intravenous bolus to be repeated after 10 minutes if unsuccessful. In cases that are unresponsive to chemical cardioversion, or when there is severe haemodynamic compromise with a heart rate above 250 beats/min, the patient should receive emergency synchronized DC cardioversion.

4. J – Tenecteplase followed by intravenous heparin infusion

This patient has had an anterior myocardial infarction that fills the criteria for thrombolysis. In most hospitals, streptokinase is the first-line thrombolytic agent. However, following administration of streptokinase, patients develop anti-streptokinase immunoglobulin G antibodies that will reduce the thrombolytic activity and can potentially trigger a severe allergic reaction if streptokinase is administered for a second time. To prevent this from happening, patients who receive streptokinase are given a card or wear a MedicAlert bracelet to warn medical staff in emergency situations.

The other major class of thrombolytic drugs is the tissue-type plasminogen activators, which include tenecteplase, alteplase and reteplase. When tenecteplase is given, it is followed by an intravenous infusion of heparin in order to improve the chance of reperfusion. The main complications of thrombolysis are bleeding, reperfusion arrhythmia, allergic reaction and hypotension. Haemorrhagic stroke is perhaps the most serious complication of thrombolysis, and occurs in approximately 0.5% of cases.

5. K – Unsynchronized DC cardioversion

This patient has ventricular tachycardia without a cardiac output, which required basic life support measures and unsynchronized DC cardioversion. In cases of cardiac arrest, you should try and look for (and manage) reversible causes.

These are indicated by the *4 Ts and 4 Hs* (Tamponade, Tension pneumothorax, Toxicity, Thromboembolism and Hyper-hypokalaemia, Hypothermia, Hypoxia, Hypovolaemia). In this case, the arrhythmia is likely to be secondary to hyperkalaemia, since there is a history of end-stage renal failure. An arterial blood gas sample will give a rapid bedside indication of the serum potassium concentration before the venous sample can be processed. Hyperkalaemia should be treated with 10 mL of intravenous calcium gluconate (10%) to protect the myocardium, followed by an intravenous insulin and glucose infusion (e.g. 10 units of Actrapid with 50 mL of 50% glucose), which forces potassium into the intracellular compartment, where it cannot influence the myocardium.

Theme 11: Gait disturbance 2

1. B – Cerebellar ataxia

The examination features of spider naevi and gynaecomastia suggest significant alcohol use. This patient is also displaying features of cerebellar dysfunction (wide-based gait and past pointing), which can be a consequence of alcohol excess. Cerebellar dysfunction results in a characteristic set of features summarized by the acronym DANISH:

Dysdiadochokinesis
Ataxia (wide-based gait)
Nystagmus
Intention tremor
Slurred speech
Hypotonicity.

Less severe degrees of cerebellar ataxia can be elicited by asking the patient to walk heel to toe.

2. C – Extrapyramidal gait

This man has difficulty walking and controlling the speed of his gait. This is typical of an extrapyramidal gait seen in Parkinson's disease. Patients find it difficult to initiate walking. They start with stuttering steps that quickly increase in frequency while decreasing in length (also known as a festinant gait). Patients with Parkinson's disease may also get 'stuck' when walking though doors ('freezing').

Festinant, from Latin *festino* = to hurry.

3. J – Trendelenburg gait

The Trendelenburg gait is caused by unilateral weakness of the hip-stabilizing lower limb abductor muscles (gluteus medius and minimus). The hip abductors prevent the pelvis from tilting down when the contralateral leg is lifted off the ground. If there is weakness of these stabilizing muscles, the pelvis sags when the opposite leg is lifted. To compensate, the trunk is swung to the other side (the side of the hip weakness) to maintain the pelvis level. Unilateral hip abductor weakness is primarily caused by damage to the superior gluteal nerve.

Freidrich Trendelenburg, German surgeon (1844–1924).

4. I – Spastic gait

This man has recently had a stroke causing a right-sided spastic hemiparesis. This results in a gait where the upper limb is held in flexion, the hip in extension and the ankle plantarflexed. Patients with spastic hemiparesis find that they need to swing their affected leg out from the hip (circumduction) to prevent it from scuffing the ground on walking.

5. F – Marche à petit pas

In view of the history of ischaemic heart disease, this man is likely to have vascular dementia. Patients who have multiple small-vessel cerebrovascular disease tend to walk with small, slow steps and instability. This is known as marche à petit pas. It is different from the festinant extrapyramidal gait of parkinsonism, as there is no acceleration or freezing. Examination of these patients may reveal signs of bilateral upper motor neuron disease (e.g. extensor plantars).

Marche à petit pas, from French = 'gait with little steps'.

Theme 12: Treatment of gastrointestinal disease

1. I – Oral rehydration therapy

Patients with diarrhoea and vomiting are at risk of becoming dehydrated and developing electrolyte imbalance, e.g. hypernatraemia or hypokalaemia. The initial management of patients without severe dehydration or electrolyte disturbance is with oral fluids, ideally in the form of oral rehydration solutions, which replace lost water and electrolytes. If oral rehydration solution is not available, the patient should be encouraged to take regular sips of water. Antiemetics may be used to reduce nausea and vomiting, but agents that stop diarrhoea should be avoided when infection is suspected. Certain groups, such as elderly people, children and those with significant comorbidity are more prone to dehydration, and should be monitored closely and given intravenous fluids if required.

2. K – Prednisolone enema

Patients with ulcerative colitis can experience regular relapses that present with fever, lethargy, high stool frequency and rectal blood loss. The acute management of rectal and distal colonic ulcerative colitis involves fluid and electrolyte management, 5-aminosalicylic acid (5-ASA)-type drugs (e.g. sulfasalazine), systemic steroids and local steroids (e.g. rectal steroid enemas such as Predfoam). Thromboembolic disease is a potential complication of active ulcerative colitis, for which prophylaxis with low-molecular-weight heparin is given. Severe and life-threatening exacerbations may require surgery.

3. F – Oesophageal stenting

Patients with metastatic oesophageal adenocarcinoma should be treated with palliative measures, as cure is impossible. Patients who experience distressing dysphagia should be considered for endoscopic oesophageal dilatation and stenting in order to relieve dysphagia and improve quality of life. Radiotherapy to debulk the tumour may be indicated, but invasive surgery such as oesophagectomy should be avoided as the risks are high and the outcomes are poor.

4. E – Lifestyle advice

Constipation can be a chronic problem that causes much discomfort and distress to the patient. It is important to consider conditions such as Hirschsprung's disease and drugs such as opiates that may predispose to constipation, but the vast majority of cases result from poor diet, inadequate fluid intake and a sedentary lifestyle. Therefore, the first-line management of constipation involves a holistic approach to the patient's lifestyle, which should include offering advice such as adapting diet to include plenty of fibre and water and encouraging regular exercise. If the constipation does not respond to lifestyle changes, a simple laxative should be considered, e.g. senna. More invasive treatment (suppositories and enemas) should be reserved for disease refractory to lifestyle changes and simple laxatives.

5. B – Infliximab

Crohn's disease was traditionally treated with the 5-ASA group of anti-inflammatory medicines, e.g. sulfasalazine. However, their ability to prevent remission has been proven to be poor. Infliximab is a monoclonal antibody to tumour necrosis factor α (TNF-α) that inhibits its action at the cellular level, thus exerting an anti-inflammatory effect. It is used in steroid-unresponsive disease to induce remission, and has shown good results so far. Other treatments used in Crohn's disease include corticosteroids, azathioprine, methotrexate, metronidazole, elemental diet and surgery as a last resort (although up to 80% of patients will require surgical intervention at some point).

Theme 13: Autoantibodies 2

1. A – Anti-centromere

2. C – Anti-Jo-1

3. B – Anti-dsDNA

4. H – cANCA

5. G – Anticardiolipin

The main autoantibodies of rheumatological disease are as follows:

- rheumatoid factor: rheumatoid arthritis
- anti-dsDNA: systemic lupus erythematosus (SLE)
- anti-Sm (anti-Smith):SLE (especially renal lupus)
- anti-Jo-1: dermatomyositis
- cANCA (proteinase 3): Wegener's granulomatosis
- pANCA (myeloperoxidase): microscopic polyangiitis

- anticardiolipin: antiphospholipid syndrome
- lupus anticoagulase: antiphospholipid syndrome
- anti-topoisomerase II (anti-SCL-70): diffuse scleroderma
- anti-centromere: limited scleroderma (CREST syndrome)
- anti-U1-RNP: mixed/overlap connective tissue disease
- anti-Ro (SS-A) and anti-La (SS-B): Sjögren's syndrome.

Theme 14: Diagnosis of endocrine disorders

1. A - Acromegaly

Acromegaly is caused by a growth hormone (GH)-secreting tumour of the anterior pituitary gland. The functions of GH include lipolysis, protein synthesis and gluconeogenesis – in other words, it is an anabolic hormone. Patients with acromegaly may present with headaches, excessive sweating, thick/oily skin, hypertrophy of soft tissues (large nose/lips/tongue and 'spade-like' hands), big viscera, prognathism (protruding lower jaw) and prominent supraorbital ridges. Other associations are carpal tunnel syndrome, diabetes and hypertension. The pituitary mass may result in features of a space-occupying lesion in the brain, i.e. an early morning headache that is worse on coughing and straining. If a GH-secreting tumour occurs in children before the bone epiphyses have fused, the long bones grow rapidly and gigantism results.

The reason why it is important to treat acromegaly is because it is associated with an increased risk of atheromatous disease and colon cancer. The diagnosis is made by measuring GH levels before and after a 75 g glucose load (an oral glucose tolerance test). Glucose normally suppresses GH secretion, but in acromegaly the glucose load has little effect. Surgical treatment is by trans-sphenoidal surgery. Medical therapy is with somatostatin analogues (such as intramuscular octreotide), which inhibit GH secretion.

2. L – Nelson's syndrome

This woman has been treated for Cushing's disease in the past. Cushing's disease is the presence of an adrenocorticotrophic hormone (ACTH)-secreting tumour in the pituitary that results in excess cortisol and features of Cushing's syndrome. The treatment of Cushing's disease is usually by removal of the primary tumour. However, in occasional cases where the tumour is occult, bilateral adrenalectomy is performed to eliminate the production of cortisol. The lack of cortisol's negative feedback on the pituitary allows the pre-existing pituitary ACTH tumour to grow rapidly. This process is known as Nelson's syndrome and occurs after 20% of bilateral adrenalectomies. The excess ACTH of Nelson's syndrome results in skin hyperpigmentation via the secretion of melanocyte-stimulating hormone.

Nelson D, Meakin J, Thorn G. ACTH-producing pituitary tumors following adrenalectomy for Cushing's syndrome. *Ann Intern Med* 1960; **52**: 560–9.

3. I – Multiple endocrine neoplasia type 1

This young patient has multiple peptic ulcers, which are suggestive of a gastrinoma, a pancreatic tumour. The brain tumour that causes lactation is a prolactinoma, a tumour of the pituitary gland. The combination of pancreatic endocrine tumours with a gastrinoma suggests multiple endocrine neoplasia (MEN) type I.

There are three types of MEN, all of which are autosomal dominant conditions. MEN type 1 (Wermer's syndrome) includes the presence of parathyroid adenomas, pancreatic islet cell tumours and pituitary adenomas. MEN type 2A (Sipple's syndrome) comprises parathyroid adenomas, medullary carcinoma of the thyroid and phaeochromocytoma. Finally, MEN type 2B (which has in the past been termed 'MEN type 3') includes the presence of the tumours of MEN type 2A with the addition of multiple mucosal neuromas of the gastrointestinal tract and a marfanoid phenotype.

Paul Wermer, American physician (1898–1975).

John Sipple, American physician (b1930).

4. E – Conn's syndrome

This woman presents with polyuria, polydipsia and muscle cramps associated with a high sodium and a low potassium. This suggests a diagnosis of Conn's syndrome. Conn's syndrome results from an aldosterone-secreting adenoma of the adrenal gland. Aldosterone causes sodium reabsorption and potassium excretion in the kidneys. Excess aldosterone results in sodium and water retention, leading to high blood pressure and oedema. Excess potassium excretion results in hypokalaemia, the features of which include muscle cramps and weakness, polyuria (secondary to renal tubular damage, i.e. nephrogenic diabetes insipidus) and polydipsia. The diagnosis of Conn's syndrome can be made by measuring serum aldosterone and renin levels – aldosterone will be raised and renin levels will be reduced due to negative feedback. It should be noted that many antihypertensive medications interfere with these hormones, so it is important to stop these for at least 6 weeks before testing. Initial management is with spironolactone, an aldosterone antagonist. Once the adenoma has been localized (using CT), it can be surgically removed.

Jerome Conn, American endocrinologist (1907–81).

5. K – Multiple endocrine neoplasia type 2B

This patient is likely to have MEN type 2B, an autosomal dominant condition characterized by phaeochromocytoma, parathyroid adenomas, medullary thyroid cancer, multiple mucosal neuromas and a marfanoid habitus (e.g. tall, arachnodactylyl, high-arched palate).

Antoine Marfan, French paediatrician (1858–1942).

Theme 15: Dermatomes 2

1. L – L5

2. E – C7

3. P – Trigeminal nerve

4. J – L1

5. F – C8

For a complete list of dermatomes, see 'Dermatomes 1' (Paper 2 Answers, Theme 12).

Index of conditions